Eradicating Blindness

Logan D. A. Williams

Eradicating Blindness

Global Health Innovation
from South Asia

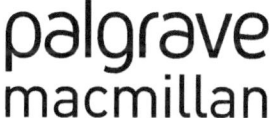

Logan D. A. Williams
Logan Williams Consultancy Services, LLC
Cumberland, MD, USA

ISBN 978-981-13-1624-1   ISBN 978-981-13-1625-8   (eBook)
https://doi.org/10.1007/978-981-13-1625-8

Library of Congress Control Number: 2018949316

Cover design: Fatima Jamadar

This Palgrave Macmillan imprint is published by the registered company Springer Nature Singapore Pte Ltd.
The registered company address is: 152 Beach Road, #21-01/04 Gateway East, Singapore 189721, Singapore

Preface

In 2006, I discovered that my mother had early-stage cataracts in both eyes. At that time, we both lived in Boulder, Colorado, where I was a graduate research assistant in the Cardiovascular Dynamics and Ultrasound Laboratory. I decided that cataract disease (and the knowledges and technologies used to address it around the world) warranted closer scrutiny. In addition to my main research project on cardiovascular ultrasound, I completed a small secondary project at CU-Boulder on the bio-mechanics of porcine natural lenses. I also performed background research in February 2007 on the nature of cataract disease and was surprised by the great number of people it affects around the world. As part of this preliminary research, I checked out the World Health Organization's information about cataracts. On their website, they had a map that showed cataract surgical rates (or how many cataract surgeries per capita) for each country in the world in 2004. The fact that the USA, Western Europe, and Australia had high cataract surgical rates was not a surprise. What was confounding (to me) about this map was that it showed that India and Nepal also had high cataract surgical rates. *I had a puzzle: Why was it that India and Nepal had such high cataract surgery rates?* With my nascent interests in knowledge and technology transfer for a social purpose, I began to determine just why these two countries, which are not as economically developed as the USA, had comparable rates of surgery. After I entered the Science and Technology Studies post-graduate program at Rensselaer Polytechnic Institute, I conducted initial doctoral dissertation fieldwork at Tilganga Institute of Ophthalmology in Nepal in 2009. Thus by starting "at home" with my mother's cataract disease diagnosis, an interesting research project was born.

Cumberland, MD, USA   Logan D. A. Williams

Acknowledgements

I would like to thank God who answered my prayers with closed doors and open doors—guiding me all of this way on a path that I never could have imagined. I also very much appreciate the prayers and encouragement from my family and friends across the globe without which I would have been unable to finish this book!

Thanks are owed to all of the ophthalmologists, engineers, managers, and other individuals that I interviewed and observed in Kenya, Nepal, India, Mexico, and the USA. My fieldwork was facilitated by the introductions from various managers that I have been privileged to meet. For example, I am obliged to Thulasiraj Ravilla (India) for e-introducing me to Samson R. Ndegwa (Kenya); this introduction smoothed the way for my interviews at the Lions SightFirst Eye Hospital, Loresho (Kenya). Once I arrived at Loresho, Peter Ndigwa was kind enough to give me a tour of the campus, introduce me to potential interviewees, and organize my volunteer internship. I similarly appreciate Nabin K. Rai's coordination of my volunteer internships in the research department at Tilganga (Nepal) and Juan Carlos Rodriguez's work in arranging my interviews at Sala Uno (Mexico). My fieldwork in India would not have been possible without the invitation from Aurolab's P. Bala Krishnan to visit the Aravind Eye Care System. Thanks also to Thulasiraj for hosting me at the Lions Aravind Institute of Community Ophthalmology (India).

My homestay family in Kathmandu (God Bless you J, D, S, R, M and N!) and my colleagues at LAICO were generous in their welcome, especially: my officemate Sanil Joseph, his wife Anuja Sanil, and their daughter Sarah Sanil; Thulsi's daughter Dhivya Ramasamy; and Dhivya's officemate Sashipriya Karumanchi Munirathnam. Thanks to Shrilakshmi Kannan and Dhivya for introducing me to potential interviewees at the Aravind Eye Hospital, Madurai (India). I continue to have fond memories of: "Melody Fridays" and teaching the Research Seminar at LAICO.

Some of my interviews in the USA would not have been possible without the e-introductions provided by John Ciccione at the American Society for Cataract and Refractive Surgery, and Jenny E. Benjamin, the director of the American Academy of Ophthalmology Museum of Vision in San Francisco, CA.

I appreciate the comments of my colleagues (specifically Thomas S. Woodson, Mark Waddell, Denver Tang, Amit Prasad, Toluwalogo B. Odumosu, Dean Nieusma, Sharlissa Moore, Daniel Menchik, Les Levidow, Anna Lamprou, Abby Kinchy, Christopher Henke, Steve J. Gold, Sara Fingal, Kevin Elliott, Jubin Cheruvelil, Cliff Broman, Kean Birch, James Bergman, Rich Bellon, Javiera Barandiaran, and Atsushi Akera) on chapters as I revised my dissertation into this book manuscript. Dissertation comments from my mentor, Ron B. Eglash, made me more sensitive to the economic and organizational practices of non-profits. The work of my mentor, David J. Hess, on industrial transition movements, provoked the insight of dual socio-technical regimes that I develop in this book. I especially want to thank Sean Valles for his chapter-by-chapter comments—I can only hope that I did a good job of coherently and selectively incorporating these suggestions into the manuscript. I was significantly encouraged by those conference participants who commented on an early draft of Chapter 6 at "Science and Technology Studies in South Asia" in May 2010, especially my discussant Deboleena Roy.

Audra Wolfe at The Outside Reader and my first two anonymous referees showed me the potential of transforming an early draft of this book into something more interesting. Finally, I appreciate Linda Nathan at LogosWord Designs, LLC, for copyediting an early draft of the manuscript.

Collecting empirical data for this book was directly supported by: a Short-Term Travel to Collections Award from the Lemelson Center at the National Museum of American History–Smithsonian Institute; a Council of American Overseas Research Centers Multi-Country Fellowship; a National Science Foundation DDIG (No. 1153308); and a Rensselaer Polytechnic Institute HASS Fellowship. The data collection was indirectly supported by the Council of Women World Leaders Environmental Policy Fellowship. Any opinions, findings, and conclusions or recommendations expressed in this material are mine and do not necessarily reflect the views of any of the financial supporters.

Parts of this book, especially Chapters 1 and 2, draw from the following journal articles:

Williams, Logan D. A. 2013. "Three Models of Development: Community Ophthalmology NGOs and the Appropriate Technology Movement." *Perspectives on Global Development and Technology* 12 (4): 449–75.

Williams, Logan D. A. 2018. "The South Asian Origins of the Global Network to Eradicate Blindness: WHO, NGOs, and Decentralization." *Endeavour* 42 (1): 27–41.

Contents

1   Introduction   1

2   Origins of an Autonomous Global Network
to Eradicate Blindness   37

3   Balancing the Scales: Appropriate Technology
and Social Entrepreneurship   77

4   Witnessing Rural Blindness: Standardizing
Benchmarks from Eye Camps   111

5   A Laboratory of Our Own: Technology Diffusion
from the Incumbent Regime   145

6   The Hard Case of White Cataracts: Appropriation
of Surgical Science   181

7   Training the New Cadre: Translation of Interlocking
Innovations   217

8   Evidence-Based Medicine: Contesting the Phaco-Regime   253

9   Conclusion: Innovation from Below   289

10   Appendix A: The Extended Case Method and Global
      Ethnography   315

11   Appendix B: The Robin Hood Model   333

Organizational Charts for Four Community
Ophthalmology Units   353

Glossary of Common Ophthalmology Surgical Terms   359

Index   363

List of Figures

Fig. 1.1   An emergent radical rule-set, multiple niches supporting
            interlocking innovations in finance, science and technology,
            and coexistence of dual regimes in the landscape   23
Fig. 3.1   Aravind Eye Hospital Outpatient Building (the first
            building on the central campus of Aravind Eye Care
            System in Madurai) which G. Srinivasan built
            floor-by-floor over five years as funds allowed
            (Photo by Logan D. A. Williams)   91
Fig. 5.1   Checking IOL surface quality under a microscope at
            Tilganga-FHIOL in Kathmandu, Nepal (Photo by Logan
            D. A. Williams)   171
Fig. 7.1   Entrance to the Lions Aravind Institute for Community
            Ophthalmology which shows a drawing of Gandhi to the
            right of the doorway and a bust of Sri Aurobindo
            centered between the open doors (Photo by Logan
            D. A. Williams)   226
Fig. 8.1   Drawing of my observation in the Aravind "Free Hospital"
            (Walk-in Hospital) Operating Theater. I stood by the
            instruments window and ophthalmic assistants came past
            me every few minutes to the window near my left shoulder
            to drop off a tray, with its set of used instruments, so they

could be quickly sterilized and used again
(Williams 2012, July 16)   268

Fig. 9.1   Coexistence of dual regimes, SICS v. Phaco, in the
differentiated landscape. Each of the two regimes has the
typical dimensions: Dimension 1 Technology; Dimension 2
Markets, user practices; Dimension 3 Culture, symbolic
meaning; Dimension 4 Infrastructure; Dimension 5
Industry; Dimension 6 Policy; and Dimension 7 Scientific
knowledge   297

Fig. 11.1   New building on campus of Tilganga Institute of
Ophthalmology (Photo by Logan D. A. Williams)   334

Fig. 11.2   Bright windows shine light onto the patient walking
ramp between ground floor and first floor in the Lions
SightFirst Eye Hospital, Loresho, Premchandbhai
foundation wing (Photo by Logan D. A. Williams)   341

Fig. 11.3   Reception desk at Sala Uno (Photo by Logan
D. A. Williams)   346

List of Tables

Table 3.1 Two main types of social enterprise organizations (partially adapted from Alter [2003], Jalali [2008], Monroe-White [2014]) 80

Table 3.2 Diverse revenue sources pay for expenses at the Aravind Eye Care System (India) 93

Table 3.3 Comparing percentages of paying versus subsidized (or non-paying) patients in the cost recovery models across four community ophthalmology units in 2012 101

Table 7.1 Ranking countries using GDP (PPP) per capita; in the world system, core countries have low number ranks while peripheral countries have high number ranks (Central Intelligence Agency 2012; United Nations Development Programme 2017) 230

Table 11.1 Diverse revenue sources pay for expenses at Tilganga Institute of Ophthalmology (Nepal) 336

Table 11.2 Diverse revenue sources pay for expenses at the Lions SightFirst Eye Hospital, Loresho (Kenya) 340

Table 11.3 Diverse revenue sources pay for expenses at Sala Uno (Mexico) 345

1

Introduction

On a Saturday afternoon in April 2011, an ophthalmologist speaking at the Unite for Sight Global Health and Innovation Conference described his observation of two eye clinics in the global south. During his slide show of photographs, he commented that the first Ghanaian eye clinic was "a one stop shop for eye disease" with a "systems approach" featuring two surgeons performing surgery simultaneously in the same surgical theater, a well-organized flow of patients, and the use of a microsurgical technique to correct blindness from cataract disease. A cataract is the clouding (opacity) of the eye's natural lens; like the mist from a waterfall, a cataract inside the eye obscures light and detail causing visual impairment or blindness.

I was already aware that the groundbreaking microsurgical technique developed at Tilganga Institute of Ophthalmology (Kathmandu, Nepal) results in very good patient outcomes despite the fact that expensive suture thread is not required to stitch the incision closed. Nor is this particular microsurgery disrupted by the rolling electricity blackouts that are frequent in some countries with overloaded electrical grids. As I listened, other parts of this systems approach were sharpening into focus: a radical aseptic technique to prevent pathogens from

© The Author(s) 2019
L. D. A. Williams, *Eradicating Blindness*,
https://doi.org/10.1007/978-981-13-1625-8_1

contaminating the surgical theater and unique labor-intensive logistical practices for the surgical theater. The speaker pointed out it was a "very efficient flow system that even by American standards is quite admirable." His comment, while appreciative, still manages to make the standards developed by ophthalmologists in the global south seem Other. He firmly places those clinics in a network of ophthalmologists broadly focused on population eye health. This network is subordinate as compared to the dominant network of ophthalmologists narrowly focused on individual eye health. His rhetoric also carefully delineated the boundaries between medical practices that are good for the global south versus what is good for the USA.

A live report from the 2010 Asia-Pacific Academy of Ophthalmology Congress in Beijing also emphasized the work of Aravind Eye Care System (Madurai, India) and Tilganga. This live report highlighted a growing scientific controversy in ophthalmology—the dispute between proponents of two different microsurgical techniques to restore eyesight clouded by cataract (Anonymous 2010). The incumbent microsurgical technique was made by an American ophthalmologist in New York City; the challenger microsurgical technique was made by a Nepalese ophthalmologist in Kathmandu. Before this September meeting, ophthalmologists, engineers, and managers at Aravind and Tilganga had spent many years creating South Asian eye healthcare institutions. These experts contested the definition of what true cataract blindness means in terms of visual acuity worldwide and helped to redefine blindness as a public health problem that is avoidable or preventable. Additionally, they performed the operations research, health education outreach, and community-building activities to make poor rural patients aware that blindness is often a preventable or solvable problem. They utilize evidence-based medicine to challenge the incumbent regime's cataract microsurgical technique because of its high cost. After they created the alternative microsurgical technique, they then performed the research necessary to validate this alternative technique as an appropriate option, both scientifically and economically viable, for poor patients.

Throughout this book, I will develop a theoretical framework for socio-technical transition called the dual regime thesis. In order to define this novel transition pathway, I will summarize existing literature on the multi-level perspective in transition studies, demonstrate the relationship of this literature to my case of community ophthalmology, and also develop the concepts of interlocking innovations, contestation, and systemic technology choice. In this book, I argue that community ophthalmology professionals are an example of systemic technology choice. Systemic technology choice illustrates a new shift in the global appropriate technology movement, where there is an emerging form of high-technology innovation that responds to the needs of low-income people. Unlike the previous appropriate technology movements, this new approach to development emphasizes systems thinking, where activists believe that technology transfer is the transfer of an appropriate system of artifacts, values, norms, and ideology.

The dual regimes emerge in part because of interlocking innovations: a novel constellation of context-appropriate processes or products in science, technology, and management connected to each other by a shared ideology. Interlocking innovations circulate through diffusion, appropriation, and translation to address problems of poverty in low-income countries. These interlocking innovations travel on a global stage to other less economically developed countries and even to the economic centers of the world economy. Finally, contestation explains how, in order to move from below, some actors use new forms of science and technology to challenge existing knowledge hierarchies and that this is a normal and productive part of scientific knowledge building and technology transfer. These concepts add a newer theorization of how knowledge and technology circulate as part of socio-technical system change to transition studies (Geels 2005; Smith et al. 2016), the political sociology of science (Hess et al. 2016), and feminist postcolonial science studies (Harding 2009; Pollock 2014).

In this chapter, I provide an overview of the goals of this book. The book's central argument is that the multi-level perspective in transition studies cannot be used to explain endogenous development of science and technology in the global south, unless we account for the occasional development of dual regimes. Endogenous development in this case includes a novel microsurgical technique used for high-volume, low-cost care for poor people in the global south that is supported by further innovations in surgical theater management techniques, low-cost technologies, and finance. This model is being successfully exported to other countries in the south.

The remainder of this introductory chapter has the following structure: Sect. 1.1 discusses the book's purpose to introduce South Asia as having multiple sites of low-cost innovation in the global field of ophthalmology; I describe connections between the problem of blindness, epistemology, and innovation from below. Next, Sect. 1.2 introduces the problem of avoidable blindness in more detail, including the startling facts that make this problem noteworthy; meanwhile, I also present the theoretical framework of multi-level perspective with socio-technical regimes. Scholars from science and technology studies, business, evolutionary economics, and, the government of the Netherlands, use this theoretical framework to think through science and technology adoption and governance issues (Geels 2002; Smith 2002). Section 1.3 describes the historical origins and current practitioner understanding of technology transfer, modern development, and appropriate technology in the global south. Next, Sect. 1.4 returns to the multi-level perspective and evaluates its limitations for understanding socio-technical change in the global south. Consequently, Sect. 1.5 introduces a new theoretical framework, the dual regime thesis, in more detail. Finally, Sect 1.6 concludes by summarizing Chapters 2–8.

1.1   Science, Technology, and Innovation from Below

The purpose of this book is to demonstrate how India and Nepal have emerged as sites of innovation in low-cost, high-volume cataract surgery. Cataract disease causes 51% of avoidable blindness worldwide, approximately 20 million out of a total of 39 million blind people (Pascolini and Mariotti 2012). This disease predominantly affects an older, low-income, and rural demographic (Pascolini and Mariotti 2012). While the causes are unknown, there is an increase in cataract incidence with age worldwide, where 1 in 5 people over the age of 55 years will have at least one eye with a cataractous lens (Pascolini and Mariotti 2012). The good news is that, in industrialized nations where prospective patients have regular access to eye health care, an outpatient surgical procedure can skillfully and quickly correct cataracts.

The bad news is that the infrastructure to address this problem in low-income rural communities around the world is largely absent. While significant gains have been made since the first efforts of rural ophthalmologists started in the early 1960s, there are still not enough trained ophthalmologists or hospitals to fight the problem as the average population age increases and likewise the incidence of age-related cataract disease. An exception to this bad news lies within two countries in South Asia, India and Nepal. India and Nepal are not known for being innovative in health and medicine. Still, in 2004, both countries had high cataract surgical rates, a measurement of surgeries performed per million people with blindness due to cataract (WHO 2004).

Ophthalmology experts from around the world are beginning to look to India and Nepal for models in efficiency and cost cutting in health services delivery. Each country contains many high-volume eye hospitals that are circulating blind patients from rural through urban areas and making them sighted.

In this book, I focus on ophthalmology institutions providing a valuable eye health service to the most disadvantaged in their communities, while utilizing an approach that maximizes their self-sufficiency and self-governance. The four high-volume eye hospitals I describe include: non-profit Aravind Eye Care System in India (est. 1976); non-profit Tilganga Institute of Ophthalmology in Nepal (est. 1992); non-profit Lions SightFirst Eye Hospital, Loresho in Kenya (est. 1998); and for-profit Sala Uno in Mexico (est. 2011). In the back of the book, you will find their organizational charts. Each high-volume eye hospital provides access to primary, secondary, or tertiary levels of eye health care.

The lowest level of eye health care, primary, involves vision screenings and eyeglasses (on par with a US optical shop). Secondary eye care centers involve all the care provided at the primary level as well as outpatient cataract surgery and a few other limited services. This is similar to a private clinical ophthalmologist affiliated with an outpatient surgical center in the USA. Finally, tertiary eye care centers provide a wide range of subspecialties in eye health care including: cataracts, cornea, retina, orbit and oculoplasty, glaucoma, uvea, low vision, pediatric ophthalmology, and neuro-ophthalmology. At this level, the care provided is similar to that of an ophthalmology department in a large US hospital, but several times larger. Through endogenous development (i.e., locally initiated, self-reliant development, see Malunga and Holcombe 2014), they have successfully produced their innovations to meet local needs. Experts in India and Nepal have endogenously developed a socio-technical system of linked innovations in science, management, finance, and technology. They challenged the status quo in ophthalmology to address their mission to provide eye health care to poor rural patients around the world.

The Aravind Eye Care System in southern India and the Tilganga Institute of Ophthalmology in Kathmandu, Nepal, are unique among the many eye hospitals in India and Nepal. These two eye hospitals are well known globally for their high-volume, high-quality cataract surgeries that poor patients receive for free or for a nominal fee. Their work is cutting edge in its focus on increasing surgical infrastructure and decreasing surgical costs for eye diseases. Additionally, around the world, Aravind and Tilganga are known for their novel innovations, which include surgical techniques, surgical theater management practices, and the production of low-cost ophthalmic technologies. Furthermore, they have disseminated their innovations to other eye hospitals in South Asia and around the world. To illustrate this, I will discuss two additional eye hospitals in this book: the Lions SightFirst Eye Hospital, Loresho in Nairobi, Kenya, and Sala Uno in Mexico City, Mexico. Additionally, Aravind and Tilganga disseminate their innovations to industrialized countries such as Australia, Finland, and the USA (see Chapter 5, 8, and 9).

The example of South Asian eye hospitals addressing infrastructure needs for controlling eye disease holds valuable insights for our understanding of social entrepreneurship and science and technology transfer in global public health. The work of these organizations helps illuminate issues of economic justice through systems of appropriate technology in global public health, including (1) funding models; (2) the formal and informal relationships through which flows capital, science, and technology. These southern high-tech experts circulate their novel surgical sciences, management practices, and ophthalmic technologies from below, that is, from a position of low socioeconomic and geo-political status in the global field of science (Hwang 2008; Worthington 1993).

As I designed my research study, I deliberately made the choice to interview those from "below"—persons marginalized in some relationship of power. In this study, focusing on "sciences from below" (Harding 2008) indicates an attention to science and technology produced by people who have, in recent times or in the history of Western imperialism, been marginalized at the periphery of science and technology production. Thus, my study uses empirical content derived predominantly from the ophthalmology units that I studied in countries with less social and economic power than Western nations in transnational arenas.

Therefore, in this book, the users and producers of science and technology from below are primarily from less economically developed countries (LEDCs). Other commonly used terms that refer to a similar set of sovereign states include less developed countries, global south, non-Western countries, developing countries, the third world, and low-income countries. I prefer the term less economically developed countries because it is comparative, relational, and points to a specific power relationship that is based on global domestic product (GDP) per capita Purchasing Power Parity (PPP). The broader term of developing country dismisses the ancient history, education, artisan culture, and religion preserved for many centuries in active, every day, sites in Nepal and India. For example, the ancient art of Nepalese pagoda architecture was transferred to China in the 1270s when the emperor invited Arniko to create the White Stupa Temple (Miaoying Temple) in Beijing (Singh and Bhuju 2001). The narrower term, less economically developed country, keeps the comparative element, but points toward the uneven accumulation of economic privilege in some countries over others that is a direct result of past colonial projects and recent globalization of finance (Escobar 1994; McMichael 2010; Pieterse 1991, 2000; Wallerstein 1974), including poverty capital (Roy 2010). The word economic development invokes capital, jobs, incomes, and taxes. The precision of the term means that it raises fewer inappropriate comparisons about lack of culture and lack of values. By using the term less economically developed country, I am attempting to avoid causally associating economic privilege with epistemic privilege or scientific prestige (although often these forms of privilege go hand-in-hand; see Englander 2014).

Usually, questions about the creation and transfer of innovative science and technology start with research in core countries of the world-system that already have a high degree of economic and epistemic privilege. In contrast, my research started with the assumption that innovative science and technology can and does start from persons (or countries) in marginalized (or peripheral) positions of power. I started this global ethnography (Burawoy 1998, 2000) with two questions:

1. What explains the emergence of alternative high-tech solutions combined with social enterprise to address a set of problems common to the rural poor in less economically developed countries instead of wealthy countries?
2. How are these innovations produced in less economically developed countries being disseminated throughout the region and around the world?

For more details about my methodology, please see Chapter 10, which describes my process of multi-sited, extended case method global ethnography (Burawoy 1998, 2000).

While acknowledging the importance of marginalized standpoints for creating new innovation, this book does not celebrate such knowledge and insight as inherent to resource-constrained individuals, organizations, or states. Essentializing creativity as a characteristic of impoverished people is irresponsible (Birtchnell 2011, 2013). Such celebratory discourse overlooks the asymmetry (between innovators in well-resourced versus poverty-stricken areas of the world) that shapes the necessity for the poor to innovate in spite of the risks to themselves and their livelihoods (Birtchnell 2009).

This book avoids such celebratory discourse; instead, it explores the structural opportunities and constraints for innovation from below. I unpack the historically contingent emergence of innovative, community ophthalmology eye clinics and eye hospitals in the global south. Contrary to the dominant twentieth-century policy narrative among international development professionals, my study of South Asia's development and distribution of self-organized high-tech innovation reveals that subordinate networks of high-tech experts from less economically developed countries have the potential for both innovation and development in global fields of science.

The subordinate experts in this book are community ophthalmology professionals: community eye healthcare workers, ophthalmologists, hospital managers, epidemiologists, optometrists, paramedics, and other allied health professionals. They typically provide eye health services to a large number of poor, blind and low-vision patients, and track population-wide outcomes. Likely as a result, their pattern of spending on technologies, consumables, etc., skews toward high volume and low cost. The eye health services provided by community ophthalmology professionals ranges from simple screening for vision problems to more complex surgical correction for eye diseases. Frequently, but not always, community ophthalmology professionals are embedded in international networks.

US ophthalmologist, Dr. Patricia E. Bath first defined the term community ophthalmology in her 1976 presentation to the American Public Health Association meeting in Miami, Florida, as "the discipline of blindness prevention utilizing the methodologies of public health, community medicine and clinical ophthalmology" (Bath 1978, 1913 citing Bath 1976). She was the first to coin this term in the peer-reviewed scientific literature written in English (Bath 1976, 1978, 1979). In 1970, primary health care was a newly imagined agenda inspired by Chinese barefoot doctors and propagated through the World Health Organization (WHO) 1978 Alma-Ata Declaration (Chorev 2012, 66–79; Xu and Hu 2017, 143; WHO Executive Board, 55 1974). Dr. Bath made integrating eye health care into primary health care the cornerstone of her new program of community ophthalmology (Bath 1976, 1978, 1979). This was a controversial argument for her to make to the US public health community and the US ophthalmology community In the 1970s and 1980s.

1.2   Blindness and Cataract Surgery as a Socio-Technical Regime

Of the many diseases that affect human health around the world, blindness is important to study because it affects such a large number and has such a devastating impact on identities and livelihoods. Blindness in Asia is interesting for a variety of reasons. The first couching surgery to correct blindness due to cataract was first performed in southern India more than two-thousand years ago (Elliot 1917; Wilson 1988, 3). Seventh-century records from China show Indian men with couching needles (Deshpande 2000, 371). Thus, South Asia appears to be an important site over time for investigating and treating eye diseases.

Cataract disease causes most of the avoidable blindness globally and therefore has been the focus of programmatic efforts by multilateral agencies such as the World Health Organization and by international non-governmental organizations such as the International Agency for the Prevention of Blindness and the Lions Clubs International Foundation. After cataract disease, the non-communicable disease of glaucoma causes the second highest number of patients with blindness at 8%. Trachoma is one of several other eye diseases that cause blindness. At present, trachoma and other diseases that damage the cornea of the eye account for only 7% of avoidable blindness (Pascolini and Mariotti 2012). As a communicable disease, trachoma is widely known because of the highly publicized efforts of several civil society organizations (e.g., Sight Savers International and the James E. Carter Center Trachoma Control Program) working over many decades to address this disease in Africa. Eye diseases that damage the cornea can often be corrected through surgery. Eye bank technicians excise intact corneas from the donated eyes of deceased persons, and ophthalmologists then surgically implant the corneas into patients to restore their sight.

Cataract disease likewise requires surgery for restoring sight. Therefore, the efforts of eye hospitals such as Tilganga and Aravind have focused on creating human and physical infrastructures to meet the demand for cataract surgery. As part of their work, they created a new surgical technique for cataract called small incision cataract surgery (see Chapter 6).

I discuss five types of cataract surgery in this book. These include intracapsular cataract extraction (ICCE), extracapsular cataract extraction (ECCE), phacoemulsification (Phaco), mini-nuc, and small incision cataract surgery (SICS). Every surgery performed to remove a cataract is a derivative of either ICCE or ECCE (see the Glossary). Each cataract surgery involves, at minimum, removing the opacified (or clouded) natural lens (typically a diameter of 8–9 mm) from the eye. As time passes, the innovations in surgical technique, and advances in ophthalmic products (called consumables), result in: smaller incisions, fewer costly sutures, shorter recovery periods, and better visual outcomes for the patients who undergo cataract surgery.

My initial example of an incumbent socio-technical regime in the global field of ophthalmology is phacoemulsification. A system builder and the inventor of the phacoemulsification probe, Dr. Charles D. Kelman, found to his chagrin that government policies and regulations are key to the growth of any socio-technical regime. In clinical ophthalmology, one might compare the phacoemulsification probes of ophthalmologists to the drills of dentists—an ubiquitous and taken-for-granted tool for quickly restoring health to their patients. For the field of ophthalmology, the common idea is that Phaco is the gold standard for cataract surgery (Hillman 2017). This, however, was not always true. Before Phaco was the gold standard, ICCE was the gold standard in cataract surgery (see Chapters 2 and 5).

Dr. Kelman had to argue with his peers in the field of ophthalmology in the 1970s in order to convince them of the utility of his new ECCE-derived phacoemulsification technique. In 1973, US federal regulators decided that no Medicare payments should be made to any ophthalmologists who were using phacoemulsification, as it was deemed an experimental procedure (Ocular Surgery News U.S. Edition 2004; Hillman 2017). This was bad news for phaco: medicare payments were a significant source of income for ophthalmologists performing cataract surgery on an aging US population.

Dr. Kelman is an example of a heroic inventor who had to work as an opinion leader (see Rogers 2003); he had to convince his peers that his new surgical technology practice was useful and could provide better outcomes for patients than the conventional procedure of the time. He was successful; by the early 1980s, Phaco went into clinical trials and US medical schools quickly adopted it for training ophthalmologists (Ocular Surgery News U.S. Edition 2004).

A socio-technical regime includes elements such as: governmental regulation; economic capital; technological artifacts; networks of experts; an education pipeline of technicians in training; and other supporting social, economic, and technical infrastructures (Geels 2002; Hughes 1994). A socio-technical regime is large and embedded in a socio-technical landscape (Geels 2002; Hughes 1987, 1994). The socio-technical landscape is the environment external to the socio-technical regime, to include macroscale politics, values, culture, and economics as well as the physical environment (Geels and Schot 2007). This book looks closely at global networks of medical experts, biomedical companies, and users. Therefore, the socio-technical landscape physically stretches worldwide and operates through globalization (Ritzer 1996; Worthington 1993).

The socio-technical regime, over time, wields increasing influence over the development of new technologies. Historian Thomas Hughes (1987, 62) suggests that, "Radical inventions, if successfully developed, culminate in technological systems." A socio-technical system grows through the efforts of system builders who build networks. Additionally, the socio-technical regime grows through economies of scale and scope. Economies of scale decrease the unit cost per product because of the efficient production of a high volume of products. In economies of scope, the same flexible equipment (or people) can make a variety of products efficiently and therefore attracts the design of new products (Hughes 1994). For example, using phacoemulsification involves one-time costs in the form of training and the purchase of the machine. However, it also involves repeated costs in the form of ophthalmic consumables, consistent electricity supply, and maintenance. Within the Phaco-regime, economies of scope arise from training infrastructure that has developed in teaching hospitals around the world to train ophthalmology residents to perform surgery. Economies of scope also involve employing biomedical engineers, instrument technicians, ophthalmologists, and ophthalmic assistants to design, repair, use, and clean expensive phacoemulsification surgical equipment.

The Phaco-regime is dominated by multinational firms and physicians located geo-politically in the global north, to include: Apollo Optical Systems (New York), Bausch & Lomb Surgical (California), Johnson & Johnson Vision (Florida), STAAR Surgical (California), Carl Zeiss Meditech (Germany), Ophtec (Netherlands), and Hoya Vision Care (Japan). One of the market leaders in ophthalmic consumables and equipment is Alcon, Inc. (Data Monitor 2008; Medical Devices and Surgical Technology Week 2006). Alcon is a company that produces ophthalmic consumables as the second largest division of Novartis. It also purchased CooperVision (California) and through that company owned Cavitron Equipment Corp. (New York), which was the original manufacturer of the Kelman-Cavitron phacoemulsification probe (Hillman 2017).

Originally, Alcon was founded in Texas—its name shortens and combines the two founders' family names. Presently, Alcon is headquartered in Switzerland (Novartis 2013). It employs 1550 employees in research and development spread across laboratories in the global north and specifically in Japan, the USA, Spain, and Switzerland (Data Monitor 2008). As is typical of a multinational company, Alcon has manufacturing facilities all over the world, including in Belgium, Ireland, Germany, the USA, and Switzerland (Data Monitor 2008). In these facilities, Alcon produces a variety of ophthalmic consumables, instruments, and equipment. These include pharmaceuticals (e.g., eye drops and glaucoma medication), consumer products (e.g., contact lenses), and surgical products and equipment (e.g., intraocular lenses, glaucoma and retina stents, phacoemulsification machines). Alcon's most popular product is the foldable AcrySoft® intraocular lens (Data Monitor 2008).

Socio-technical regimes have momentum: As time increases, and the socio-technical system grows, the landscape that used to shape it has less influence, while the regime becomes more entrenched, ossified, and stable. With this stability, it is harder for the socio-technical regime to change its technological trajectory (Hughes 1987, 1994; Geels 2002, 2005; Geels and Schot 2007). This momentum is visible by the waning of societal influence on the elements of the system and the waxing of the system's influence in shaping societal problems and outcomes (Hughes 1987, 1994).

The Phaco-regime has momentum in the global field of ophthalmology. Multinational companies such as Alcon demonstrate the momentum of the Phaco-regime. For example, Alcon features largely in philanthropy: it regularly donates equipment to various eye units around the world. Thus, it is likely that Aravind and other eye institutions in less economically developed countries count Alcon among their international partners. Additionally, as a multinational company, Alcon's sales are global, with the larger share, 52.3%, outside of the USA. Indeed, 15.5% of Alcon's sales are from emerging markets, e.g., Brazil, India, China, and so forth (Data Monitor 2008). The global sales of products by multinational companies such as Alcon, Zeiss, and Hoya help to increase accumulation of capital in the global north. Ophthalmologists and wealthy patients in the global south may benefit from these products on an individual basis, but there is no corresponding national economic development in less economically developed countries.

Meanwhile, many international development practitioners are interested in a general model of endogenous technological development that actually works for countries in the global south. Two concerns among postcolonial science and technology studies, especially among subaltern historians of science, are to provincialize Europe (Anderson 2002; Arnold 2005; Chakrabarty 1995; McNeil 2005) while demonstrating the complexity of intercultural exchanges of knowledge and technology (Fan 2012; Raj 2010).

This book addresses these two concerns by offering a general theoretical model and correlating concepts. Firstly, by conceptualizing interlocking innovations, the book describes the production of linked innovations in technique, product, and process. Secondly, by conceptualizing contestation, the book explains how challengers from niches in the global south contest global knowledge hierarchies in a socio-technical regime under the control of incumbents in the global north. Finally, by describing the general theoretical model, the dual regime thesis, the book explains the emergence of a global socio-technical regime from a particular region of the world, South Asia, which has grown in scale and scope to encompass many countries of the global south.

1.3   Scaling Up Development in Appropriate Technology

Several theories account for science, technology, and international development; the majority have technology transfer as a major component. Historian of science, George Basalla's diffusion thesis (1967), states that science and technology transfers from Empire to Colony (the West to the Rest). This diffusion thesis is, unfortunately, implicit to many development experts' work involving science and technology transfer. As a result of their experience rebuilding Europe through the US Marshall Plan, such experts as early as 1948 began to believe that they could extend this plan to successfully transfer technology to the less economically developed countries in the non-West or global south (Seely 2003, 13). The invisibility of Basalla's thesis among development experts means that the directionality of technology transfer from a wealthy industrialized global north to a less economically developed (but historically and culturally developed) global south is rarely questioned (Pollock 2014). As a result, alternative forms of development are underexplored.

After withdrawing their imperial forces from colonies, Western nations emphasized linear and incremental change through progressive stages of technological implementation in economic development projects within their former colonies. This theory of national economic and social change has had a different scientific basis over time, but typically highlights a Western definition of linear progress through diffusion (Pieterse 1991). Like many theories, developmentalism was created from the perspective of those in power, in this case, Western development experts (Pieterse 1991).

Scholars studying international development have critiqued developmentalism (Escobar 1994; Pieterse 1991, 2000). Beginning in the 1970s, dependency theory has long challenged developmentalism, saying that,

> the economic structures of contemporary underdeveloped countries is .... the result of being involved in the world-economy as a peripheral, raw material producing area, or as [Andre Gunder] Frank puts it for Chile, 'underdevelopment ... is the necessary product of four centuries of capitalism itself'. (Wallerstein 1974, 392)

The work of Frantz Fanon has been a strong influence on dependency theorists. Fanon was a psychiatrist and African liberation activist who had earlier argued that the "Third World literally created the Modern World" (Ouaissa 2015 citing Fanon 1961, 58). Many of the successes of the First World, or the global north, comes at the rarely discussed cost of extracting resources (mineral, epistemic, agricultural, etc.) from the Third World or the global south (Harding 2008).

Dependency theory points toward why high-technology transfer from the global north to the global south tends to fail. Typically, such high-technology transfer is one way, local capacity is not developed, culture and values are not considered, and, most importantly, the power dynamics between countries that shape directionality of science and technology flow remain unaltered. The types of projects that international development experts typically conduct continue to originate primarily from government agencies or development organizations in the global north and are disseminated, one way, to other institutions or agencies in the global south (Packard 1997; Pollock 2014). Likewise, health technology transfer is typically unidirectional from the global north to the global south or from urban to rural areas (WHO Executive Board, 55 1974). The diffusion thesis remains alive and well because there is a strong-thread of technological determinism in Western development aid (Cherlet 2014; Visvanathan 2015 [2001]).

Despite opposing evidence and theoretical critique, developmentalist ideology persists among international development professionals, nationalists, and wealthy philanthropists (individuals and institutions). The myth of linear modern development permeates all discussions of national economic development. Fanon furthermore suggested that, because they believe this myth, those in authority (elites from both the global north and the global south) are not attentive to the power structures of exploitation, extraction, and racism that have characterized past colonialism and continue to characterize neoliberal globalization (Grosfoguel and Cervantes-Rodríguez 2002, xxv–xxvii; Ouaissa 2015 citing Fanon 1961, 98). Instead, development practitioners point toward the outcomes of these unequal power structures—the various deficits, and lacks—and misidentify them as the problem that a linear international development program can solve (Escobar 1994; Nieusma 2007).

The unfortunate result is that, despite small gains, this developmentalist model often fails because it addresses peoples' needs temporarily and haphazardly.

The appropriate technology movement, started by the British economist Ernst F. Schumacher in the late 1960s, offers another critique of diffusion. Schumacher advanced a different perspective on matching societal needs to technological design and transfer (Kaplinsky 2011; Seely 2003, 19). Influenced by Gandhian and Burmese Buddhist philosophies that he encountered in South Asia, Schumacher was interested in small-scale, locally produced industry (Willoughby 1990; Schumacher 1973). Such industry is appropriate for places with a large population density and thus a large labor surplus (Schumacher 1973). Therefore, Schumacher (1973) argued that appropriate technology should be labor intensive instead of capital intensive. Schumacher's argument was important, and credible, but did not adequately interrogate the conflicts between appropriate technology and existing social structures, values, and norms.

Existing social structures enable elites to accumulate wealth and power through the growth of large-scale, low-labor socio-technical systems such as energy infrastructure. These same social structures put elites in control of the corporations responsible for both large-scale and small-scale technology transfer. However, Schumacher failed to critique these social structures (Varma 2003). Moreover, the appropriate technology movement did not consider that transferring technology involves transferring culture and values (De Castro 1997; Parthasarathy 2006, 352).

Once international development experts ran into problems caused by differences in culture and values, they became more thoughtful about the social underpinnings of technology transfer activities (Seely 2003, 13, 19). The Sussex Manifesto, published by the United Nations in 1970, was heavily influenced by the appropriate technology movement and the work of Schumacher. It served as a pivotal document that deemphasized technology transfer and instead stressed the importance of systematic build-up of endogenous science and technology production capabilities in less economically developed countries (Ely and Bell 2009; Kaplinsky 2011).

Thus, the internal tensions of the appropriate technology movement directly relate to the economic and social logics of who consumes appropriate technology versus who accumulates wealth produced through disseminating appropriate technology (Kaplinsky 1990). This implicates: models of entrepreneurship, corporate structure, and the circulation of science and technology.

Previous theories of innovation based in social movements or civil society organizations (Hess 2007; Smith et al. 2016; Vasi 2011) have described persons in a subordinate position of power challenging existing global structural inequality by producing and distributing innovation to meet an ideological goal. However, this previous work does not provide a generalized model of socio-technical change. The next section introduces the current theory on socio-technical change using the multi-level perspective and some its shortcomings. This is followed by a section which introduces a general theoretical framework for how a socio-technical regime, originates from a less economically developed country to serve the needs of the poor, develops and uses context-appropriate high technology, and exists in the global south in parallel to a different socio-technical regime that addresses the same socio-technical problem in the global north.

1.4   Multi-level Perspective in Transition Studies of the Global South

Early work in sociology of technology focused on highlighting the importance of studying non-humans in addition to humans (Callon 1984; Bruno Latour writing as Jim Johnson 1988). Studying the relationship between humans and artifacts was essential to understand how user groups shape the development and diffusion of particular technologies (Pinch and Bijker 1987; Kline and Pinch 1996). This scholarship illuminated how the many linkages between various actors (e.g., humans, non-humans, organizations and infrastructures) form into a seamless web or large technological system (Hughes 1987). This early scholarship demonstrated that non-humans, humans, and the social world are inextricably intertwined.

As sociology of technology was incorporated into management studies of innovation, a central concern emerged of how to study change in such systems of interlinked: users, emerging technologies, regulatory policies, entrenched infrastructures, etc. Scholars were very interested in how large technological systems transition over time to incorporate new and emerging technologies (Geels 2002, 2005, 2014). Transition studies scholars use a suite of concepts that evaluate change over time across multiple levels through mutual shaping between landscapes, socio-technical regimes (elsewhere called socio-technical systems; see definitions in Sect. 1.2), and niches.

Now that the multi-level perspective has been around for more than a decade, several scholars are interested in how this framework can explain different types of socio-technical change in the global south (Furlong 2014; Osunmuyiwa and Kalfagianni 2016; Power et al. 2016). This transitions theory scholarship provides a multi-level perspective, but the analyses thus far have primarily been about socio-technical regimes at the level of nation-states (Osunmuyiwa and Kalfagianni 2016). One exception (see Power et al. 2016) evaluates south-south cooperation between the emerging power block of BRIC nations (the less economically developed countries of Brazil, Russia, India, and China) and two African countries (Mozambique and South Africa).

Furlong suggests that multiple incremental innovations can coexist together over many years in the dilapidated water supply infrastructure of Columbia as a socio-technical regime characterized by disrepair (Furlong 2014, 141–43; Henke 1999). Her example, because of its longevity and emphasis on incremental innovation, contradicts previous research where multiple radical innovations briefly coexist until one becomes dominant (Geels and Schot 2007, 408–9). Instead, Furlong (2014) argues that disrepair has its own particular momentum in a socio-technical regime. This momentum occurs through the interests, concerns, and actions of human users as they are enabled and constrained by artifacts, resources, companies, and government regulations. Furthermore, Furlong (2014) usefully points to a consistent irregularity: in many countries of the global south, often there are coexisting physical infrastructures to address the same technical problem.

Furlong's (2014) scholarship highlights an underlying problem with the multi-level perspective: the implicit Eurocentrism embedded in the founding case for the theoretical framework. Geels (2002) first demonstrated the multi-level perspective with the case of the expansion of the worldwide shipping industry after the war between Britain and its American colonies. The story of a former colony gaining market share and navigating mercantile capitalist international trade has unexplored themes of national sovereignty and anti-dependency. Uncovering such embedded postcolonial relationships might be useful for explaining technological change in the global south. Previously, development discourse has defined such former colonies and less economically developed countries of the global south as dependent on the wealthier nations of the global north. As a counterpoint, this book offers a case of innovation that is arising outside the West, thereby disputing the one-way direction for global science and technology flow typically assumed by experts.

Furlong's (2014) scholarship challenged the understanding of socio-technical system transitions as moving from one singular regime to a new singular regime. This book further extends this line of inquiry by examining the conditions where a global landscape shifts from supporting one dominant regime to supporting two dominant regimes, each with their own geographically delineated, but economically intertwined, areas of control. I suggest a new socio-technical system transition pathway: coexistence of dual (incumbent and challenger) regimes.

Coexistence of dual regimes begins with actors who are challenging the incumbent regime. These challengers have an emergent radical rule-set that shapes their orientation toward new technologies, sciences, beliefs, missions, and business models to address a profoundly large market failure. Their efforts to address this market failure result in interlocking innovations that scale up to become a new socio-technical regime that does not replace the incumbent regime, but operates alongside it in the landscape.

The dual regime thesis suggests that, because of the uneven development of science and technology globally, especially between wealthy countries of the global north and less economically developed countries of the global south, it is possible to have two regimes that are both dominant in different geographic regions of the world. The two regimes interact with each other, but one controls the technological trajectories of innovations in one geo-politically prescribed area, while the other controls the technological trajectories of innovations in a second, different geo-politically prescribed area.

The dual regime thesis accounts for how two socio-technical regimes can simultaneously be ideologically in opposition to each other, and coexist in the socio-technical landscape. Through the dual regime thesis, this book will continue to explore the nature and boundaries of a socio-technical regime, and whether a global socio-technical regime must also be physically located worldwide (Worthington 1993).

1.5 General Theoretical Framework: Dual Regime Thesis

This book offers a general theory, the dual regime thesis, to explain the emergence, in less economically developed countries, of alternative high-tech solutions combined with social enterprise to address a particular problem of the rural poor, and the distribution of these innovations throughout the region and around the world. The example of community ophthalmology professionals and their systemic technology choice demonstrates how to bridge the two main approaches to science and technology selection: capital intensive and low labor versus cost-efficient and labor intensive.

In this book, I will describe dual regimes as a new technology transition pathway in the multi-level perspective of socio-technical change. This adds to previous work by Geels and Schot (2007) who outlined the following four transition pathways,

> **reconfiguration**: emphasizes internal changes in how a regime utilizes linked incremental innovations for economic reasons;
> **transformation**: highlights internal changes, but this time in a regime's policies and rules that shape future technological trajectories in response to advocacy from outsiders and fringe groups;

technological substitution: demonstrates how a mature radical innovation emerging from a niche accumulates more niches, and grows to replace the incumbent regime with a new one; and lastly; and

dealignment and realignment: reveals how an incumbent regime is destabilized and in the vacuum it leaves behind, multiple niche-protected radical innovations compete until one emerges as dominant and grows into a new regime that replaces the incumbent regime.

There are some similarities between these four transition pathways (Geels and Schot 2007; Slayton and Spinardi 2016). The first two pathways, reconfiguration and transformation, emphasize stability in the landscape and internal change in the incumbent regime; the incumbent regime is then renewed. In contrast, instability in the landscape triggers the last two pathways, technological substitution and dealignment and realignment, which then create a new regime that replaces the old one. All four transition pathways start and end with one socio-technical regime. The new transition pathway I will describe, coexistence of dual regimes, starts with the incumbent regime and ends with dual regimes.

Challengers with an emergent radical rule-set scale up interlocking innovations through diffusion and appropriation. The interlocking innovations accumulate niches through translation and then, through contestation, fracture the singular incumbent regime, which splits into dual regimes. In Fig. 1.1, the three small clusters of arrows represent multiple niches, each nurturing an innovation. The autonomous social network supporting these niches has its own emergent radical rule-set. The three solid lines, one starting in each niche and moving upward, represent how the innovations are centered around this emergent radical rule-set as they interlock multiple, complimentary knowledge and artifacts composed of incremental, radical, and sub-system innovations. Similar to any other socio-technical regime, the incumbent socio-technical regime, STR, is defined by seven points for its seven dimensions: dimension 1 technology; dimension 2 markets, user practices; dimension 3 culture, symbolic meaning; dimension 4 infrastructure; dimension 5 industry; dimension 6 policy; and dimension 7 scientific knowledge (Geels 2002).

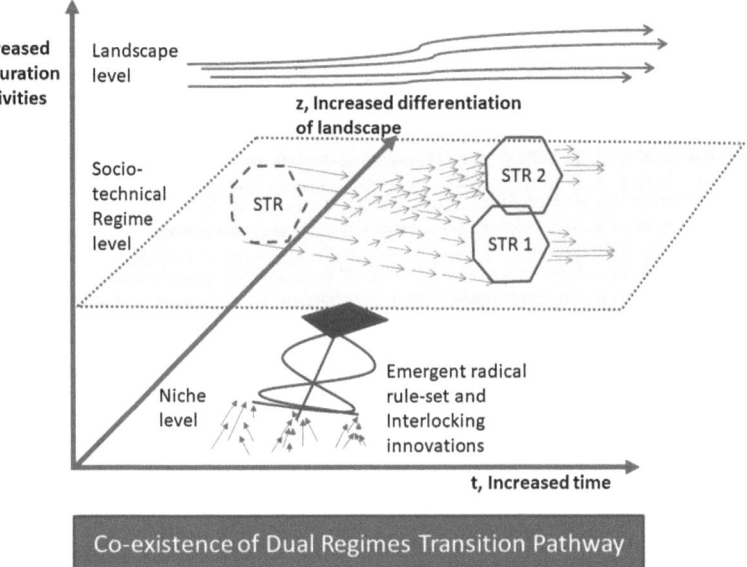

Fig. 1.1 An emergent radical rule-set, multiple niches supporting interlocking innovations in finance, science and technology, and coexistence of dual regimes in the landscape

In Fig. 1.1, the interlocking innovations accumulate niches across geo-political areas of the landscape and become black boxed with: a market of nonusers from the incumbent regime, an emergent radical rule-set, and innovations in finance, science and technology. In particular, an early financial innovation is key because the incumbent regime resists the emergent radical rule-set and is not inclined to support the novel scientific and technical innovations in the niches. The interlocking innovations contest and fracture the incumbent socio-technical regime, forming the challenger socio-technical regime STR2 that coexists with the incumbent regime STR1. At the meso-level of socio-technical regimes, both STR1 and STR2 solve the same technical problem, but operate in different geo-political areas of the world.

Several features of the dual regime thesis make it a distinctive way of theorizing technological change in socio-technical systems. The most significant is that the dual regime thesis results in dual regimes (the incumbent and the new); this outcome makes it a unique transition pathway in the transition studies literature. Dual regimes form in part by accommodating the interests of nonusers (Winner 1980, Wyatt 2003) and non-producers of the incumbent regime. The challengers to the incumbent regime, in this case, community ophthalmology professionals, deliberately focus their limited resources (influence, funds, time, etc.) and attention on addressing the needs of nonusers, e.g., rural poor blind patients. Expert non-producers who act as consumers of science and technology in the incumbent regime then become producers in the new second regime that emerges. In this case, ophthalmologists and engineers in the global south then create their own surgical sciences, technology products, organizational practices, and finance models. This demographic of nonusers and non-producers was previously unacknowledged in the incumbent regime, but now occupy important places in the new second regime.

A second distinctive feature of the dual regime thesis is its relevance for considering the politics of transferring a large technological system versus the politics of transferring an artifact (Winner 1980). This is especially important when considering technology for development. As past literature has shown (see above), both proponents of technology for development and advocates of appropriate technology for development have suffered the same blind spot: They have been unable to envision how to mass produce high-quality, low-cost goods for the working poor without increasing wealth inequality between the rich corporation owners and poor laborers. This blind spot across multiple scales of analysis arbitrates unjust outcomes for: poor laborers versus rich corporation owners; poor rural areas versus wealthy urban areas; poor versus wealthy people within urban areas; and less economically developed countries versus wealthy industrialized nations. The dual regime thesis helps us to consider the politics of transferring a socio-technical system because it emphasizes the importance of collective action-based industrial transitions. While epistemic and design conflicts are typical of industrial transition movements (Hess 2016), I argue that for challengers creating a new regime, these conflicts are multiple, simultaneous, and interwoven.

Some scholars might maintain that the coexistence of dual regimes is not a new transition pathway, but instead a reconfiguration. The two pathways are similar because they both emphasize economic reasons for the diffusion of linked incremental innovations from an old niche to a new regime. However, the dual regime thesis differs from reconfiguration primarily because it still involves the development of radical innovations.

Other transition studies scholars might argue that the coexistence of dual regimes is really just another example of dealignment and realignment. In both pathways, the challengers recognize that their radical emergent rule-set and technological trajectory do not match the incumbent regime. However, in the dual regime thesis these challengers create and circulate interlocking innovations to create a new second overlapping, parallel regime instead of replacing the dominant regime with a new regime.

The third distinctive feature of the dual regime thesis is the importance of multiple modes of science and technology circulation where knowledge and artifacts are transferred, e.g., diffusion, appropriation, translation, and contestation. The multiple modes of science and technology circulation have different power dynamics and directions of travel. In the dual regime thesis, diffusion and appropriation are concurrent, while translation occurs later after the development of interlocking innovations. Meanwhile, contestation occurs at the same time as the three other modes of circulation until the fracture point is reached in an incumbent regime to produce dual regimes. Consequently, the dual regime thesis definitively highlights that technological change in socio-technical systems is co-constructed with science and technology circulation.

1.6   Conclusion: Chapter Summaries

Jamison and Hård (2003) argue that scholars studying technological change need to be attentive to how the different social science and humanistic scholarly traditions shape the sites, objects, and practices being studied. They have characterized scholarly studies of technological change as three types of story lines: economists studying production and products; sociologists studying mediators and networks; and historians and anthropologists studying users and sites (Jamison and Hård 2003). In many ways, this book is an attempt to interweave these types of storylines together, to tell a story of science and technology circulation that pays attention to users in different sites who are mediating production and moving products through networks. Endogenous and context-appropriate science and technology production and circulation are significant; this story counters the more common narrative of Western technology transfer as development aid.

In answer to my first research question about the emergence of alternative high-tech solutions combined with social enterprise, Chapters 2 through 4 describe the origins of community ophthalmology organizations, and their models of social enterprise, while later Chapters 5 through 6 provide more detail on their local production and global circulation of science and technology.

In Chapter 2, I describe how community ophthalmology professionals in the global south began to create an expert social network that would later challenge clinical ophthalmologists practicing phacoemulsification in the incumbent regime. The community ophthalmology appropriate technology movement emerged in South Asia and has strong connections to the earlier eradication of smallpox. Chapter 3 illuminates how Indian and Nepalese community ophthalmologists made a model of social entrepreneurship that later supported the creation of novel technological innovations. By recounting the origins of eye hospitals in India and Nepal, I illuminate how their unique finance model allows community ophthalmologists to maintain their economic ideology, which diverges from that of clinical ophthalmology. This resulted in the provision of quality health care to low-income patients for a minimal (subsidized) fee or no fee. Chapter 4 describes how, over time, community ophthalmology professionals learned how to increase local community support for their efforts, while simultaneously developing standardized practices to further their goal of eradicating and controlling blindness. I expand the concept of scientific witnessing to account for community ophthalmology professionals' habit of equating objective scientific practice with providing health care.

These first four chapters emphasize the network building and community embeddedness that created protective spaces in India and Nepal for the emerging autonomous global network to create niche innovations. Later community ophthalmologists continued their work with the endogenous production of technologies such as intraocular lenses (see Chapter 5) and novel surgical sciences such as small incision cataract surgery (see Chapter 6). This involved the circulation of science and technology.

In response to my second research question about the distribution of innovation throughout the region and around the world, Chapter 5 on diffusion and Chapter 6 on appropriation primarily describe north-south, and south-south science and technology circulation. Later, Chapter 7 on translation and Chapter 8 on contestation primarily describe south–south and south–north circulation. In this exemplary case of the creation of the network to control and eradicate blindness, interlocking innovations circulated from South Asia outward.

The diffusion of biomedical prosthetics from the global north to the global south meant debates about appropriate technology and technical sovereignty. In Chapter 5, I discuss the implicit anti-developmentalist ideology that emerged from the work of Indian and Nepalese community ophthalmology professionals to create local biomedical manufacturing laboratories. In contrast to adopting manufacturing technologies from the global north, Chapter 6 describes how South Asian community ophthalmology professionals adapted and reinvented the surgical science of extracapsular cataract extraction to make it into a microsurgical technique. I argue that their radical innovations in finance, standards, technologies, and science linked together to form interlocking innovations where context-appropriate changes in the science shape and are shaped by other changes in technology and management practices. Different eye units simultaneously created multiple models of low-cost, high-quality eye health care for the masses of unreached rural poor.

In Chapter 7, Indian and Nepalese institutions increasingly gained global visibility and stature as they translated interlocking innovations while training other community ophthalmology professionals in the global south. I trace the global movement of management practices, medical consumables, surgical sciences, and capital through medical professionals, managers, technologists, and consultants circulating between community ophthalmology units in Nepal, India, Kenya, and Mexico. The eye units in India and Nepal are particularly interested in disseminating their innovations both locally and to international colleagues. They offer reasonably priced (or free) educational materials, training courses, and consultations. In Chapter 8, Indian and Nepalese community ophthalmologists created new operating theater management practices and aseptic techniques as part of challenging knowledge hierarchies. I describe the feminist standpoints of community ophthalmologists as they politely insist on their scientific sovereignty to clinical ophthalmologists both domestic and foreign.

The community of ophthalmology professionals I describe are deliberate in their technology choices. In their resolve to combat avoidable blindness, they have embraced advocacy, health education, social entrepreneurship, and the production and circulation of science and technology. In Chapter 9, I offer to the multi-level perspective on socio-technical change a general theoretical model, the dual regime thesis, and associated concepts. I also argue that the production and dissemination of science and technology are better understood as concurrent processes.

In Chapter 2, I will describe the origins of a social network and appropriate technology movement which formed around the radical goal to provide accessible, affordable, and appropriate eye health care for blind patients.

References

Anderson, Warwick. 2002. "Introduction—Postcolonial Technoscience." *Social Studies of Science* 32 (5–6): 643–58.

Anonymous. 2010. "APACRS Eye World Asia-Pacific Meeting Reporter: Reporting Live From the 25th APAO Congress Bejing, September 16–20, 2010." *Eye World Magazine*, September 20. Retrieved August 21, 2011. http://www.apacrs.org/edm/APAO/mr/web_09202010.htm.

Arnold, David. 2005. "Europe, Technology, and Colonialism in the 20th Century." *History and Technology: An International Journal* 21 (1): 85–106.

Basalla, George. 1967. "The Spread of Western Science." *Science* 156: 611–22.

Bath, Patricia Era. 1976. "Rationale for a Program in Community Ophthalmology." Paper Presented at the American Public Health Association, Miami, FL.

———. 1978. "Blindness Prevention Through Programs of Community Ophthalmology in Developing Countries." XXIII Concilium Ophthalmologicum, Kyoto, International Congress Series No. 450, 2 (May): 1913–15.

———. 1979. "Rationale for a Program in Community Ophthalmology." *Journal of the National Medical Association* 71: 145.

Birtchnell, Thomas. 2009. "From 'Hindolence' to 'Spirinomics': Discourse, Practice and the Myth of Indian Enterprise." *South Asia-Journal of South Asian Studies* 32 (2): 248–68.

———. 2011. "Jugaad as Systemic Risk and Disruptive Innovation in India." *Contemporary South Asia* 19 (4): 357–72.

———. 2013. "Pyramid or Iceberg? Problematizing the Fortune to Be Made from India's Austerity." *Marketing Theory* 13 (3): 389–92.

Burawoy, Michael. 1998. "The Extended Case Method." *Sociological Theory* 16: 4–33.

———. 2000. "Introduction: Reaching for the Global." In *Global Ethnography: Forces, Connections, and Imaginations in a Postmodern World*, edited by Michael Burawoy, Joseph A. Blum, Sheba George, Zsuzsa Gille, Millie Thayer, Teresa Gowan, Lynne Haney, Maren Klawiter, Steve H. Lopez, and Sean Riain, 1st ed., 1–40. Berkeley and Los Angeles: University of California Press.

Callon, Michel. 1984. "Some Elements of a Sociology of Translation: Domestication of the Scallops and the Fishermen of St Brieuc Bay." *The Sociological Review* 32 (1_suppl): 196–233.

Chakrabarty, Dipesh. 1995. "Postcoloniality and the Artifice of History." In *The Post-colonial Studies Reader*, edited by Bill Ashcroft, Gareth Griffiths, and Helen Tiffin, 383–90. London and New York: Routledge.

Cherlet, Jan. 2014. "Epistemic and Technological Determinism in Development Aid." *Science Technology Human Values* 39 (6): 773–94.

Chorev, Nitsan. 2012. *The World Health Organization Between North and South*. Ithaca, NY: Cornell University Press.

Data Monitor. 2008. "Alcon, Inc. SWOT Analysis." Company Report DUNS Number: 086022753. Data Monitor. EBSCOhost. http://search.ebscohost.com/login.aspx?direct=true&db=buh&AN=33082004&site=ehost-live.

De Castro, Leonardo D. 1997. "Transporting Values by Technology Transfer." *Bioethics* 11 (3–4): 193–205.

Deshpande, Vijaya. 2000. "Ophthalmic Surgery: A Chapter in the History of Sino-Indian Medical Contacts." *Bulletin of the School of Oriental and African Studies*, University of London 63 (3): 370–88.

Elliot, Robert H. 1917. *The Indian Operation of Couching for Cataract*. London, UK: H. K. Lewis and Co. Ltd. The Foundation of the American Academy of Ophthalmology Museum of Vision & Ophthalmic Heritage. San Francisco, CA.

Ely, Adrian, and Martin Bell. 2009. "The Original "Sussex Manifesto": Its Past and Future Relevance." STEPS Working Paper 27, STEPS Centre, Brighton. http://steps-centre.org/wp-content/uploads/ely-and-bell-paper-27.pdf.

Englander, Karen. 2014. "The Rise of English as the Language of Science." In *Writing and Publishing Science Research Papers in English*, edited by Karen Englander, 3–4. Dordrecht: Springer Netherlands. http://link.springer.com/10.1007/978–94-007-7714-9_1.

Escobar, Arturo. 1994. *Encountering Development*. Princeton, NJ: Princeton University Press.

Fan, Fa-Ti. 2012. "The Global Turn in the History of Science." *East Asian Science, Technology and Society: An International Journal* 6 (2): 249–58.

Fanon, Frantz. 2004 [1961]. *The Wretched of the Earth*. Translated by Richard Philcox. New York: Grove Press.

Furlong, Kathryn. 2014. "STS beyond the 'Modern Infrastructure Ideal': Extending Theory by Engaging with Infrastructure Challenges in the South." *Technology in Society* 38 (August): 139–47.

Geels, Frank W. 2002. "Technological Transitions as Evolutionary Reconfiguration Processes: A Multi-level Perspective and a Case-Study." Research Policy, NELSON + WINTER + 20, 31 (8–9): 1257–74.

———. 2005. "Conceptual Perspective on Sytems Innovations and Technological Transitions." In *Technological Transitions and System Innovations: A Co-evolutionary and Socio-Technical Analysis*, 75–102. Cheltenham, UK and Northampton, MA: Edward Elgar.

———. 2014. "Regime Resistance Against Low-Carbon Transitions: Introducing Politics and Power into the Multi-level Perspective." *Theory, Culture & Society* 31 (5): 21–40.

Geels, Frank W., and Johan Schot. 2007. "Typology of Sociotechnical Transition Pathways." Research Policy 36 (3): 399–417.

Grosfoguel, Ramón, and Ana Margarita Cervantes-Rodríguez, eds. 2002. *The Modern/Colonial/Capitalist World-System in the Twentieth Century: Global Processes, Antisystemic Movements, and the Geopolitics of Knowledge*. Westport, CT: Greenwood Press.

Harding, Sandra. 2008. *Sciences from Below: Feminisms, Postcolonialities and Modernities*. Durham, NC: Duke University Press.

———. 2009. "Postcolonial and Feminist Philosophies of Science and Technology: Convergences and Dissonances." *Postcolonial Studies* 12 (4): 401–21.

Henke, Christopher R. 1999. "The Mechanics of Workplace Order: Toward a Sociology of Repair." *Berkeley Journal of Sociology* 44: 55–81.

Hess, David J. 2007. *Alternative Pathways in Science and Industry: Activism, Innovation, and the Environment in an Era of Globalization*. Cambridge: The MIT Press.

———. 2016. *Undone Science: Social Movements, Mobilized Publics, and Industrial Transitions*. Cambridge: The MIT Press.

Hess, David J., Sulfikar Amir, Scott Frickel, Daniel Lee Kleinman, Kelly Moore, and Logan D. A. Williams. 2016. "Structural Inequality and the Politics of Science and Technology." In *The Handbook of Science and Technology Studies*, edited by Clark Miller, Laurel Smith-Doerr, Ulrike Felt, and Rayvon Fouché, 4th ed. Society for Social Studies of Science. Cambridge: The MIT Press.

Hillman, Liz. 2017. "Phaco Turns 50." *Eyeworld*, April. https://www.eyeworld.org/phaco-turns-50.

Hughes, Thomas Parke. 1987. "The Evolution of Large Technological Systems." In *The Social Construction of Technological Systems: New Directions in the Sociology and History of Technology*, edited by Wiebe E. Bijker, Thomas Parke Hughes, and Trevor J. Pinch, 51–82. Cambridge: The MIT Press.

———. 1994. "Technological Momentum." In *Does Technology Drive History? The Dilemma of Technological Determinism,* edited by Merritt Roc Smith and Leo Marx, 101–14. Cambridge: The MIT Press.

Hwang, K. 2008. "International Collaboration in Multilayered Center-Periphery in the Globalization of Science and Technology." *Science Technology & Human Values* 33 (1): 101–33.

Jamison, Andrew, and Mikael Hård. 2003. "The Story-Lines of Technological Change: Innovation, Construction and Appropriation." *Technology Analysis & Strategic Management* 15 (1): 45–59.

Johnson, Jim. 1988. "Mixing Humans with Non-humans? Sociology of a Few Mundane Artefacts." *Social Problems* 35: 298–310.

Kaplinsky, Raphael. 1990. "The Institutional Framework of Appropriate Techonology (AT) Development and Diffusion: Brick Manufacture in Three African Countries." In *The Economies of Small: Appropriate Technology in a Changing World*, 74–103. Rugby, Warwickshire, UK: Practical Action Publishing.

————. 2011. "Schumacher Meets Schumpeter: Appropriate Technology below the Radar." *Research Policy* 40 (2): 193–203.

Kline, Ronald, and Trevor Pinch. 1996. "Users as Agents of Technological Change: The Social Construction of the Automobile in the Rural United States." *Technology and Culture* 37 (4): 763–95.

Malunga, Chiku, and Susan H. Holcombe. 2014. "Endogenous Development: Naïve Romanticism or Practical Route to Sustainable African Development?" *Development in Practice* 24 (5–6): 615–22.

McMichael, Philip. 2010. *Contesting Development: Critical Struggles for Social Change.* New York: Routledge.

McNeil, Maureen. 2005. "Introduction: Postcolonial Technoscience." *Science as Culture* 14 (2): 105.

Medical Devices and Surgical Technology Week. 2006. "Frost & Sullivan Presents Alcon with Market Leadership Award." *Medical Devices and Surgical Technology Week,* April 9.

Nieusma, Dean. 2007. "Challenging Knowledge Hierarchies: Working Toward Sustainable Development in Sri Lanka's Energy Sector." *Sustainability: Science Practice and Policy* 3: 32–44. https://doi.org/10.1080/15487733.2007.11907990.

Novartis. 2013. "Alcon History and Timeline Represents How We Became the Global Leader in Eye Care." Retrieved April 28, 2013. http://www.alcon.com/about-alcon/alcon-history.aspx.

Ocular Surgery News U.S. Edition. 2004. "Visionary, Inventor Charles D. Kelman Is Dead at Age 74." *Ocular Surgery News U.S. Edition,* July 1. http://www.healio.com/ophthalmology/cataract-surgery/news/print/ocular-surgery-news/%7B0c283179-d00c-43f8-bac9-cc3c779c6e3c%7D/visionary-inventor-charles-d-kelman-is-dead-at-age-74.

Osunmuyiwa, Olufolahan, and Agni Kalfagianni. 2016. "Transitions in Unlikely Places: Exploring the Conditions for Renewable Energy Adoption in Nigeria." *Environmental Innovation and Societal Transitions.* Accessed November 10. https://doi.org/10.1016/j.eist.2016.07.002.

Ouaissa, Rachid. 2015. "Frantz Fanon: The Empowerment of the Periphery." *Middle East: Topics & Arguments* 5 (0): 100–6.

Packard, Randall M. 1997. "Visions of Postwar Health and Development and Their Impact on Public Health Interventions in the Developing World." In *International Development and the Social Sciences: Essays on the History and Politics of Knowledge,* edited by Frederick Cooper and Randall M. Packard. Berkeley and Los Angeles: University of California.

Parthasarathy, Shobita. 2006. "Reconceptualizing Technology Transfer: The Challenge of Shaping an International System of Genetic Testing for Breast Cancer." In *Shaping Science and Technology Policy: The Next Generation of Research*, edited by D. H. Guston and D. R. Sarewitz, 333–58. Madison: University of Wisconsin Press.

Pascolini, Donatella, and Silvio Paolo Mariotti. 2012. "Global Estimates of Visual Impairment: 2010." *British Journal of Ophthalmology* 96 (5): 614–18.

Pieterse, Jan Nederveen. 1991. "Dilemmas of Development Discourse: The Crisis of Developmentalism and the Comparative Method." *Development and Change* 22 (1): 5–29.

———. 2000. "After Post-development." *Third World Quarterly* 21 (2): 175–91.

Pinch, Trevor, and Wiebe E. Bijker. 1987. "The Social Construction of Facts and Artifacts: Or How the Sociology of Science and the Sociology of Technology Might Benefit Each Other." In *The Social Construction of Technological Systems: New Directions in the Sociology and History of Technology*, edited by Wiebe E. Bijker, Thomas Parke Hughes, and Trevor Pinch, 159–87. Cambridge: MIT Press.

Pollock, Anne. 2014. "Places of Pharmaceutical Knowledge-Making: Global Health, Postcolonial Science, and Hope in South African Drug Discovery." *Social Studies of Science* 44 (6): 848–73.

Power, Marcus, Peter Newell, Lucy Baker, Harriet Bulkeley, Joshua Kirshner, and Adrian Smith. 2016. "The Political Economy of Energy Transitions in Mozambique and South Africa: The Role of the Rising Powers." *Energy Research & Social Science* 17 (July): 10–19.

Raj, Kapil. 2010. "Introduction: Circulation and Locality in Early Modern Science." *The British Journal for the History of Science* 43 (Special Issue 04): 513–17.

Ritzer, George. 1996. "The McDonaldization Thesis: Is Expansion Inevitable?" *International Sociology* 11 (3): 291–308.

Rogers, Everett M. 2003 [1962]. *Diffusion of Innovations*, 5th ed. New York: The Free Press.

Roy, Ananya. 2010. *Poverty Capital: Microfinance and the Making of Development*. New York: Routledge.

Schumacher, Ernst F. 1973. *Small Is Beautiful: Economics as if People Mattered*. London: Blond & Briggs.

Seely, Bruce Edsall. 2003. "Historical Patterns in the Scholarship of Technology Transfer." *Comparative Technology Transfer and Society* 1 (1): 7–48.

Singh, Ramesh M., and Dinesh R. Bhuju. 2001. "Development of Science and Technology in Nepal." *Science Technology and Society* 6 (1): 159–178.

Slayton, Rebecca, and Graham Spinardi. 2016. "Radical Innovation in Scaling up: Boeing's Dreamliner and the Challenge of Socio-Technical Transitions." *Technovation* 47 (January): 47–58.

Smith, Adrian. 2002. "Transforming Technological Regimes for Sustainable Development: A Role for Appropriate Technology Niches?" 86. *SPRU Working Paper Series*. UK: University of Sussex. http://www.sussex.ac.uk/Units/spru/publications/imprint/sewps/sewp86/sewp86.html.

Smith, Adrian, Mariano Fressoli, Dinesh Abrol, Elisa Arond, and Adrian Ely. 2016. *Grassroots Innovation Movements*. New York, NY: Routledge.

Varma, Roli. 2003. "EF Schumacher: Changing the Paradigm of Bigger Is Better." *Bulletin of Science, Technology & Society* 23 (2): 114–24.

Vasi, Ion Bogdan. 2011. *Winds of Change: The Environmental Movement and the Global Development of the Wind Energy Industry*. New York: Oxford University Press.

Visvanathan, Shiv. 2015 [2001]. "Technology Transfer." In *International Encyclopedia of the Social & Behavioral Sciences*, edited by James D Wright, 2nd ed., 141–45. Amsterdam: Elsevier.

Wallerstein, Immanuel. 1974. "The Rise and Future Demise of the World Capitalist System: Concepts for Comparative Analysis." *Comparative Studies in Society and History* 16: 387–415.

Willoughby, Kelvin W. 1990. *Technology Choice: A Critique of the Appropriate Technology Movement*. Boulder, CO: Westview Press.

Wilson, John. 1988. "Preventing Blindness, A Retrospective." In *World Blindness and Its Prevention: Volume 3*, edited by the International Agency for the Prevention of Blindness and Carl Kupfer. New York: Oxford University Press.

Winner, L. 1980. "Do Artifacts Have Politics." *Daedalus* 109 (1): 121–36.

WHO. 2004. "Global Cataract Surgical Rates in 2004." Retrieved February 1, 2007. http://www.who.int/blindness/data_maps/CSR_WORLD_2004.jpg.

WHO Executive Board, 55. 1974. "Promotion of National Health Services: Report by the Director-General." EB55/9. Geneva, Switzerland: World Health Organization. http://apps.who.int/iris/handle/10665/148378.

Worthington, Richard. 1993. "Introduction: Science and Technology as a Global System." *Science, Technology, & Human Values* 18 (2): 176–85.

Wyatt, Sally ME. 2003. "Non-users Also Matter: The Construction of Users and Non-users of the Internet." In *How Users Matter: The Co-construction of*

Users and Technology, edited by Nelly Oudshoorn and Trevor Pinch, 67–79. Cambridge: MIT Press.

Xu, Sanchun, and Danian Hu. 2017. "Barefoot Doctors and the 'Health Care Revolution' in Rural China: A Study Centered on Shandong Province." *Endeavour*, Science, Technology, and Medicine in China's Cultural Revolution, 41 (3): 136–45.

2

Origins of an Autonomous Global Network to Eradicate Blindness

[T]here was already a very important movement underway that was begun by Sir John Wilson, then the founding Director of the Royal Commonwealth Society for the Blind (now "Sightsavers International"), who founded the International Agency for the Prevention of Blindness, IAPB...So this little network kept growing, this whole blindness prevention network with the WHO. (Dr. Alfred Sommer, Johns Hopkins University, unpublished interview, 2013)

In 1999, the International Agency for the Prevention of Blindness (IAPB) and the World Health Organization (WHO) created the "Vision 2020: The Right to Sight...the global initiative for the elimination of avoidable blindness, a joint program" (IAPB 2018a; Pascolini and Mariotti 2012). The goal of the Vision 2020 program was to prevent the predicted doubling of the number of people blind due to avoidable causes for the period of 1990–2020 (Foster and Resnikoff 2005; WHO 2009). In 2013, the sixty-sixth World Health Assembly approved the 2014–2019 Global Action Plan, which focused more concretely on steps to make eye health care universal and integrated at the primary healthcare level (IAPB 2018a; Bath 1976, 1978, 1979; WHO 2013).

© The Author(s) 2019
L. D. A. Williams, *Eradicating Blindness*,
https://doi.org/10.1007/978-981-13-1625-8_2

In this chapter, I begin to answer the puzzle with which I started my research: "Why do India and Nepal have high cataract surgical rates considering that they are less economically developed in comparison to the U.S.?" I have divided the remainder of this chapter into the following arguments: Sect. 2.1, explains some theory from sociology, history and the multi-level perspective of socio-technical system change, on the development of social networks and rules. Next, Sect. 2.2 suggests that because of war, capitalism, and colonialism, European medical professionals have long been involved in health care in South Asia. Subsequently, Sect. 2.3 reveals that the eradication of smallpox in WHO South-East Asia Regional Office was a serendipitous event that resulted in South Asia becoming the center of an autonomous global network to eradicate blindness. Section 2.4 indicates that the autonomous global network to eradicate blindness, represented by its most prominent member association, the IAPB, operates in the interstitial space between the WHO as the premier global health multilateral organization and national governments implementing blindness eradication and control programs. Section 2.5 describes how the Indian and Nepalese governments worked with NGOs to create eye health care programs, in their respective countries, that serve the rural poor. Finally, Sect. 2.6 concludes by describing the cognitive rule which continued to guide the work of the autonomous global network to eradicate blindness through appropriate and affordable methods.

2.1   Theory: Rules, Networks, and Socio-Technical Change

This chapter demonstrates that a new network of outside actors grows with a guiding principle that challenges the incumbent regime. This network develops its own expectations and vision. Social networks are an important first step for change in a socio-technical regime. Actors in the social network can act as rule users and rule makers (Geels and Schot 2007, 403). Rules in the network can be formal (e.g., regulations, standards, and laws), normative (e.g., values and norms), and cognitive (e.g., belief systems and guiding principles; see Geels 2005; Geels and Schot 2007).

The multi-level perspective draws on prior work in sociology and history of technology that has investigated networks across different scales, at the microscale of an individual laboratory and its interests (Latour 1987), the mesoscale of relevant interest groups (Bijker 1987), and the macroscale of large socio-technical systems (Hughes 1987). Similarly, prior work in sociology of health movements has demonstrated an interest in thinking through: who are the insiders and outsiders of health movement networks (Goldner 2004); and whether all health movement networks focus on challenging the classic target of the state (Hess 2007, 2016; Moore 1999, 2006). Joseph Harris (2015, 8) developed the concept of autonomous political networks to describe,

> people who share similar values and aims with respect to policy and politics and who operate in the intermediate space between dominant political actors...who occupy an assortment of occupational positions but whose relationships are characterized by regular interaction...these networks are 'autonomous' in the sense that they have their own agendas and act independently to advance them.

Harris (2015) describes how local elite physicians, who are not typically involved in politics (and are therefore outsiders), can trade on their vaunted professional objectivity and good reputation to make changes within a democratic political system. These autonomous networks of elite professionals independently advocate for social change and specific policy initiatives.

Likewise, the professionals in the autonomous global network I will describe in this chapter make similar recourse to their own expertise. However, they do not just target state governments, but additionally target the WHO. Later on in this book, you will see that they furthermore contest ophthalmology as a global field of science (Worthington 1993). As they work across geo-political borders, and the international aid divide between the global north and the global south, they are also developing a cognitive rule: the guiding principle that blindness in the human population should be eradicated if it is preventable or avoidable. This guiding principle is radical because, if these experts accomplish their goal, they will have eliminated their own jobs. Therefore, this cognitive rule is the foundation of an emergent radical rule-set that will support the challengers' work to contest the incumbent Phaco-regime in the global field of ophthalmology.

2.2 NGOs, Corporations, and Western Medicine in South Asia, the 1600s Onward

The origins of the autonomous global network to eradicate blindness offer an important opportunity to explore South Asians' significant contributions to the history of NGOs in global health. War, capitalism, and colonialism meant European medical professionals have long been involved in health care in South Asia.

One example is Nepal which was first introduced to Western modern medicine through foreign NGOs in the late 1600s, however, the Nepalese Kings and Regents tended to associate it with Western military dominance. In 1661, Catholic missionaries en route to Tibet and China first brought Western modern medicine to Nepal by establishing medical clinics in the three largest kingdoms of Kathmandu valley. From 1743 to 1768, Ghorkali King Prithvi Narayan Shah conquered or persuaded the small kingdoms inside Kathmandu valley to become one Hindu kingdom under his reign, despite attempted interference by the British East India Company (Manandhar 2005; Marasini 2003; Rankin 2004). This interference prompted His Majesty's Government of Nepal to expel the Catholic monks, but not before a wounded Ghorka prince was treated by a Capuchin Franciscan monk in 1763 for an eye injury received during war (Marasini 2003). After King Prithvi's death in 1775, his heir and oldest son, King Pratap Singh Shah, died in 1777 from smallpox after a two-year reign (Marasini 2003). Consequently, King Prithvi's younger son, Prince Bahadur Shah, acted as regent and continued his father's unification campaign outside the Kathmandu valley. This monarchy existed until 2008 when the government shifted to a federal republic. By the late 1700s, small Christian missions were engaged in Nepal without the administrative influence of large mercantile capitalist corporations like the British East India Company.

The British East India Company was interested in using Nepal as a route to China but was stymied at first by the Ghorkali kings. Later in the 1770s, the Ghorkali kings embarked upon a program to make Ghorkali their kingdom's official language (Hachhethu 2003). As a feudal kingdom, they were concerned with protecting their sovereignty. This guided their wary interactions with the British as the Ghorkali kings observed how the British East India Company ruled the many principalities of India through their diplomatic residencies. Earlier in their diplomatic relations with the British, Nepal blocked British trade to China through the major trans-Himalayan south to north route that runs from India through Kathmandu and into Tibet (Rankin 2004, 95; von der Heide 2012).

While the British failed to rule in Nepal, they did introduce Western medicine to the country (Marasini 2003; Heydon 2011). The British East India Company (and later British India) established residencies (1801–1804 and 1816–1923) to attempt indirect rule in Nepal as they had with Indian princely states (UK and Nepal 1923; Manandhar 2005). Having acquired better facility with mountain warfare through their skirmishes in North India, the British triumphed in the Anglo-Nepalese war (Rankin 2004). Therefore, in the 1816 treaty of Sugauli, the kingdom of Nepal turned over one-third of its territory to the British (including some Terai "plains" lands and the state of Sikkim). Nepal also began supplying Ghurka soldiers who fought against Indians to secure strategic sites for the British East India Company in the Indian princely states (Manandhar 2005; Rankin 2004).

Western cultural influence is demonstrated by the first modern Western hospital built in Nepal. While some Nepalese kings (Shahs) and hereditary prime ministers (Ranas) focused on building infrastructure for the country, many were occupied instead with conspicuous consumption and fighting each other for power. In the 1800s and 1900s, the kings visited Europe; they brought back interesting architecture, automobiles, etc., which were carried by foot into the hilly country which did not have rail until 1927 (Rankin 2004). The first hospital modeled after Western modern medicine, Prithvi–Bir Hospital, was named after the incumbent King and Prime Minister of Nepal in 1889 (Marasini 2003). The United Kingdom acknowledged Nepal's sovereignty by sending envoys (ambassadors) to the Hindu kingdom starting in 1924 (see UK and Nepal 1923).

In the mid-1960s, His Majesty's Government initiated a big plan for regionally administered health infrastructure. Once they were allowed to return to the country, Christian missions started establishing Nepalese hospitals in 1954 and the first domestic NGO hospital in 1958. By 1963, Nepal had 34 hospitals and 102 health centers as part of a healthcare scheme by His Majesty's Government Ministry of Health. In 1964, the government began regionalizing the comprehensive, multi-specialty hospitals in seven of fourteen zones across Nepal (Marasini 2003). This initiative required trained medical personnel.

Before the late 1980s, most Nepalese doctors were first educated in India. Many Nepalese institutions trained technicians and nurses (but not physicians) starting in 1951. Meanwhile, Nepal sent thirty to forty medical undergraduate students to train in India every year—some of whom never returned. In 1974, the Nepal Ministry of Health was concerned about this brain drain (WHO Regional Office for South-East Asia, Twenty-Seventh Session 1974). Once the first teaching hospital was established in 1986, Nepalese medical undergraduate students could train in medicine domestically (Marasini 2003).

In contrast to the kingdom of Nepal, British India and the mercantilist British East India Company fought many wars and generated substantial public health infrastructure before giving India independence in 1947. British East India Company ruled India indirectly through the three presidencies and the northwestern province starting in the late 1700s. The British East India Company set up the first medical departments with 234 surgeons across the three presidencies in 1785 (Mushtaq 2009). In the Madras presidency (now the state of Tamil Nadu, and parts of Andhra Pradesh, Karnataka, Kerala and Orissa), the second eye hospital in the world started by Europeans, Madras Eye Infirmary, was created in 1819 (Madras Medical College, n.d.). After the Indian Rebellion, Britain ruled the Indian colony directly starting in 1858.

British India started creating public health commissions in each province in 1870. These were created in part to decrease the attrition rate of Army soldiers: 69 deaths out of every 1000 (Mushtaq 2009; Johnson 2008). Meanwhile, the Madras Eye Infirmary was renamed the Government Ophthalmic Hospital by the British Crown in 1888

(Madras Medical College n. d.). Western ophthalmologists learned from Indian itinerant eye surgeons in the late 1800s. A historical account of this knowledge transfer was written by the former Government Ophthalmic Hospital superintendent, Lt. Colonel R. Henry Elliot, in his post-retirement book (Elliot 1917). In 1896, the Indian Medical Service concentrated administrative power from three earlier medical departments, one per each presidency (Mushtaq 2009).

In the early 1900s, British India also tended to see high infectious eye disease rates, specifically trachoma, among its cataract surgery patients (Smith 1910, 102). While in the Indian Medical Service, Lt. Colonel Henry Smith practiced intracapsular cataract extraction surgery for years on tens of thousands of Indian patients in the northwestern province of Panjab (now the state of Punjab). Lt. Colonel Smith wrote an educational textbook at the request of US and European ophthalmologists who used his popular technique (Smith 1910, v). Dr. Derrick T. Vail, a professor of Ophthalmology at the University of Cincinnati (USA), created the illustrations for the textbook based on the sketches he made when he observed Col. Smith at work.

Smith believed his version of ICCE was very efficacious and caused fewer complications than the more popular ECCE technique (Smith 1910, 5). He compared the results for ECCE, where in 14% of cases the eye was lost, to his own results with ICCE where in 1% of cases the eye was lost (Smith 1910, 103). European ophthalmologists in the early 1900s knew the cataracts Smith operated on were predominantly mature cataracts (Smith 1910, 5). Immature cataract was more prevalent in European communities; therefore, these European ophthalmologists questioned him about the relevance of his technique to their community (Smith 1910, 5). Applying Smith's ICCE technique to immature cataract would reduce the potential negative impact of the patient's deteriorating vision (Smith 1910, 5). Dr. Alfred Knapp gave an account in the US journal the *Archives of Ophthalmology* that describes Smith's work performing 104 surgeries (Knapp 1908, 13). Together, Smith's book and Knapp's journal article show the legacy of cataract surgery at Jullundur Hospital in Panjab under British rule.

It is unknown how Col. Smith's technique spread from India and became popular in the USA and Europe. Its popularity was short-lived, innovation scholars write that the ICCE technique was in use until the 1970s when it was displaced by ECCE and the intraocular lens developed by British ophthalmologist Harold Ridley (Metcalfe et al. 2005; see Chapter 5).

British India was interested in democratic peripheral governments demonstrated by their deliberate movement of political and administrative authority from the central government to the peripheral government (Arnold 2005; Packard 2016; Mushtaq 2009). The Indian Medical Service was devolved to provincial governments in 1919 and again in 1935 (Mushtaq 2009). By 1941, British India had 2.2 million blind (Nair 2017). Before independence from Britain in 1947, India had a high rate of blindness due to the smallpox virus, which damages different parts of the eye (Rathinam and Cunningham 2010; Rogers 1944).

The British administrative apparatus also impacted the governance of India's public health infrastructure (Mushtaq 2009). After Indian independence, the separate departments of Public Health and Medicine were combined into one Department of Health and Medical Services under the new central government. However, public health professionals and clinical medical professionals drew strong boundaries around their areas of expertise and authority. Meanwhile, the state and district governments did not use the funds provided by the Ministry of Health as intended for "health for all" (rural and urban). Instead, they usually tended to set up health infrastructure in areas with strong political supporters (Bhattacharya 2006). Therefore, at the local level, the combination of political favoritism, expertise-boundary drawing, and financial shortages meant that it was difficult to implement the five-year plans for health and medical service ordered by the central government (Bhattacharya 2006).

2.3   WHO Defines Blindness as a Global Health Problem and Creates the IAPB, 1965–1975

The eradication of smallpox in South Asia was a serendipitous event that resulted in South Asia becoming the center of an autonomous global network to eradicate blindness. Dr. Nicole Grasset, a Swiss-French epidemiologist, and Dr. Lawrence Brilliant, a US internist, first met when she employed him to work at WHO South-East Asia Regional Office to eradicate smallpox in India in 1972 (Fenner et al. 1988; Rubin 2000; Marseille 1994; Willard et al. 2010). In an unpublished interview, Suzanne Gilbert (2010) noted that the complete eradication of smallpox from human populations worldwide provided the initial "climate of optimism" for a blindness eradication program (Wilson 1988, 3; IAPB 1986, 27–29; WHO Regional Office for South-East Asia, Twenty-Eighth Session 1975). This is likewise clearly indicated in letters sent from the WHO Prevention of Blindness and Deafness program and from Dr. R. P. Pokhrel in Nepal to celebrate SEVA's twenty-five years of service (SEVA 2003). Medical professionals involved in rural and public health ophthalmology felt confident to propose a program to eradicate blindness worldwide. These professionals worked through various NGOs.

Before any blindness eradication programs were launched, John F. Wilson began his many years-long mentorship of Indian ophthalmologist Dr. Govindappa Venkataswamy. They met in 1965 while both were attending an ophthalmology meeting on rehabilitating the blind in New York City (Manikutty and Vohra 2004). This began a decades-long friendship.

John F. Wilson was a blind British lawyer. A minister's son, he suffered from chemical burns in a school laboratory when he was twelve years old that caused permanent blindness (Martin 1999; Mehta and Shenoy 2011, 57–66). Before meeting Dr. Venkataswamy, Wilson had long been active in member associations for the blind including the World Council for the Welfare of the Blind. Under his purview, the Royal Commonwealth Society for the Blind accomplished considerable work in former British colonies in Asia and Africa during the 1950s and 1960s to address infectious trachoma and, therefore, was highly esteemed by ophthalmologists and public health professionals worldwide (Mehta and Shenoy 2011, 57–66).

During this same time period, Dr. Venkataswamy was a well-regarded ophthalmologist in southern India. He was responsible, in 1956, for heading an ophthalmology department in a government hospital and, in 1961, for implementing community-based eye health outreach in the southern state of Tamil Nadu (Mehta and Shenoy 2011, 61–62). Dr. Venkataswamy had significant achievements—especially considering he suffered pain from rheumatoid arthritis since the beginning of his medical career before Indian independence. Despite his accomplishments, he sometimes felt unconfident because of his caste and race (Manikutty and Vohra 2004; Mehta and Shenoy 2011, 64; Venkataswamy 1992). Before Wilson met Dr. Venkataswamy, the latter already presided over "the growing network of eye camps all over Tamil Nadu and had developed a network of friends and well-wishers across India who empathized with his passion for providing good quality affordable eye care" (Manikutty and Vohra 2004, 3).

In addition to Dr. Venkataswamy and Wilson, the WHO was beginning to recognize blindness as a severe threat to global health. A report published by the WHO in 1966 described sixty-five different definitions of blindness, as defined by various member-states. At the 22nd World Health Assembly in 1969, resolution WHA 22.29 requested the WHO Director-General study the extent and causes of blindness, propose new activities to cure blindness, and collaborate with other organizations including non-governmental organizations (WHA, 22, 1969, 2).

This interest in collaboration with NGOs was not as distinctive as it seems. The World Health Assembly frequently urged the WHO to coordinate with non-governmental organizations around key programmatic areas (WHA, 1, 1948; WHA, 25, 1972; WHA, 28, 1975; WHA, 31, 1978). Over time, the WHO has coordinated many programs with NGOs (World Health Organization Office of External Coordination 1990), while decreasing the number of staff in Geneva and maintaining staff size in regional offices. For example, two-thirds of the WHO staff were based in six regional offices in 1967, and this decreased slightly to 60% of staff in 1993 (see Siddiqi 1995, 55).

Meanwhile, Wilson was trying to refocus Dr. Venkataswamy from working regionally in Tamil Nadu, to eliminate blindness nationally in all of India. When Dr. Venkataswamy recounted their friendship, he said,

> You see, as an eye doctor, I was not thinking of a national programme or a global programme…I just wanted to be a good doctor and operate on the people who came to me—whoever I could reach…. John saw I

was working with the community, he thought, 'Now here is a fellow who can be gradually molded to work at the national or international level'. (Mehta and Shenoy 2011, 64)

Therefore, Dr. Venkataswamy indicates in the quote above that mentorship from Wilson, including the social networks that Wilson brought him into, expanded his self-confidence that what he was doing in Tamil Nadu was valuable across all of India and, perhaps, around the world as well.

In 1969, the Royal Commonwealth Society for the Blind began the "Eyes of India" campaign, which Wilson credited with leading to: (1) new procedures for treating blindness on a large scale in the rural areas of India, and (2) influencing the Indian government's National Programme to fight blindness (Wilson 1988, 3).

The WHO was still gathering data from member-states about the causes of blindness in 1970. As part of fulfilling his duties after resolution WHA 22.29, the WHO Director-General sent a questionnaire to all member countries, soliciting information on the state of blindness within each country in March 1970—just two months before the 23rd World Health Assembly (WHA, 25 and Candau 1972). Two years later, he reported his results: There were, at minimum, 8.5 million people confirmed with blindness in 41 countries around the world; and this was on the same order of magnitude as previous estimates of 10 million people with blindness worldwide (WHA, 25 and Candau 1972, 5). In his report to the 25th World Health Assembly in provisional agenda item 2.6, Dr. Candau argued that infectious causes of blindness had decreased over time and diseases such as smallpox no longer contributed to blindness at the same high level that they did in 1943 when the first worldwide data were recorded (WHA, 25 and Candau 1972, 5, 13). Throughout the report, he acknowledged the role of UNICEF in assisting the WHO to address trachoma in Asia, Africa, and Europe, as well as the importance of nonprofit non-governmental organizations such as the Royal Commonwealth Society for the Blind in fighting infectious causes of blindness such as onchocerciasis in former British colonies in Asia and Africa. However, in this report, the Director-General expressed the desire to move away from the WHO's work on understanding disease etiology (origins and causes) to future work on disease prevention and cures.

With the many different national definitions of blindness, further standardization and clarity of technical details for preventing and curing blindness were required (WHA, 25 and Candau 1972, 5). Therefore, Dr. Candau proposed that a Study Group on the Prevention of Blindness was necessary to provide more detailed technical information to inform the need for a comprehensive "public health ophthalmology" program (WHA, 25 and Candau 1972, 1, 16). The Director-General ended his report by suggesting that more collaboration was necessary with organizations such as UNICEF that are internal to the United Nations as well as external non-governmental organizations (WHA, 25 and Candau 1972, 16).

The Indian delegation to the 25th World Health Assembly in 1972 then proposed that WHO intensify technical and educational assistance to member-states. This assistance would support national programs to prevent blindness and medical education for ophthalmologists. The secretariat of the WHO and the Government of India (with the support of the third Prime Minister of India, Indira Gandhi) drafted resolution WHA 25.55 which the assembly unanimously approved (Kupfer and McManus 2009, 164; WHA, 25 1972).

While the global program to eradicate blindness was proposed and the idea circulated worldwide at the 25th World Health Assembly in May 1972, some believe the idea first originated in Israel in the 1960s (Wilson 1988, 3). Scottish-Israeli Professor Isaac Michaelson convened the first scientific meeting on public health ophthalmology in Jerusalem in 1971 (IAPB 2016; Mooreville 2016). In August, just a few months after WHA 25.55 was proposed, a special issue of the *Israel Journal of Medical Sciences* on "public health ophthalmology" was published. The special issue promoted the idea of a global program to eradicate blindness and featured an article by Dr. Venkataswamy, among other ophthalmologists from around the world (Wilson 1988; Venkataswamy 1972).

A few months later in November 1972, approximately 24 people met at the WHO in Geneva to convene the Study Group about preventing and curing the problem of blindness. The Study Group included leaders in public health ophthalmology from around the world, including: Dr. A. E. Maumenee, Director of The Wilmer Institute at Johns Hopkins Hospital in Maryland, USA, and Dr. G. Venkataswamy, Professor of Ophthalmology at Madurai Medical College in India. Dr. W. J. Holmes (USA) represented the International Association for the Prevention of Blindness. Meanwhile, John F. Wilson represented both the Royal Commonwealth Society for the Blind and the World Council for the Welfare of the Blind as a member of the Study Group secretariat (WHO 1973). Therefore, the idea of a global program to eradicate blindness was taken up worldwide in 1972 at the World Health Assembly, in scientific journals, and among nonprofit, non-governmental organizations around the world. Dr. Venkataswamy was later recognized for his work fighting avoidable blindness by the Indian government with the Padma Shri award in 1973 (Mehta and Shenoy 2011).

Of the many diseases that cause blindness, this Study Group identified cataract disease as a target for an international program, saying that such a program would likely have a "massive impact in the countries concerned" because cataract surgery was advanced enough to be practical and justifiable at a large scale (WHO 1973). The Study Group also advocated for the creation of an international coordinating body for blindness in addition to national ophthalmic health services (WHO 1973).

Dr. Marcelino G. Candau retired from the WHO in July 1973 after 20 years shaping the organization as its second and longest serving Director-General (26 World Health Assembly 1973). The new Director-General, Dr. Halfdan Mahler (Denmark), participated in the WHO SEARO meeting in New Delhi shortly after his inauguration and was lauded by the various national representatives to the Regional Committee for his decision to participate in their 25th anniversary celebration (WHO Regional Office for South-East Asia 1975). At the 25th anniversary celebration, the Regional Director of WHO SEARO, Dr. V. T. Herat Gunaratne (Sri Lanka), commented on the office's status as the first regional office ratified by member-states at the WHA. He also praised the South-East Asia Region's progress toward eliminating smallpox and becoming more self-sufficient in biomedical laboratory analysis and vaccine production over the years.

Dr. Mahler's remarks were less congratulatory. He reflected that the world was watching what the WHO would do with the resources the member-states had provided. Dr. Mahler cautioned that the small-pox eradication program could make or break the WHO as a functional organization. Then, he requested that WHO SEARO escalate their smallpox efforts because they had "the biggest share of the work to accomplish" with 88% of the world's cases. The speeches from other WHO SEARO officials, other UN organization officials, and representatives from NGOs and member-states continued through the anniversary meeting. Only one member-state, Indonesia, spoke publically about their concern for blindness as one of several problems WHO SEARO should focus on addressing in the next twenty-five years. Indonesia's agenda did not include smallpox as they had already eradicated it (WHO Regional Office for South-East Asia 1975; Henderson 2008).

In addition to speaking publically at the celebration, Dr. Mahler also participated in the regional committee meeting. Considering that his public speech focused on the troubling elements of WHO's regional structure, his request that WHO be considered a coordinating instead of implementing partner was met with more skepticism, especially by the alternate representative from Indonesia, Dr. Peter Patta Sumbung (Chief of Bureau for Special Affairs, Department of Health, Jakarta). Yet Dr. Sumbung was supportive of Dr. Mahler's idea of making WHO health services contextually based in local needs (WHO Regional Office for South-East Asia, Twenty-Sixth Session 1973, 54–57).

Overall, a large concern at this meeting was how the regional member-states would eradicate blindness. The representative from Nepal, Dr. G. S. L. Das (Deputy Director-General, Ministry of Health, Kathmandu), asked what was being done about blindness due to xerophthalmia (nutritional deficiency of Vitamin A) and cataract since both were prevalent in SEARO. The response from the Regional Director indicated that a consultant had been hired by WHO SEARO to further investigate the magnitude of blindness in the region (WHO Regional Office for South-East Asia, Twenty-Sixth Session 1973, 54–57).

Based on this meeting, Dr. Mahler noted in his annual report that in 1973, some of the 11 member-states within the WHO South-East Asia

Region, especially Bangladesh, Burma, and India, seemed to be progressively more interested in consulting, advising, and training services from the WHO. The member-states wanted to assess requirements and resources for preventing blindness and restoring sight due to cataract and glaucoma (WHO and Halfdan Mahler 1974, 33; 1975, 73). WHO consultants also helped design or conduct blindness surveys in the Eastern Mediterranean Region and the European Region (WHO and Mahler 1974, 33). These preliminary assessments were later expanded to Nigeria in 1974 and Guatemala in 1975 (WHO and Mahler 1975, 73; WHO and Litsios 2008, 297).

By the end of 1973, the WHO Executive Board had already established official relations with nonprofit, non-governmental member associations related to blindness and ophthalmology including, e.g., International Association for Prevention of Blindness, International Federation of Ophthalmological Societies, International Organization against Trachoma, and the World Council for the Welfare of the Blind (WHO and Mahler 1974, 33, 317). The Director-General specifically noted that, "[c]ontacts with nongovernmental organizations were intensified during the year" as a deliberate act by the WHO to both provide and receive technical assistance and support as concerned the problem of blindness (WHO and Mahler 1974, 33).

With a push from Dr. Mahler, in October 1974, members of the International Association for the Prevention of Blindness Executive Committee finalized the constitution of the new restructured International Agency for the Prevention of Blindness (IAPB) while attending the American Academy of Ophthalmology and Otolaryngology meeting in Dallas, Texas (WHO and Mahler 1975, 73; WHO and Litsios 2008, 209; IAPB 1995 [1974]). On January 1, 1975, the World Blind Union and the International Council of Ophthalmology joined together in turn with individual ophthalmologists and representatives from other member associations related to the problem of blindness. Together, they formed the new International Agency for the Prevention of Blindness (which succeeded the pre-existing International Association for the Prevention of Blindness). The IAPB's purpose is to eradicate blindness through a global program "with an emphasis on underserved communities" (IAPB 1995 [1974], 1). In the IAPB Constitution, Article II function "a" is specifically related to the coordinating role of IAPB with the United Nations (IAPB 1995 [1974], 1). The WHO Director-General argued that the IAPB, as the new collaborating NGO for the WHO Prevention of Blindness program, would enable a program expansion and more efficient use of resources (WHO and Mahler 1975, 73).

Importantly, the restructured IAPB was founded by organizations, not just individuals. The IAPB was started by premiere ophthalmologists from low-income and wealthy nations. The IAPB's membership composition is unique because, from the very beginning, its executive board included the leading non-governmental agencies advocating for blind people, the leading non-governmental agencies advocating for the prevention of blindness, individual medical professionals with unique and specialized expertise (epidemiology and virology in addition to the sub-specialties of ophthalmology), and officials from the WHO (IAPB 1982, 1995 [1974]). The members elected Sir John Wilson as their first president.

2.4   IAPB Shapes WHO, Governments, and NGOs, 1975 Onward

Starting in 1975, the IAPB became a large, nonprofit, member organization focused on eradicating and controlling the diseases of avoidable blindness. The IAPB serves as a proxy for the autonomous global network to eradicate blindness. As such, the IAPB operates in the interstitial space between the WHO, as the premier global health multilateral organization, and national governments and NGOs, as the implementers of blindness eradication and control programs. However, to be effective, the IAPB had to build up its membership of technical experts along with its ability to influence standards and policy in the WHO, national governments, and NGOs.

Above, I described how the WHO directed the administrative structure of IAPB as an organization. Next, I will further substantiate that the optimism of eradicating smallpox in South Asia directly resulted in the WHO Prevention of Blindness program. The WHO Prevention of Blindness program and the IAPB co-constructed each other (Raj 2006).

This meant that members of IAPB had opportunities in advisory groups, consultation groups, and co-coordinated meetings to shape WHO policies to address blindness, as well as vice versa.

While still undergoing its restructuring under the leadership of Wilson, members of the IAPB helped push India to start the first national blindness control program. John F. Wilson received the title of "Sir" when he was knighted in England in 1975 (Martin 1999). Sometime before the 28th World Health Assembly, a visit by Sir Wilson and Dr. Venkataswamy to "the ministry" ended up becoming a request that Prime Minister Indira Gandhi provide support for a national organization to control blindness (Manikutty and Vohra 2004; Mehta and Shenoy 2011, 57–66). A survey by the Indian government in 1974 had indicated that the prevalence of avoidable blindness was 1.38% of the population (Planning Commission 2002). Therefore, a centralized program was considered necessary by the Prime Minister.

Later in May 1975, Sir John F. Wilson, in his new role as President of IAPB, presented his plea before the 28th World Health Assembly first technical Committee A that the WHO coordinate national programs to prevent blindness (WHO Regional Office for South-East Asia, Twenty-Eighth Session 1975, 94). His request was made more convincing by his revelation that the IAPB had already coordinated thirty national committees to work on the issue of blindness (WHO and Mahler 1976). The World Health Assembly plenary subsequently approved resolution WHA 28.54 which requested that Director-General Mahler: continue and expand efforts to fight blindness; continue work with NGOs on funding and other resources; and begin work with member-states to set up national programs "especially aimed at the control of trachoma, xerophthalmia, onchocerciasis and other causes and to introduce adequate measures for the early detection and treatment of other potentially blinding conditions such as cataract and glaucoma" (Kupfer and McManus 2009, 164; WHA, 28 1975). This resolution formed the basis for creating the new technical cooperation program (Kupfer and McManus 2009, 164; WHO and Mahler 1978, 118).

At the subsequent 28th WHO SEARO meeting in August, the regional committee trailed the World Health Assembly's resolution on the Prevention of Blindness (WHA 28.54) with their own resolution:

SEA/RC28/Rl0. The representative from India, Mr. Gian Prakash (Secretary, Ministry of Health and Family Planning, New Delhi), made everyone aware the Indian Ministry of Health and Family Planning's Central Council had already resolved that "the problem of blindness should be tackled under a national scheme" (WHO Regional Office for South-East Asia, Twenty-Eighth Session 1975, 90). Therefore, the Government of India requested technical assistance in the form of: visual aids for the blind and 5280 ophthalmology equipment kits for primary health centers (WHO Regional Office for South-East Asia, Twenty-Eighth Session 1975, 90; WHO and Mahler 1978).

India started the National Program for Prevention of Visual Impairment and Control of Blindness in 1976. The new program subsumed its earlier National Trachoma Control program (Preobragenski and Gupta 1964). The National Program for Prevention of Visual Impairment and Control of Blindness was started without funding from the WHO which instead provided technical assistance and advice (Planning Commission 2002; Wilson 1987). The Indian program to control blindness was unique because it was problem-oriented, not disease-oriented (Agarwal 1977; WHO and Mahler 1978). As the first national blindness eradication program in the world, it set the standard for later such programs to be coordinated instead of implemented by the WHO. Dr. Agarwal's vision for the program combined the definition of public health ophthalmology from the WHO blindness study, with Dr. Bath's emphasis on integrating eye health care into primary health care from her 1976 presentation (Agarwal 1977; Bath 1976, 1978, 1979; WHO 1973).

As had long been planned, the theme of WHO's World Health Day in 1976 was "Foresight Prevents Blindness." In that same year, the WHO organized an inter-regional meeting in Baghdad, Iraq, to discuss the causes of blindness and the requirements to address it, including the development of human resources and eye health infrastructure (WHO and Mahler 1978; UNOStamps 2008). In 1976 and 1978, Dr. Grasset and Dr. Brilliant were still employed by WHO SEARO when it held meetings, set new goals, and set a new budget to tackle blindness.

Meanwhile, in Delhi in 1976 and 1978, the WHO SEARO held meetings about blindness in South-East Asia to: identify the causes, assess the regional magnitude, and determine an eradication strategy. The WHO SEARO meeting about blindness in 1978 brought together ophthalmologists from around the region with WHO staff and therefore was a key event linking WHO SEARO smallpox staff, Dr. Nicole Grasset and Dr. Larry Brilliant, with Dr. R. P. Pokhrel, an ophthalmologist from Nepal. In order to address blindness in the region, WHO SEARO wanted to: pinpoint the causes, calculate the extent, create a strategy, and monitor and assess the results (WHO, and Regional Office for South-East Asia 1978, 79). Likely resulting from the goals identified in these meetings, $839, 300 USD was proposed for the WHO SEARO 1980–1981 budget to address blindness issues (WHO, and Regional Office for South-East Asia 1978).

At the restructured IAPB's first general assembly in 1978 in the UK, it was clear that the IAPB was regionalized imitating the WHO's administrative structure. The name, general assembly, mirrors the World Health Assembly, but the function is different. The IAPB General Assembly is where NGOs, individuals, national-member committees, and regional committee chairs report progress in meeting the charge that WHO has given the IAPB to eradicate blindness. The WHO sets policy on combating blindness (in consultation with and informed by organizations such as International Council of Ophthalmology, IAPB, and Helen Keller International). In contrast, the IAPB works at a variety of levels to support governmental and non-governmental programs implementing this policy and collect data about the results (WHO and Mahler 1978).

To start, the IAPB had eight regional committees, and this was composed of fifty-six national committees (IAPB 1982). This was deliberately modeled after the six WHO regional offices (see World Health Organization Office of External Coordination 1990; IAPB 2018a). While in 1978 there were eight IAPB regional committees, in 1990 there were six; finally, in 2018, there were seven because IAPB divided the Americas into North America and Latin America (IAPB 2018b). The IAPB organized an international general assembly every four years. In between, the regional committees and national committees organized their own conferences on blindness. Hence, from its beginning, the IAPB functioned as the most prominent member association for ophthalmology professionals interested in eradicating blindness. With this restructuring, this international nonprofit, non-governmental organization served as an ancillary to the WHO according to the resolution WHA22.29 proposed under Director-General Candau.

At the IAPB's first general assembly, Dr. Patricia E. Bath was elected as an alternate on the executive board (Patricia E. Bath, Personal Communication with Author, "IAPB 1st General Assembly Program, UK, July 8 1978" March 24, 2011). Meanwhile, Dr. Bath was passionate in believing that community ophthalmology methods would mitigate and reduce avoidable blindness; she introduced her programs in Africa and Asia with the help of colleagues like Professor Taj Kirmani from Pakistan and the IAPB regional chair for Africa, Professor C. O. Quarcoopome from Ghana (Bath 1978; Bath et al. 1983).

Finally, at IAPB's behest, WHO started the Prevention of Blindness program in 1978 (IAPB 2004, 2016; WHO 2016). In 1980, the same year that the WHO officially declared smallpox eradicated, the WHO Program for the Prevention of Blindness staff in Geneva, Switzerland, grew from one to two people and was finally assigned its own budget of $2.3 million USD (The International Agency for the Prevention of Blindness, and Carl Kupfer 1988, 9).

The autonomous global network's different definitions for community-based ophthalmology over time highlighted the widespread interest and urgent nature of the burden of avoidable blindness. The global network of professionals interested in eradicating blindness participated in the second IAPB meeting in New Delhi (IAPB 1986). At this meeting, Dr. Venkataswamy defined community ophthalmology by pointing to Director-General Candau's earlier call for a public health ophthalmology (IAPB 1986). In the late 1970s and early 1980s, there were pockets of ophthalmologists at premiere institutions around the world (e.g., Johns Hopkins University and the University College London) becoming interested in so-called public health ophthalmology or rural ophthalmology. This idea of creating dedicated ophthalmology programs to "reach the unreached" emerged along with the global network to eradicate blindness in the 1970s to the late 1980s. US ophthalmologist Dr. Carl Kupfer, who founded the US National Institutes of Health National Eye Institute in 1968 as its first director, defined public health ophthalmology as a new way of delivering eye health care that includes "preventative, curative and promotive activities" (Kupfer 1987). He commended the British ophthalmologist, Dr. Barrie Jones, as a pioneer in the field of public health ophthalmology in the UK. Dr. Jones was also known for coining the phrase "the burden of avoidable blindness" (Leaver 2009; Wilson 1987, 158). Dr. Syed Modasser Ali published the first English-language book developing practical guidance for creating community ophthalmology programs through a local press in Bangladesh. The book was reviewed by a colleague of Dr. Barrie Jones at the University College London (Johnson 1989). Thus, there was a large, international groundswell of governmental, non-profit, and private eye clinics focused on serving the underserved (Johns 1990). The 1986 IAPB general assembly in India is one point in the historical trajectory of this international network and social movement. Along this trajectory, the IAPB began by observing at WHO, before shifting to influencing the creation of the WHO Prevention of Blindness program and finally to serving as its advisor and ancillary. The jointly run Vision 2020 program exemplifies how WHO has delegated some decision-making, management, and financial authority to IAPB which acts as a multilateral organization.

2.5   NGOs Control Blindness in India and Nepal, 1992 Onward

Similar to the WHO, Indian and Nepalese national governments also worked with NGOs to create eye health care in their respective countries.

In the 1970s, Nepal began to decentralize healthcare services (Chand and Kharel 2015). At that time, Nepal had very few eye care professionals. Prominent among them was Dr. Ram Prasad Pokhrel; in 1974, he was one of nine founders of Nepal Eye Hospital which started simply in a suite of three rooms at the Tripureshwor Guest House in Kathmandu. Importantly, it was the first private eye hospital in Nepal, established through an NGO called Nepal Eye Hospital

Management Committee. Most of the personnel from the eye department of Prithvi–Bir hospital joined Nepal Eye Hospital. As an NGO,
the Nepal Eye Hospital has always been financially supported by His
Majesty's Government and later the Federal Democratic Republic of
Nepal (Pokhrel 2003).

Dr. Pokhrel had the ambitious goal of providing eye health care for
all people in Nepal, despite the fact that he had few financial resources
for his work. His goal was also complicated by Nepal's terrain; its foothills and mountains frequently made moving health personnel, equipment, and supplies difficult. Even with these known impediments, from
the time he started the Nepal Eye Hospital and onward, Dr. Pokhrel
was trying to make social connections to create plans for eye care for the
entire country (Pokhrel 2003).

Three years after smallpox was officially eradicated in India,
Dr. Pokhrel, "the father of ophthalmology in Nepal," met Dr. Nicole
Grasset at the second seminar on blindness held in 1978 at the WHO
SEARO in New Delhi, India (Pokhrel 2003). Dr. Grasset, flush with
success from having eradicated smallpox in South Asia, was interested
in a new five-year plan—this time to combat blindness (IAPB 1982,
28; Marseille 1994, 155). However, this plan was not enthusiastically
adopted by leaders in ophthalmology in India who attended the meeting (Marseille 1994, 155). There was one person in the crowd who
was keenly interested. After Dr. Pokhrel presented his work, he and
Dr. Grasset had time during a lunch break in the WHO SEARO cafeteria
to discuss human resources and funding streams for a proposed national
program of eye care for Nepal (Marseille 1994, 155; Pokhrel 2003).

That same year, SEVA Foundation started in Waldenwoods,
Michigan, US. Founders Dr. Larry Brilliant and Girija Brilliant,
DrPH, created a new organization focused on Dr. Nicole Grasset's
goal to eradicate blindness in five years (SEVA 1998). Other long-
term friends of the Brilliants, such as counterculture activist and
entertainer Wavy Gravy and spiritual teacher and former Harvard psy-
chology Professor Ram Dass, also helped with SEVA's work (Pokhrel
2003; SEVA 1998). Many of them had learned from the Indian guru
Neem Karoli Baba before his death in 1973. Therefore, they named
their organization the Sanskrit word for "service"—a key theme in the

guru's teachings. When Steve Jobs, the founder of Apple, read about Larry Brilliant's work on smallpox in India, he remembered meeting him at the ashram in India in the early 1970s and wrote SEVA Foundation its first check for $5000 USD (Wingfield 2013). This first check spurred others' donations, and SEVA Foundation was able to raise $20,000 USD in a relatively short amount of time in order to fund operations (Wingfield 2013).

The SEVA Foundation was not started entirely by Westerners. Importantly, that first meeting in December 1978 also included Dr. Govindappa Venkataswamy who not only attended yearly, but also remained on the advisory board for fifteen years (Pokhrel 2003; SEVA 1998). Dr. Pokhrel also remained involved with SEVA as he was commencing his new eye healthcare program in Nepal.

Starting in the late 1970s, Nepal created a privatized, decentralized, eye healthcare system utilizing civil society organizations. In 1978, Dr. Pokhrel became one of nine founders of the newly formed His Majesty's Government subcommittee, Nepal Netra Jyoti Sangh (Nepal National Eye Society). From 1979 to 1980, Dr. Grasset, Dr. Larry Brilliant, University of Michigan graduate student Suzanne Gilbert, and Nepalese ophthalmologists Dr. Sanduk Ruit and Dr. R. P. Pokhrel, along with many other Western and South Asian researchers, performed the pretest survey in five sites in Nepal and then the full National Blindness Survey (Brilliant et al. 1985; Pokhrel 2003). They found that blindness prevalence in Nepal was 0.84%, primarily due to cataract disease and trachoma (Brilliant et al. 1985). This was one of the first national surveys of blindness ever conducted and became a model for how to conduct future such surveys in the global south. Thus, we see that, very early on, the SEVA Foundation was involved in epidemiological research for community ophthalmology in Nepal.

In 1979, SEVA was invited by His Majesty's Government of Nepal (facilitated through Dr. Pokhrel), in coordination with the WHO Program for the Prevention of Blindness, to initiate the Nepal Blindness Prevention and Control Project (Brilliant et al. 1985).

Armed with more detailed information after a visit with Dr. Pokhrel at Nepal Eye Hospital in Kathmandu, Dr. Grasset went looking for donations from her many contacts in Europe to support blindness eradication in Nepal (Pokhrel 2003). Dr. Pokhrel (2003) writes that, in 1980, "resources came from Norway, Sweden, and the Netherlands follow[ed] by AG fund." These funders had a stipulation—they wanted to channel the funds through the two-year-old WHO Prevention of Blindness Program (Marseille 1994; Pokhrel 2003). Therefore, Dr. Pokhrel (2003) and Grasset together were an important part of channeling the newly awarded resources from the WHO Prevention of Blindness program in 1980 to support the creation of eye health human resources in Nepal.

The Nepal Blindness Prevention and Control Project orchestrated by SEVA involved domestic and foreign NGOs and agencies providing funds and expertise. Domestic NGOs and donors included: Nepal Netra Jyoti Sangh, Golchha Charity Trust, Khedia Charity Trust, and the Khetan Family. Meanwhile, international NGOs and government development agencies included: Christoffel Blinden Mission (West Germany), Norwegian Church Aid, Swiss Red Cross, Operation Eye Sight Universal (Canada), Seva Service Society (SEVA Foundation's sister society in Canada), Operation Eye Camp Himalaya (the Netherlands), Association for Ophthalmic Cooperation in Asia (Japan), and Japanese International Cooperation Agency (NNJS 2015; Pokhrel 2003; SEVA 1987).

Over time, it became clear that Dr. Grasset's ambitious five-year plan would not be successful. There were not enough eye hospitals or enough community ophthalmology personnel to conduct cataract surgeries. While both eye hospitals and personnel were increasing, they still could not keep pace with the backlog of patients needing cataract surgery. The WHO stood firm in its commitment to coordinating instead of implementing health care; it refused to provide additional funding and, instead, cut existing funding. Frustrated by WHO's inability to commit resources to reducing blindness in Nepal, Dr. Grasset resigned from WHO in 1983 (Marseille 1994, 163).

When the WHO withdrew from the Nepal Blindness Prevention and Control Project, SEVA was asked by Dr. Pokhrel in 1984 to be responsible for all eye care in Nepal's Lumbini zone (the birthplace of Buddha; Marseille 1994). Accepting this responsibility required a change in their internal organizational structure (Marseille 1994). Founding members of SEVA Foundation overlapped with the Hog Farm entertainment activist commune in California and were dedicated to service and radical social change. However, SEVA had to become more centralized and money-focused in order to best provide support for the Nepal Blindness Prevention and Control Project (Marseille 1994, 157).

The overall structure of eye health care in Nepal became increasingly decentralized. From 1961 to 2008, the Nepalese Panchayat administrative structure involved 14 zones and 75 districts. In 1980, Nepal Netra Jyoti Sangh transitioned to become a domestic NGO that still predominantly received funding from the Nepalese government (NNJS 2015). In the early 1980s, Nepal Netra Jyoti Sangh included specialty eye hospitals built in every 1–2 zones—each independently run by a different foreign NGO such as Swiss Red Cross, Norwegian Church Aid, or German Christoffel Blinden Mission (Marseille 1994, 160, 162; Marasini 2003). Dr. Pokhrel and the Nepalese government provided general guidance. Therefore, eye health care for Nepalese patients looked very different depending upon which eye hospital was implementing it. Each eye hospital had different orientations toward rural eye education, rural screening for eye disease, cataract surgical technique (Europeans tended to favor ICCE while Americans tended to favor ECCE), role of ophthalmic assistants, and role of foreign versus Nepalese ophthalmologists (Marseille 1994, 160, 162). The distinct structure of eye health care in Nepal was therefore likely difficult for the WHO to replicate. However, it was also very flexible, and the government of Nepal did not need to spend extensive funds to provide high-quality eye health services to its constituents because it relied on autonomous and independently funded foreign NGOs—a win for Dr. Pokhrel. Unfortunately, even after increasing cataract surgeries from approximately 300 in 1982 to 22,000 in 1989, existing ophthalmologists had not reached a high enough surgical volume to address the backlog of patients with cataract disease, especially as this backlog grew every year with the aging population (Marseille 1994, 160).

From 1985 to 2003, no multi-specialty zonal hospitals were established in Nepal (Marasini 2003). The instability of civil war (1996–2006) prevented many infrastructure projects and health services (Chand and Kharel 2015). An external review by a WHO consultant found that, in Nepal, many private hospitals (both for-profit and non-profit) were not fulfilling their government-mandated mission to serve the underserved. Instead, they were using the relaxation of tariff imports provided by the government to subsidize the services for patients who already could afford to pay (Pokharel 2001). Two counterexamples of this in 2012 were: Lumbini Eye Hospital run by SEVA Foundation and Tilganga Institute of Ophthalmology run by Dr. Ruit and his domestic NGO, Nepal Eye Program. Both Nepalese institutions are well known in both northern India and Nepal for high-quality, high-volume cataract surgery for the poor.

The structure of eye health care in India made a similar shift from centralized to decentralized, but this shift did not begin until the 1990s. The first ten years of Indira Gandhi's National Program for Prevention of Visual Impairment and Control of Blindness came to an end in 1986, at which time blindness prevalence was again surveyed in India. Disappointingly, this three-year study ending in 1989 found that the blindness prevalence was the same as in 1974: 12 million people in India were blind with 80% of this blindness due to cataract disease (Planning Commission 2002; Jose and Bachani 1995). This same prevalence involved both positive and negative news. The positive news was increased rates for eye screening and cataract surgery (1.9 million cataract surgeries annually). The negative news was that community ophthalmology professionals could not keep up with the increased numbers of adults living longer and developing cataracts (up to 3.8 million cataracts annually; see Jose and Bachani 1995). After the Indian government determined that the initial National Program for Prevention of Visual Impairment and Control of Blindness had not reduced blindness, they revamped their efforts.

The cataract surgical rate from 1989 to 1990 was low at 1,342 per million (Murthy et al. 2008). As an addition to the existing National Program for Prevention of Visual Impairment and Control of Blindness, funds were solicited by the Government of India from the International Development Association of the World Bank, for a new program called the Cataract Blindness Control Project that would occur from 1994 to 2003 (Ocular Surgery News Asia Pacific Edition 2002). The Cataract Blindness Control Project paid for ophthalmic consumables, equipment, and to train surgeons in the newer technique of cataract surgery: extra capsular cataract extraction with intraocular lens implantation (Ocular Surgery News Asia Pacific Edition 2002). The remittances provided by the Indian government through the Cataract Blindness Control Project were specifically targeted to the seven southern states (Uttar Pradesh, Madhya Pradesh, Andhra Pradesh, Rajasthan, Maharashtra, Tamil Nadu, and Orissa) that together were responsible for 66% of avoidable blindness in India and 25% of avoidable blindness in the world (Jose and Bachani 1995; Planning Commission 2002; Ocular Surgery News Asia Pacific Edition 2002).

After a pilot program organized by the Danish International Development Agency was successful, in 1992, the Ministry of Family Health and Welfare decentralized the National Program for Prevention of Visual Impairment and Control of Blindness by creating District Control of Blindness Societies (DCBS) (Jose and Bachani 1995). The DCBSs are civil society organizations that serve as autonomous agencies with ability to fund-raise but without ability to own property. DCBSs are comprised of district government officials, government hospital representatives, medical college representatives, and NGO representatives (Jose and Bachani 1995; Planning Commission 2002). Various government, NGO, and for-profit hospitals receive remittances from DCBSs for outreach eye camp patients to receive free eye health care (Planning Commission 2002). Sentinel Surveillance Units embedded into government hospitals and medical colleges collect data for the Indian government on the impact of those remittances on cataract surgical rates in the country (Planning Commission 2002).

In 2002, the Indian government determined the Cataract Blindness Control Project had indeed reduced blindness. The results of the 2001–2002 survey examining the impact of the Cataract Blindness Control Project showed improvement. In comparison with 1986, when cataract disease represented 80% of avoidable blindness in India, in 1999 cataract disease only represented 55% of avoidable blindness in India (Planning Commission 2002).

The 2002 World Bank report on India's Cataract Blindness Control Project highlighted the importance of NGOs which provided 30% of eye health care in India and provided "the most cost-effective option for cataract surgery ... at INR 1,297, as compared [to] the cost in a private facility at INR 5,440" (World Bank 2002, 7). The World Bank (2002) recognized just how important NGOs had become in India for providing eye health care to rural and poor patients who would not otherwise benefit from eye health care.

The people of South Asia have long been a part of blindness investigation and treatment (Nair 2017). Now both India and Nepal are known for high-quality eye hospitals and well-trained ophthalmic personnel. Furthermore, some of the most well-known eye institutions in the world are located in South Asia, e.g., Aravind Eye Care System in Tamil Nadu, India, L. V. Prasad Eye Institute in Telangana, India, and Tilganga Institute of Ophthalmology in Nepal. These influential NGOs, as well as others such as SEVA Foundation and the Royal Commonwealth Society for the Blind, are coordinated by the IAPB. They are central to an autonomous global network dedicated to eradicating and controlling blindness.

2.6 Conclusion: The Emerging Cognitive Rule to Eradicate Blindness

From the 1960s to the 1990s, a global network focused on eradicating blindness clearly emerged from South Asia. The eradication of smallpox by the WHO South-East Asia Regional Office brought Western epidemiologists to the region and proved a tipping point for international interest in a global program to eradicate avoidable blindness. Arguably, in the late 1970s, there was a conversion of economic and social resources from the disease of smallpox to the diseases of avoidable blindness.

The health ministries of India and Nepal worked with NGOs to create eye health care in their respective countries; these NGOs especially focused on the eye healthcare needs of the rural poor. The development of the autonomous global network to eradicate and control blindness involved changing a European- and American-led smallpox vaccination team in India into dollars (but not doctors or infrastructure) for surveying avoidable blindness in Nepal. The general structure of eye health care that followed in India and Nepal was decentralized. Indian eye health care relied heavily on domestic NGOs and remuneration from the District Control of Blindness Societies (parastatal organizations). In Nepal, various foreign non-governmental organizations funded eye health units in specific districts; they were coordinated by the domestic NGO, Nepal Netra Jyoti Sangh.

Ophthalmology, optometry, paramedic, epidemiology, management, and other professionals have formed an autonomous global network (Harris 2015). This network is dedicated to eradicating and controlling blindness; it developed in both the wealthy industrialized nations of the global north and the less economically developed nations of the global south around the discourse of treating the "burden of avoidable blindness" by providing eye health services that are "affordable, accessible and appropriate" (Leaver 2009; IAPB 1994, 1986). Two key differences make this autonomous global network distinct in the global field of ophthalmology: first, its cognitive rule of eradicating and controlling blindness, and second, its geo-political origins in nation-states on the periphery (Nepal) and semi-periphery (India) of the world-system. As such, the autonomous global network dedicated to eradicating and controlling blindness is on the economic periphery of scientific knowledge production compared to the dominant network of clinical ophthalmologists located in urban centers around the world.

In the next chapter, I will explain how this autonomous global network created a novel finance model and built niches to create appropriate technology for the rural masses of blind and visually impaired patients.

References

Agarwal, L. 1977. "National Programme for Prevention of Visual Impairment and Control of Blindness." *Indian Journal of Ophthalmology* 25 (4): 1–5.

Arnold, David. 2005. "Europe, Technology, and Colonialism in the 20th Century." *History and Technology: An International Journal* 21 (1): 85–106.

Bath, Patricia Era. 1976. "Rationale for a Program in Community Ophthalmology." Paper presented at the American Public Health Association, Miami, FL.

————. 1978. "Blindness Prevention through Programs of Community Ophthalmology in Developing Countries." XXIII Concilium Ophthalmologicum, Kyoto, International Congress Series No. 450, 2 (May): 1913–15.

————. 1979. "Rationale for a Program in Community Ophthalmology." *Journal of the National Medical Association* 71: 145.

Bath, Patricia E., C. O. Quarcoopome, and Taj H. Kirmani. 1983. "Community Ophthalmology Plan for Underserved Populations." *ACTA XXIV International Congress of Ophthalmology* 2: 13–17.

Bhattacharya, Sanjoy. 2006. "Universalist Claims Selective Upgrades The Complexities of Health Policy Reformulations in India 1947–1960." In *Expunging Variola: The Control and Eradication of Smallpox in India, 1947–1977*, 12–44. New Delhi: Orient Longman.

Bijker, Wiebe E. 1987. "The Social Construction of Bakelite: Toward a Theory of Invention." In *The Social Construction of Technological Systems: New Directions in the Sociology and History of Technology*, edited by Wiebe E. Bijker, Thomas Parke Hughes, and Trevor J. Pinch, 155–82. MIT Press.

Brilliant, L. B., R. P. Pokhrel, N. C. Grasset, J. M. Lepkowski, A. Kolstad, W. Hawks, R. Pararajasegaram, G. E. Brilliant, S. Gilbert, and S. R. Shrestha. 1985. "Epidemiology of Blindness in Nepal." *Bulletin of the World Health Organization* 63 (2): 375–86.

Chand, Priyankar Bahadur, and Ramesh Kharel. 2015. "Politics of Primary Health Care in Nepal." In *Health for All: The Journey of Universal Health Coverage*, edited by Alexander Medcalf, Sanjoy Bhattacharya, Hooman Momen, Monica Saavedra, and Margaret Jones, 35–44. Hyderabad, Telangana, India: Orient Blackswan.

Elliot, Robert H. 1917. *The Indian Operation of Couching for Cataract.* London, UK: H. K. Lewis and Co. Ltd. The Foundation of the American Academy of Ophthalmology Museum of Vision & Ophthalmic Heritage. San Francisco, CA.

Fenner, Frank, Donald Ainslie Henderson, Isao Arita, ZdenEk JeZek, and Ivan Danilovich Ladnyi. 1988. "Chapter 15: India and the Himalayan Area." In *Smallpox and Its Eradication, History of International Public Health*. Geneva: World Health Organization.

Foster, Allen, and Serge Resnikoff. 2005. "The Impact of Vision 2020 on Global Blindness." *Eye* 19 (10): 1133–35.

Geels, Frank W. 2005. "Conceptual Perspective on Sytems Innovations and Technological Transitions." In *Technological Transitions and System*

Innovations: A Co-evolutionary and Socio-Technical Analysis, 75–102. Cheltenham and Northampton, MA: Edward Elgar.

Geels, Frank W., and Johan Schot. 2007. "Typology of Sociotechnical Transition Pathways." *Research Policy* 36 (3): 399–417.

Goldner, Melinda. 2004. "The Dynamic Interplay between Western Medicine and the Complementary and Alternative Medicine Movement: How Activists Perceive a Range of Responses from Physicians and Hospitals." *Sociology of Health & Illness* 26 (6): 710–36.

Hachhethu, Krishna. 2003. "Democracy And Nationalism: Interface Between State And Ethnicity In Nepal." *Contributions to Nepali Studies* 30 (2): 21–252.

Harris, Joseph. 2015. "Who Governs? Autonomous Political Networks as a Challenge to Power in Thailand." *Journal of Contemporary Asia* 45 (1): 3–25.

Henderson, Donald A. 2008. "Smallpox: Dispelling the Myths. An Interview with Donald Henderson." *Bulletin of the World Health Organization* 86 (12): 909–88.

Hess, David J. 2007. *Alternative Pathways in Science and Industry: Activism, Innovation, and the Environment in an Era of Globalization.* Cambridge, MA: The MIT Press.

———. 2016. *Undone Science: Social Movements, Mobilized Publics, and Industrial Transitions.* Cambridge, MA: The MIT Press.

Heydon, Susan. 2011. "Medicines, Travellers and the Introduction and Spread of 'Modern' Medicine in the Mt Everest Region of Nepal." *Medical History* 55 (4): 503–21.

Hughes, Thomas Parke. 1987. "The Evolution of Large Technological Systems." In *The Social Construction of Technological Systems: New Directions in the Sociology and History of Technology*, edited by Wiebe E. Bijker, Thomas Parke Hughes, and Trevor J. Pinch, 51–82. Cambridge, MA: The MIT Press.

IAPB. 1982. "International Agency for the Prevention of Blindness 2nd General Assembly, New Horizons, Washington, DC. October 24–28, 1982." GVERI Resources Collection Box No. ORG-20. Govindappa Venkataswamy Eye Research Institute, Aravind Eye Care System, Madurai, India.

———. 1986. "International Agency for the Prevention of Blindness 3rd General Assembly, A Decade of Progress, New Delhi, India December 6–11, 1986." GVERI Resources Collection Box No. ORG-20. Govindappa

Venkataswamy Eye Research Institute, Aravind Eye Care System, Madurai, India.

————. 1990. "International Agency for the Prevention of Blindness 4th General Assembly, Sustainable Strategies—Agenda for the 1990s, Kenyatta International Conference Center, Nairobi, Kenya, November 11–15, 1990." GVERI Resources Collection Box No. ORG-20. Govindappa Venkataswamy Eye Research Institute, Aravind Eye Care System, Madurai, India.

————. 1994. "International Agency for the Prevention of Blindness 5th General Assembly, Towards Affordable, Accessible, Appropriate Eye Care, International Conference Center, Berlin, Germany, May 8–13, 1994." Berlin, Germany: International Agency for the Prevention of Blindness. GVERI Resources Collection Box No. ORG-20. Govindappa Venkataswamy Eye Research Institute, Aravind Eye Care System, Madurai, India.

————. 1995 [1974]. "IAPB Constitution." West Sussex: International Agency for the Prevention of Blindness. GVERI Resources Collection Box No. ORG-20. Govindappa Venkataswamy Eye Research Institute, Aravind Eye Care System, Madurai, India.

————. 2004. "Introduction: What Is IAPB?" IAPB-What Is IAPB. http://www.iapb.org/wat_iapb.htm.

————. 2016. "IAPB History." IAPB History | International Agency for the Prevention of Blindness. http://www.iapb.org/about-iapb/iapb-history.

————. 2018a. "VISION 2020: The Right to Sight- IAPB." International Agency for the Prevention of Blindness. 2018. https://www.iapb.org/vision-2020/.

————. 2018b. "IAPB Regions." IAPB. 2018. https://www.iapb.org/iapb-regions/.

International Health Conference. 1948. "WHO Constitution." In *Summary Report on Proceedings, Minutes and Final Acts of the International Health Conference Held in New York from 19 June to 22 July 1946*, 100–9. New York: United Nations, World Health Organization, Interim Commission. http://www.who.int/iris/handle/10665/85573.

Johns, Alan. 1990. "The International Agency for the Prevention of Blindness and Non-Governmental Organisations: An Effective Network." *International Ophthalmology* 14 (3): 227–30. https://doi.org/10.1007/BF00158323.

Johnson, Gordon J. 1989. "Community Ophthalmology. By Syed Modasser Ali, pp. 144. Tk.150. Anamoy: Bangladesh. 1985." *The British Journal of Ophthalmology* 73 (7): 583.

Johnson, Ryan. 2008. "Tabloid Brand Medicine Chests: Selling Health and Hygiene for the British Tropical Colonies." *Science As Culture* 17 (3): 249–68.

Jose, R., and Damodar Bachani. 1995. "World Bank-Assisted Cataract Blindness Control Project." *Indian Journal of Ophthalmology* 43 (1): 35.

Knapp, Alfred. 1908. "On Extraction of Cataract in the Capsule: Report of a Visit to Major Henry Smith in Jullunder, India." *Arch Ophthalmol* 190 (37): 13–15. San Francisco, CA: The Foundation of the American Academy of Ophthalmology Museum of Vision & Ophthalmic Heritage.

Kupfer, Carl. 1987. "Public Health Ophthalmology." *The British Journal of Ophthalmology* 71 (2): 116–17.

Kupfer, Carl, and Edward H. McManus. 2009. *History of the National Eye Institute: 1968–2000*. Bethesda, MD: National Institutes of Health National Eye Institute.

Latour, Bruno. 1987. *Science in Action: How to Follow Scientists and Engineers Through Society*. Cambridge, MA: Harvard University Press.

Leaver, Peter. 2009. "Obituaries: Professor Barrie R. Jones CBE Bsc (NZ) FRCS (Eng) FRCP (Lon) Hon FRACS." Retrieved February 25, 2013. http://www.moorfields.nhs.uk/Healthprofessionals/MoorfieldsAlumni Association/Alumninews/Obituaries.

Madras Medical College. n.d. "Madras Medical College ::: ASSOCIATED INSTITUTIONS: Regional Institute of Ophthalmology Institution History." Directorate of Medical Education, Government of Tamil Nadu. Accessed February 22, 2018. http://www.mmc.ac.in/mmc/content_page. jsp?sq1=eye&sqf=404.

Manandhar, Tri Ratna. 2005. "British Residents at the Court of Nepal During the 19th Century." *Voice of History* 20 (1): 5–22.

Manikutty, Sankaran, and Neharika Vohra. 2004. *Aravind Eye Care System: Giving Them the Most Precious Gift*. Ahmedabad: Indian Institute of Management.

Marasini, Babu Ram. 2003. "Health and Hospital Development in Nepal: Past and Present." *Journal of Nepal Medical Association* 42 (149): 306–11.

Marseille, Elliot. 1994. "Intraocular Lenses, Blindness Control, and the Hiding Hand." In *Rethinking the Development Experience: Essays Provoked by the Work of Albert O. Hirschman*, edited by Lloyd Rodwin and Donald A. Schön, 147–75. Washington, DC and Cambridge, MA: Brookings Institution and Lincoln Institute of Land Policy.

Martin, Douglas. 1999. "J.F. Wilson, 80, Whose Work Saved Millions From Blindness." *The New York Times*, December 6, sec. World. http://www. nytimes.com/1999/12/06/world/jf-wilson-80-whose-work-saved-millions-from-blindness.html.

Mehta, Pavithra K., and Suchitra Shenoy. 2011. *Infinite Vision: How Aravind Became the World's Greatest Business Case for Compassion.* San Francisco, CA: Berrett-Koehler Publishers.

Metcalfe, J. Stanley, Andrew James, and Andrea Mina. 2005. "Emergent Innovation Systems and the Delivery of Clinical Services: The Case of Intra-Ocular Lenses." *Research Policy* 34 (9): 1283–304.

Moore, Kelly. 1999. "Political Protest and Institutional Change: The Anti-Vietnam War Movement and American Science." In *How Social Movements Matter,* edited by Marco Giugni, Doug McAdam, and Charles Tilly, 10: 97–118. University of Minnesota Press.

———. 2006. "Powered by the People: Scientific Authority in Participatory Science." In *The New Political Sociology of Science: Institutions, Networks, and Power,* edited by Scott Frickel and Kelly Moore. Madison: University of Wisconsin Press.

Mooreville, Anat. 2016. "Eyeing Africa: The Politics of Israeli Ocular Expertise and International Aid, 1959–1973." *Jewish Social Studies* 21 (3): 31–71.

Murthy, G. V. S., Sanjeev K. Gupta, Neena John, and Praveen Vashist. 2008. "Current Status of Cataract Blindness and Vision 2020: The Right to Sight Initiative in India." *Indian Journal of Ophthalmology* 56 (6): 489.

Mushtaq, Muhammad Umair. 2009. "Public Health in British India: A Brief Account of the History of Medical Services and Disease Prevention in Colonial India." *Indian Journal of Community Medicine: Official Publication of Indian Association of Preventive & Social Medicine* 34 (1): 6–14.

Nair, Aparna. 2017. "'They Shall See His Face': Blindness in British India, 1850–1950." *Medical History* 61 (2): 181–99.

NNJS. 2015. "Nepal Netra Jyoti Sangh (NNJS)." http://nnjs.org.np.

Ocular Surgery News Asia Pacific Edition. 2002. "India's Government Tackles Challenges of Eye Care." *Ocular Surgery News Asia Pacific Edition,* March. http://www.healio.com/news/print/ocular-surgery-news-europe-asia-edition/%7B718ad951-a6e3-403d-9f92-9c34e8c06c72%7D/indias-government-tackles-challenges-of-eye-care.

Packard, Randall M. 2016. *A History of Global Health Interventions into the Lives of Other Peoples.* Baltimore: Johns Hopkins University Press.

Pascolini, Donatella, and Silvio Paolo Mariotti. 2012. "Global Estimates of Visual Impairment: 2010." *British Journal of Ophthalmology* 96 (5): 614–18.

Planning Commission. 2002. "Annual Plan 2003–04: Chapter 4 Human and Social Development." Annual Five Year Plans. New Delhi, India: Government of India. http://planningcommission.nic.in/plans/annualplan/ap0304pdf/ap0304_ch4.pdf.

Pokharel, Bhojraj. 2001. "Decentralization of Health Services." SEA-HSD-245 2000. New Delhi, India: World Health Organization, Regional Office for South-East Asia.

Pokhrel, Ram Prasad. 2003. *Reaching the Unreached: Three Decades of Struggle in Nepal.* Kathmandu: International Forum. Retrieved April 30, 2009 (http://www.rppokhrel.com/index.php?pageid=pub).

Preobragenski, V. V., and U. C. Gupta. 1964. "The National Trachoma Control Programme in India." *Journal of the All-India Ophthalmological Society* 12 (July): 68–73.

Raj, Kapil. 2006. *Relocating Modern Science: Circulation and the Construction of Knowledge in South Asia and Europe, 1650–1900.* New Delhi: Permanent Black.

Rankin, Katharine N. 2004. *The Cultural Politics of Markets: Economic Liberalization And Social Change In Nepal.* Toronto: University of Toronto Press.

Rathinam, S. R., and E. T. Cunningham. 2010. "Vitiligo Iridis in Patients with a History of Smallpox Infection." *Eye* 24 (10): 1621–22.

Rogers, Leonard. 1944. "Smallpox and Vaccination in British India during the Last Seventy Years." *Proceedings of the Royal Society of Medicine* 38 (November): 135–39.

Rubin, Harriet. 2000. "Dr. Brilliant vs. the Devil of Ambition." *Fast Company*, September 30. Retrieved February 1, 2012. http://www.fastcompany.com/41704/dr-brilliant-vs-devil-ambition.

SEVA. 1987. *Progress Report 1987.* Chelsea, MI: SEVA Foundation. GVERI Resources Collection Box No. ORG-14. Govindappa Venkataswamy Eye Research Institute, Aravind Eye Care System, Madurai.

———. 1998. "An Evolving Vision of Service, 1978–1998." GVERI Resources Collection Box No. ORG-14. Govindappa Venkataswamy Eye Research Institute, Aravind Eye Care System, Madurai.

———. 2003. "SEVA's Silver Anniversary Concert." GVERI Resources Collection Box No. ORG-14. Govindappa Venkataswamy Eye Research Institute, Aravind Eye Care System, Madurai.

Siddiqi, Javed. 1995. "Part II Attempts to Build a Decentralized Universal Health Organization." In *World Health and World Politics: The World Health Organization and the UN System*, 53–122. University of South Carolina Press.

Smith, Henry. 1910. *The Treatment of Cataract.* Calcutta, India: Thacker, Spink & Co. The Foundation of the American Academy of Ophthalmology Museum of Vision & Ophthalmic Heritage, San Francisco, CA.

The International Agency for the Prevention of Blindness, and John Wilson, eds. 1980. *World Blindness and Its Prevention: Volume 1.* Oxford: Oxford University Press.

The International Agency for the Prevention of Blindness, and Carl Kupfer, eds. 1988. *World Blindness And Its Prevention: Volume 3.* New York: Oxford University Press.

United Kingdom, and Nepal. 1923. "Treaty between the United Kingdom and Nepal Together with Note Respecting the Importation of Arms and Ammunition into Nepal." 31. Treaty Series. London: His Majesty's Stationery Office. http://treaties.fco.gov.uk/treaties/treatyrecord.htm?tid=11170&pg=2.

UNO Stamps. 2008. "World Health Day 1976–Foresight Prevents Blindness." *UNO Stamps,* February 6. Retrieved March 17, 2012. http://www.unos-tamps.nl/subject_world_health_day_1976.htm.

Venkataswamy, Govindappa. 1972. "Public Health Ophthalmology within the Nations. India." *Israel Journal of Medical Sciences* 8 (8): 1066–68.

———. 1992. "Spiritual Consciousness and Healing: An Interview with Govindappa Venkataswamy." By Missy Daniel. *Second Opinion* 18 (1): 68–81.

von der Heide, Susanne. 2012. "Linking Routes from the Silk Road through Nepal–The Ancient Passage through Mustang and Its Importance as a Buddhist Cultural Landscape." In *International Association of Silk Road Universities 2nd International Conference Archi-Cultural Translations through the Silk Road,* 613: 353–359. Nishinomiya, Japan: Mukogawa Women's University. http://www.mukogawa-u.ac.jp/~iasu2012/proceedings.html.

WHA, 1. 1948. First World Health Assembly, Geneva 24 June–24 July 1948: Plenary Meetings: Verbatim Records: Main Committees: Summary of Resolutions and Decisions. Geneva: World Health Organization. http://www.who.int/iris/handle/10665/85592.

WHA, 22. 1969. "Draft Second Report of the Committee on Programme and Budget." A22/P&B/21. WHA22. Geneva: World Health Organization. http://apps.who.int/iris/handle/10665/144305.

WHA, 25. 1972. Twenty-Fifth World Health Assembly, Geneva, 9–26 May 1972: Part I: Resolutions and Decisions: Annexes. Geneva: World Health Organization. http://www.who.int/iris/handle/10665/85850.

WHA, 25 and M. G. Candau. 1972. "Provisional agenda item 2.6 Prevention of Blindness: Report by the Director-General." A25/10. WHA25. Geneva: World Health Organization. http://www.who.int/iris/handle/10665/145459.

WHA, 26. 1973. "Dr. M. G. Candau, Director-General Emeritus." WHA26. Geneva: World Health Organization. http://www.who.int/iris/handle/10665/92035.

WHA, 28. 1975. Twenty-Eighth World Health Assembly, Geneva, 13–30 May 1975: Part I: Resolutions and Decisions: Annexes. Geneva: World Health Organization. http://www.who.int/iris/handle/10665/86022.

WHA, 31. 1978. Thirty-First World Health Assembly, Geneva, 8–24 May 1978: Part I: Resolutions and Decisions: Annexes. Geneva: World Health Organization. http://www.who.int/iris/handle/10665/86043.

WHO. 1973. "The Prevention of Blindness: Report of a WHO Study Group." 518. World Health Organization Technical Report Series. Geneva: World Health Organization. http://apps.who.int/iris/bitstream/10665/38222/1/WHO_TRS_518_eng.pdf.

———. 2009. "WHO Prevention of Avoidable Blindness and Visual Impairment." Retrieved April 30, 2009. http://www.who.int/blindness/en/.

———. 2013. Universal Eye Health: A Global Action Plan 2014–2019. Geneva: World Health Organization. http://apps.who.int/iris/handle/10665/105937.

———. 2016. "Prevention of Blindness and Visual Impairment Historical Perspective." WHO | Historical Perspective. http://www.who.int/blindness/history/en/.

WHO and Halfdan Mahler. 1974. The Work of WHO, 1973: Annual Report of the Director-General to the World Health Assembly and to the United Nations. OFFICIAL RECORDS OF THE WORLD HEALTH ORGANIZATION 213. Geneva: World Health Organization. http://apps.who.int/iris/handle/10665/85868.

———. 1975. The Work of WHO, 1974: Annual Report of the Director-General to the World Health Assembly and to the United Nations. OFFICIAL RECORDS OF THE WORLD HEALTH ORGANIZATION 221. Geneva: World Health Organization. http://www.who.int/iris/handle/10665/85882.

———. 1976. The Work of WHO, 1975: Annual Report of the Director-General to the World Health Assembly and to the United Nations. OFFICIAL RECORDS OF THE WORLD HEALTH ORGANIZATION 229. Geneva: World Health Organization. http://www.who.int/iris/handle/10665/86025.

———. 1978. The Work of WHO, 1976–1977: Annual Report of the Director-General to the World Health Assembly and to the United Nations. OFFICIAL RECORDS OF THE WORLD HEALTH ORGANIZATION 243. Geneva: World Health Organization. http://apps.who.int/iris/handle/10665/86039.

World Health Organization Office of External Coordination. 1990. "Directory of Nongovernmental Organizations in Official Relations with the World Health Organization." Geneva: World Health Organization. http://www.who.int/iris/handle/10665/59634.

WHO and Socrates Litsios. 2008. THE THIRD TEN YEARS OF THE WORLD HEALTH ORGANIZATION: 1968–1977. Geneva: World Health Organization. http://www.who.int/global_health_histories/who-3rd 10years.pdf.

WHO Regional Office for South-East Asia. 1975. "25th Anniversary of the WHO Regional Organization for South-East Asia, 1948–1973." New Delhi, India: World Health Organization, Regional Office for South-East Asia. http://apps.searo.who.int/pds/ShowDetails.asp?Code=B3768.

———. 1978. "WHO Regional Office for South-East Asia Proposed Programme Budget for 1980–1981." SEA/RC31/3. Regional Committee Meeting 31 Ulan Bator, 22–28 August 1978. Geneva: World Health Organization. http://www.who.int/iris/handle/10665/129873.

WHO Regional Office for South-East Asia, Twenty-Sixth Session. 1973. "Report and Minutes of the Twenty-Sixth Session of the WHO Regional Committee for South-East Asia, New Delhi, 18–24 September, 1973." New Delhi, India: World Health Organization, Regional Office for South-East Asia.

WHO Regional Office for South-East Asia, Twenty-Eighth Session. 1975. "Report and Minutes of the Twenty-Eighth Session of the WHO Regional Committee for South-East Asia, New Delhi, 25–30 August, 1975." New Delhi, India: World Health Organization, Regional Office for South-East Asia.

Willard, Nedd, Poppy Willard, and R. Pararajasegaram. 2010. "Dr. Nicole Grasset A Retrospective." SEVA Foundation. Retrieved February 1, 2013. http://www.seva.org/site/DocServer/Dr_Nicole_Grasset_Retrospective. pdf?docID=1141.

Wilson, John. 1987. "Clearing the Cataract Backlog." *The British Journal of Ophthalmology* 71 (2): 158–160.

———. 1988. "Preventing Blindness, A Retrospective." In *World Blindness and Its Prevention: Volume 3*, edited By the International Agency for the Prevention of Blindness and Carl Kupfer. New York: Oxford University Press.

Wingfield, Nick. 2013. "A Gift From Steve Jobs Returns Home." *New York Times*. Bits Blog. November 20. http://bits.blogs.nytimes.com/2013/ 11/20/a-gift-from-steve-jobs-returns-home/.

World Bank. 2002. "India—Cataract Blindness Control Project." 25232. Washington, DC: The World Bank. http://documents.worldbank. org/curated/en/238341468752788935/India-Cataract-Blindness-Control-Project.

Worthington, Richard. 1993. "Introduction: Science and Technology as a Global System." *Science, Technology, & Human Values* 18 (2): 176–85.

3

Balancing the Scales: Appropriate Technology and Social Entrepreneurship

Rich people agree to support poor people because they are the family members, they are the neighbors – they are [the] same citizens. Another issue is equity in distribution of services. (Mr. Nabin K. Rai, MPA, Tilganga Institute of Ophthalmology, unpublished interview, 2012)

During his seventeen-minute TedIndia talk in 2009, Thulasiraj Ravilla described Aravind Eye Care System's origins by emphasizing founder Dr. Venkataswamy's attention to creating "building blocks" that nurtured radical innovations to help the poor. Thulasiraj bookended the talk at the beginning (3:25 minutes) and the end (16:23 minutes) with a quote from Dr. Venkataswamy who says, "When you grow in spiritual consciousness, we identify with all that is in the world so there is no exploitation. It is ourselves we are helping. It is ourselves we are healing" (TedIndia 2009). In addition to appearing in the TedTalk, this quote also appears everywhere in Aravind: on signs in hallways, on internal reports and communications, and on the Web site requesting donors to get involved in Aravind Eye Foundation. It reminds Aravind staff, Dr. Venkataswamy's family members (upper-level administrators), and friends of Aravind (volunteers and donors) that the overarching ethos

© The Author(s) 2019
L. D. A. Williams, *Eradicating Blindness*,
https://doi.org/10.1007/978-981-13-1625-8_3

of the institution is sarvodaya, good for all (Lingam 2013; Virmani and Lépineux 2016).

For the autonomous global network to meet the audacious goal of eye health care for all, starting in the 1970s they needed to build various programs and facilities using scarce resources. While each community ophthalmology professional operated in a specific and unique historical, geo-political, economic, biophysical, and psychosocial context, a particular need they all shared at the time was for funding to fulfill their goal. They solved this problem by creating a novel model of social entrepreneurship which utilizes fees charged to the rich to subsidize care for the poor. In this cost recovery model, high-income patients pay market rates, while those who cannot afford to pay receive free or subsidized eye health care.

This finance model was initiated in the late 1970s by Dr. Venkataswamy, his family members, and employees at the Aravind Eye Care System in India. It developed over time through experimentation into a robust social entrepreneurship model that can easily maintain its strategic objective to treat as many patients as possible (Seelos 2014, 13). The British folktale hero's vision of balancing the scales seems apropos here; perhaps this is why Dr. Venkataswamy's sister, Dr. Natchiar, identified the Aravind model as a "Robin Hood model" (Natchiar et al. 1994, 1998; Natchiar and Kar 2000). This strategic objective fits well with the large autonomous global network's cognitive rule to eradicate blindness globally.

Multiple scholarly, entertainment and news media have discussed and celebrated the Robin Hood model, including: case studies by business scholars (Manikutty and Vohra 2004); case studies and conference presentations by community ophthalmology professionals (Coleman 2011; Tabin 2007; TEDIndia 2009); radio programs (Ydstie 2011); and news and magazine articles (Mahadevan 2007; Rosenberg 2013; Rubin 2001). In effect, combining a business-like approach of running an eye hospital to make a profit, with a social mission of eradicating blindness, has resulted in the long-term financial stability necessary to enable institutions to fulfill this social mission for the foreseeable future. This is the opposite of what US mechanical engineering professor K. Mark Bryden refers to as "drive by development" (2011). Instead, David Green, a social entrepreneur and friend of Aravind, refers to it as a "middle way to capitalism"

(Bandarage 2013; Ydstie 2011; Schumacher 1973). This middle way to capitalism has, starting in the 1990s, been taken up by many other eye hospitals and eye clinics in less economically developed countries around the world.

This model of social entrepreneurship's identification with a British folk hero points to British colonialism's impact on Dr. Venkataswamy's experiences and spirituality as a youth and young physician. British colonialism perpetuated imbalanced power dynamics that molded his self-identity and relationships with colleagues in the global field of ophthalmology. Many years later, the current asymmetric power dynamics between the industrialized countries of the global north and the less economically developed countries of the global south continues to shape the relationships between NGOs that are community ophthalmology institutions in the global north and the global south. In some ways, the tension between the global north and the global south is incorporated into the Robin Hood model which can partially be explained by theories created by both northern economist Schumpeter and southern activist (and lawyer) Gandhi.

In this chapter, I particularly focus on explaining the Robin Hood model of social entrepreneurship developed by Aravind in southern India and adopted or appropriated by the Tilganga Institute of Ophthalmology (Nepal), the Lions SightFirst Eye Hospital—Loresho (Kenya), and Sala Uno (Mexico). Each community ophthalmology unit started with a mission to eradicate avoidable blindness. Dr. Venkataswamy originally was snubbed by his local colleagues and potential investors and donors. Therefore, Aravind developed self-sufficiency and self-rule to continue operating while only peripherally embedded in local networks of capital. The Robin Hood model emerged in the late 1970s through historical contingencies and by Dr. Venkataswamy's strong emphasis on sarvodaya (good for all), swadeshi (self-sufficiency), and swaraj (self-rule) at the Aravind Eye Hospital. Tilganga in Nepal, Loresho in Kenya, and Sala Uno in Mexico each learned about the Robin Hood model from Aravind and, from the beginning of their operations, attempted to be self-sufficient by creating their own version (see Chapter 11). Thus, these four organizations can be separated into two social enterprise organization types: the first is a nonprofit NGO with income generating activities, e.g., Aravind, Tilganga, and Loresho; the second is a legal business with a social mission and the example is Sala Uno. In Table 3.1, I describe the two types of social enterprises in more detail. By using the Robin Hood Model, an eye hospital can circumvent Kaplinsky's dilemma: the ideological tensions in scaling-up appropriate technology.

This chapter's goal is to explore how a network of expert professionals started social entrepreneurial organizations and began to create a solution to Kaplinsky's dilemma. For the remainder of this chapter, the structure is as follows: First, Sect. 3.1 elucidates theory about appropriate technology niche from the multi-level perspective in transitions studies. Next, Sect. 3.2 explains Kaplinsky's dilemma, the theoretical and practical impasse that occurs when appropriate technology activists try to scale up appropriate technology to benefit the rural masses. I also demonstrate that Gandhi's philosophy of technology can point a way out of this dilemma. Section 3.3, describes the origins of Aravind Eye Care System to illustrate how community ophthalmology professionals simultaneously created a novel financial model for cost recovery and a set of cognitive and normative rules in a new appropriate technology niche. Subsequently, Sect. 3.4 explains how the guiding principle of sarvodaya, or good for all, works as a cognitive rule to circumvent Kaplinsky's dilemma; Finally, the chapter conclusion, Sect. 3.5, summarizes how this impacts our understanding of the politics of socio-technical systems.

Table 3.1 Two main types of social enterprise organizations (partially adapted from Alter [2003], Jalali [2008], Monroe-White [2014])

Characteristics of type of social enterprise organization	Nonprofit, non-Governmental Organization with income generating activities	Socially responsible business
Motive	Mission	Profit
Accountable to	Stakeholder	Shareholder
Profit dispersal	Reinvested in social programs or overhead	Redistributed to shareholders
Orientation of objectives	Social	Social
Legal status	Nonprofit or charitable trust	Business
Example from community Ophthalmology Organizations in this book	Aravind (India); Tilganga (Nepal); Loresho (Kenya)	Sala Uno (Mexico)

3.1   Theory: Appropriate Technology Niche

In this chapter, I argue that challengers to the incumbent regime created their first radical innovation, a finance model, as they formed their own appropriate technology niches. The disparity between their economic ideology of "enoughness" and the incumbent regime's economic ideology of "growth" compelled them to create their own finance model. Community ophthalmology professionals created a niche while simultaneously creating a novel financial model. Niches are usually created by a government, nonprofit organization, or firm that nurtures radical innovations through a process of learning by doing (Geels 2002). There are two main types of niches: market niches and technology niches (Geels 2005a). However, it is possible to have alternative niches. For example, music niches combine the characteristics of both market and technology niches (Geels 2007). Therefore, in its broadest definition, "niches may have general relevance, allowing survival of deviance from the mainstream" (Geels 2007, 1428–29).

Market niches form a protective space that improves existing technologies, seeks out new users, and relies on existing formal market institutions (Geels 2005a, 79–80). Market niches best serve to create incremental innovations that have a new special application, a new market of users, or a new special-purpose performance (Geels 2005a, 79–80). When pursuing incremental innovations, market niches tend to follow the incumbent regime's technological trajectory. Their engagement with existing formal market institutions makes market niches very stable (Geels 2005a, 79–80). Since market niches focus on incrementally improving existing technologies, a large difference in economic ideology of the market niche as compared to the incumbent regime seems unlikely as this would disturb the stability for which the market niche is known.

Technology niches form a protective space that shields, nurtures, and empowers radical innovations (Smith and Raven 2012). Technology niches are protected spaces for radical science and technology to evolve, and for challengers to the incumbent regime to learn, gather support and resources, and begin developing their knowledge and products for a market of users that is initially unclear (Smith 2002; Geels 2005b; Geels and Schot 2007). Technology niches rely on public subsidies or strategic investment for that protection. In comparison with market niches, technology niches are typically more money-intensive because of their greater risk in the design and development process, and market uncertainty for the end product (Geels 2005a, 79–80). Technology niches do not follow the incumbent regime's technological trajectory. However, similar to market niches, they typically follow the economic rules of the incumbent regime.

The appropriate technology movement influences one subtype of technology niche (Smith 2002). In an appropriate technology niche, challengers to the incumbent regime form their own organizations, seek out their own users, and create their own radical innovations (Smith 2007, 429). These challengers are typically activists or other members of civil society (Seyfang and Smith 2007; Hess 2016). Actors in a niche create and are shaped by, emergent rules. These rules resonate with existing rules in the incumbent regime and attract resources and new actors to the niche, therefore, these rules help make the niche a protective space for radical innovation (Geels 2005c, 694).

However, appropriate technology niches contrast sharply with traditional technology niches because they are fundamentally in opposition to the economic ideology of the incumbent regime (Smith 2002, 7–8 [Footnote 3]; 2007, 436). Adrian Smith (2002, 7–8 [Footnote 3]) argues that a fundamental difference in a technology niche shaped by the appropriate technology movement is a change in understanding the relationship between technological transition and the economy. Instead of limitless economic growth, the appropriate technology movement focuses on limited economic growth or "enoughness" guided by desired environmental and social rules (Bandarage 2013; Schumacher 1973; Willoughby 1990). This difference in economic ideology causes incommensurability between the rules for technology and science developed inside the appropriate technology niche versus innovations developed inside the incumbent regime. The appropriate technology niche's practices and performance criteria are unappealing to the incumbent regime which has its own entrenched technological trajectory (Smith 2007, 446). This locked-in technological trajectory is largely responsible for any interactions between the incumbent regime and the emergent appropriate technology niche favoring the incumbent regime (Smith 2007, 447).

Therefore, I argue that appropriate technology niches typically combine a market niche with a technology niche that challenges the economic ideology of the incumbent regime. Appropriate technology niches both expand the defined market of users through a special application of existing and incremental technologies and challenge the technological trajectories of the incumbent regime. Due to these technology contestations, there will be a negative feedback loop between the low-status actors constructing and following the nascent rules of the appropriate technology niche and the high-status actors following and enforcing the rules of the incumbent regime.

Without a positive feedback loop of support and resources (from high-status actors within the incumbent regime) returning to it, the appropriate technology niche is unlikely to transform the incumbent regime (Smith 2002). The appropriate technology niche cannot initiate transformation of the incumbent regime without some rapprochement between their differing rules (see Smith and Raven 2012). Instead, the appropriate technology niche will likely be co-opted by the incumbent regime (Hess 2005, 2016). Alternatively, the appropriate technology niche will be entirely ignored. Therefore, the appropriate technology niche's long-term viability relies principally on the challengers' vision and advocacy; these challengers create their own market institutions and radical emergent rule-set based upon their radical economic ideology of enoughness.

3.2   Scaling-Up Appropriate Technology: Internal Tensions

Kaplinsky's dilemma illuminates the contradictory ideologies embedded in scaling-up appropriate technology.

> The policy dilemma for governments and aid donors is that maximizing AT diffusion (and the availability of cheap wage goods) in the short run may well reinforce income inequalities in the long run. (Kaplinsky 1990, 102)

Innovation studies scholar Raphael Kaplinsky spells out the tensions internal to the appropriate technology movement when it tries to employ the "Schumpeterian motor to increase the rate of diffusion of [appropriate technologies]" (Kaplinsky 1990, 102). Evolutionary economist Joseph A. Schumpeter argued that technical change drives capitalism (Kaplinsky 2011). Therefore, dedicated Fordist assembly lines and efficient Taylorist scientific management to churn out new products are best for economic growth at the firm level and the country level. Such technology production provides high wages for a few proficient workers using advanced high-technology manufacturing infrastructure to cost-efficiently fabricate new products. Some cost efficiencies shift to the consumer through a lower unit cost for the product. Shareholders accrue wealth by pressuring the firm to constantly grow its revenues.

While buying a low-cost product is good for low-income consumers, the process of mass producing low-cost products was originally critiqued by Schumacher (1973) who instead advocated labor-intensive, small-scale, appropriate technology adoption. Likewise, the resulting wealth accumulation through corporate shares by global elites is contrary to the goal of enoughness (limited growth) that is integral to the appropriate technology movement's economic philosophy. The appropriate technology movement, therefore, has internal tensions that come to light when one considers the arguments for scaling-up.

Kaplinsky's dilemma occurs when appropriate technology activists invest in privately owned firms that produce and disseminate appropriate technology. The World Bank first discussed a similar concern when internally reporting their own appropriate technology investment activities in 1976 (Willoughby 1990, 118). Recounting brick makers in three different countries in the global south, Kaplinsky (1990) found that appropriate technology investors had to make a choice between scaling-up low-cost appropriate technologies to reach the poor through capital-intensive high-technology processes, versus, sponsoring small-scale, labor-intensive artisanal production of appropriate technologies at living wages. These investors had to choose between production for the masses (Schumpeter's mass production) versus production by the masses (Gandhi's mass participation).

In the first scenario, production for the masses, such appropriate technology factories accrue wealth to the elite owner or investors. The factories also provide the poor with the ability to consume lower-cost appropriate technology products: bricks. However, few in the community benefit from being employed in the factories, which do not otherwise empower the local community socially or economically. If civil infrastructure is built from the high-quality, low-cost, locally produced bricks, then the larger community—the masses—benefit directly from local brick production. But this benefit is based upon government or civil society intervention and is not guaranteed.

In the second scenario, production by the masses, only a few laborers in the community benefit from living wages as they locally produce a high-quality product on a small scale. Their product's high cost (or scarce supply) may put it out of reach for the masses—their rural neighbors and friends. Also, because they are small-scale entrepreneurs (perhaps in the informal economy), they may not be included in the elite networks of educated businessmen that could help them develop management and business adaptation strategies to plan how to keep their small business robust over the long term.

Therefore, Kaplinsky's dilemma for scaling-up appropriate technology can be summarized as follows: On the one hand, using the capitalist market system has the short-term benefit of providing more jobs to the local poor and increasing the access to low-cost high-quality goods for the local poor; on the other hand, since the wealthy local elite own the businesses, in the long term, this solution increases the elites' wealth and thus reinforces income inequality. Therefore, scaling-up appropriate technology is unlikely to achieve the triple impact of remediation and conservation (the environmental good), equitable product and service distribution (the social good), and equitable economic growth at both firm and individual levels (the financial good).

Kaplinsky's dilemma for appropriate technology investors relates to a tangential critique Fanon had for liberation activists in Africa engaged in nation building after colonial power withdrew in the 1960s. Fanon foresaw that such local elites would rhetorically challenge the unequal distribution of resources caused by historical colonialism, while failing to address how their own access to global capital perpetuated these inequalities between themselves and other indigenous groups (Grosfoguel and Cervantes-Rodríguez 2002, xxv–xxvii; Ouaissa 2015 citing Fanon 1961, 98). For examples of Fanon's prediction realized in Ethiopia, Kenya, Senegal, Burkina Faso, and Zimbabwe, please see Cheru (1997) and Hwami (2016).

The dilemma of up-scaling appropriate technology for endogenous development through capital-intensive mass production versus labor-intensive mass participation was also present in Zambia as the country gained independence from Britain in 1964 and the new government implemented different technology transfer schemes for rural development (Bowman 2011). Such a strategy of scaling-up appropriate technology, with its inherent tensions, has likely been present in many different development projects.

I argue that Gandhian philosophy of science and technology proffers a way to move forward in scaling-up appropriate technology. Mohandas Karamchand Gandhi's philosophy of science and technology is not Luddism; it is a critique of modernity and industrialization's impact on the poor (Ninan 2009). Capital-intensive mass fabrication of Indian-grown cotton into British-made textiles unfairly accumulated technological expertise and wealth in Britain while leaving India with poorly clothed impoverished people. Gandhi advocated swadeshi (self-sufficiency; Bhatt 1982) by frequently alluding to romanticized images of traditional rural peasants and encouraging khadi (homespun cotton). His purpose was to remind Indians that they had a proud history that existed before British colonialism and that they could move forward independently without British rule or British goods (Arnold 2000a; Tidrick 2006, 140). Gandhi highlighted and emphasized nationally across India what the revolutionary Aurobindo Ghose was enacting for the swadeshi "self-sufficiency" manufacturing movement in the eastern state of West Bengal (Tidrick 2006, 201).

Gandhi additionally advocated decentralization in order to put more power into the hands of the local people (Ninan 2009; Ojha 2013). Swaraj means "self-rule" and many proponents of this philosophy started their own large factories and other industries (Arnold 2000a, b; Bhatt 1982). The prominent activists Gandhi and Aurobindo espoused the South Asian philosophies of swadeshi and swaraj as part of their push for Indian independence from the British government.

Decentralization and deregulation are tenets of neoliberal globalization (Harvey 2005). In Gandhian philosophy of science and technology, decentralization is in the service of local people having power to sustain traditional cottage industry and agriculture (Bhatt 1982). This contrasts with neoliberal globalization, where decentralization perpetuates multinational companies' ability to inexpensively conduct research and development, and manufacture products, and thus to increase revenues. Therefore, the projected technology policies are different between swaraj, which would increase endogenous development, and neoliberal globalization, which would increase foreign direct investment.

Any technology policy requires understanding the circulation of capital to support services, manufacturing, etc., for economic development. Ultimately, market capitalism under neoliberal globalization makes individually owned property and capital accumulation the ultimate goal (Harvey 2005). It takes individual rational choice to the extreme with the rational economic actor (Foucault 2008, 226). Therefore, collective understandings of ownership are not considered rational.

Socialism instead focuses on collective ownership. In many cases, socialism attempts to avoid the private exploitation of labor by encouraging state-owned industry not privately owned industry (Bhatt 1982). Gandhian philosophy of science and technology has a nonviolent ethos that rejects the state, the ultimate wielder of violence, as a safekeeper of the collective good (Bhatt 1982). Instead, Gandhian philosophy of science and technology suggests that the best owner is a community, cooperative, or collective (Bhatt 1982); this is another example of decentralization. Finally, if choosing between the violence of a state-owned enterprise, and the wealth inequality of an elite-owned enterprise, Gandhian philosophy argues for the latter (Bhatt 1982). In this case, the wealthy elite owner should serve as a trustee, distributing his or her surplus wealth to the masses (Bhatt 1982; Diwan 1987). Through elite-trusteeship, there is an negative relationship between economic privilege versus other forms of power (Diwan 1987).

Sociologist Anup Ninan suggests that "The proximity of production and use is a major concern of Gandhian understanding of technology, as it is symmetrically integrated into the decentralized, self-reliant and autonomous village economy" (Ninan 2009, 189). This suggests a place of rapprochement between market capitalism under neoliberal globalization and the Gandhian philosophy of science and technology. The market practices of an efficient assembly line and flexible specialization are both features of the modern decentralized, self-sufficient, and autonomous corporate entity (Piore and Sabel 1984). Such market practices might be paired with a new ethic of sarvodaya, or, good for all, but especially the most disadvantaged and marginalized (Bhatt 1982; Lingam 2013). In summary, a Gandhian approach to scaling-up appropriate technology works through either community ownership or elite trusteeship and involves decentralization, self-reliance (swaraj), self-sufficiency (swadeshi), and careful reflection and action on what is good for all, but especially the most disadvantaged (sarvodaya).

The Robin Hood model of social entrepreneurship utilized by community ophthalmology organizations pairs Fordist assembly lines and Taylorist scientific management with a Gandhian approach to scaling-up appropriate technology. By using this model, each organization succeeds in being economically viable and ethically sound within its local context, with various levels of structural decentralization and collective ownership of resources. Aravind, Loresho, Tilganga, and Sala Uno follow the Robin Hood model of social entrepreneurship. In a nutshell, this means that each has diversified their revenue stream in order to pay for their expenses to remain financially viable over the long term, while using surplus income to fulfill their self-imposed obligations to poor patients. In the next section, I will only describe the development of the Robin Hood Model at Aravind. More information about how the Robin Hood model works in the other institutions is available for your perusal in Chapter 11.

3.3   Aravind Eye Care System and the Robin Hood Model

Aravind Eye Care System's inception demonstrates swadeshi (self-sufficiency), swaraj (self-rule), and sarvodaya (good for all, but especially the most disadvantaged). The Aravind Eye Care System was explicitly influenced by Sri Aurobindo's spiritual leadership and implicitly influenced by Gandhian philosophy. Sri Aurobindo's name means lotus in the Bengali tongue shared by eastern India and Bangladesh. The institution's name, Aravind, also means lotus flower in the Tamil language shared by southern India and Sri Lanka. This sacred Hindu flower is also the national flower of India.

Dr. Govindappa Venkataswamy and his family members started the Aravind Eye Care System in 1976. They formed Govel Trust and serve on its executive board. The Govel Trust is a charitable trust that is tax exempt under Section 35AC of the 1961 Indian Income Tax Act, similar to a charitable organization under section 501 c 3 the US Internal Revenue code. The Govel Trust operates Aravind Eye Care System and its subsidiaries which, by 2012, included: multiple eye hospital campuses in the in the southern state of Tamil Nadu, a research center named after Dr. Venkataswamy, a manufacturing facility and several eye banks (see the organizational chart in the back of the book).

Initially, Dr. Venkataswamy planned to rely upon loans to start Aravind; however, he quickly had become self-sufficient after being denied a loan and being unable to raise donations. Dr. Venkataswamy taught and practiced medicine at the local government's Erskine Hospital (now the Government Rajaji Hospital) in Madurai. After retiring in 1976, he opened his own eleven-bed eye hospital. Dr. Venkataswamy and his family used personal funds to start the NGO; this is an example of local investment. His original goal was to create a charitable institution that would provide free eye health care for all patients. Despite Dr. V's stature in the Indian ophthalmology community (see Chapter 2), no one was interested in providing donations for his new eye hospital. Some were suspicious that he was intending to pad his own pockets for his retirement. Embarrassed by the reception that he received from potential donors and local banks, but still determined to move forward, Dr. Venkataswamy started the hospital inside his brother G. Srinivasan's home with money from a mortgage on his own home.

Aravind demonstrates swaraj (self-rule) because its staff members were Dr. Venkataswamy's family members and therefore the institution was sociopolitically autonomous (although, like many organizations, internally patriarchal and autocratic). G. Srinivasan was the civil engineer who constructed and managed the hospital. His sister, Janaky Ramaswamy, cared for everyone's children (Mehta and Shenoy 2011). Dr. Venkataswamy's four clinical officers included: his youngest sister, Dr. G. Natchiar, and her husband, Dr. P. Namperumalsamy; Dr. Namperumalsamy's younger sister, Dr. P. Vijayalakshmi, and her husband, Dr. M. Srinivasan (Mehta and Shenoy 2011). A few years later in 1981, Thulasiraj Ravilla (Dr. Venkataswamy's niece's husband) came to manage the hospital. When the five clinical officers first started working in their new hospital (see Fig. 3.1), it was a second (and unpaid) job. Aravind Eye Hospital had no funds, but Dr. Venkataswamy told them to do the work and the money would follow. His confidence was very frustrating for his siblings, who (unlike their single brother) had children they were not seeing because of long work hours, and bills to pay in order to support those children (Dr. Natchiar speaking in Krishnan 2004). Surprisingly, time proved him correct. Cost recovery at Aravind evolved to its sliding scale fee structure of today (Natchiar and Kar 2000). This sliding scale fee structure not only allows for economic self-sufficiency for Aravind Eye Care System, it also demonstrates a commitment to good for all.

Aravind Eye Care System additionally demonstrates sarvodaya by providing three tiers of service geared toward different income levels and geographic areas. At any hospital within the Aravind Eye Care System, there are three tiers of service that have their own physical spaces (either separate wings within the same building, or separate buildings within the same hospital campus). At the Aravind Eye Care System, the camp hospital is the bottom level or first tier of service and provides completely free care for patients. Camp patients are typically transported from rural outreach eye screening camps (see Chapter 4). Aravind does not demand proof of low-income status from these camp patients; instead they use social norms to ensure that high-income patients do not make a pretense of poverty. For example, at the camp hospital all the patients will receive free surgery and free food, but there are no beds on the floor just mats for sleeping. The staff at Aravind believes it is unlikely that these patients feel disturbed by these sleeping arrangements, since they are typical of what the patients have in their own rural homes. Remittances

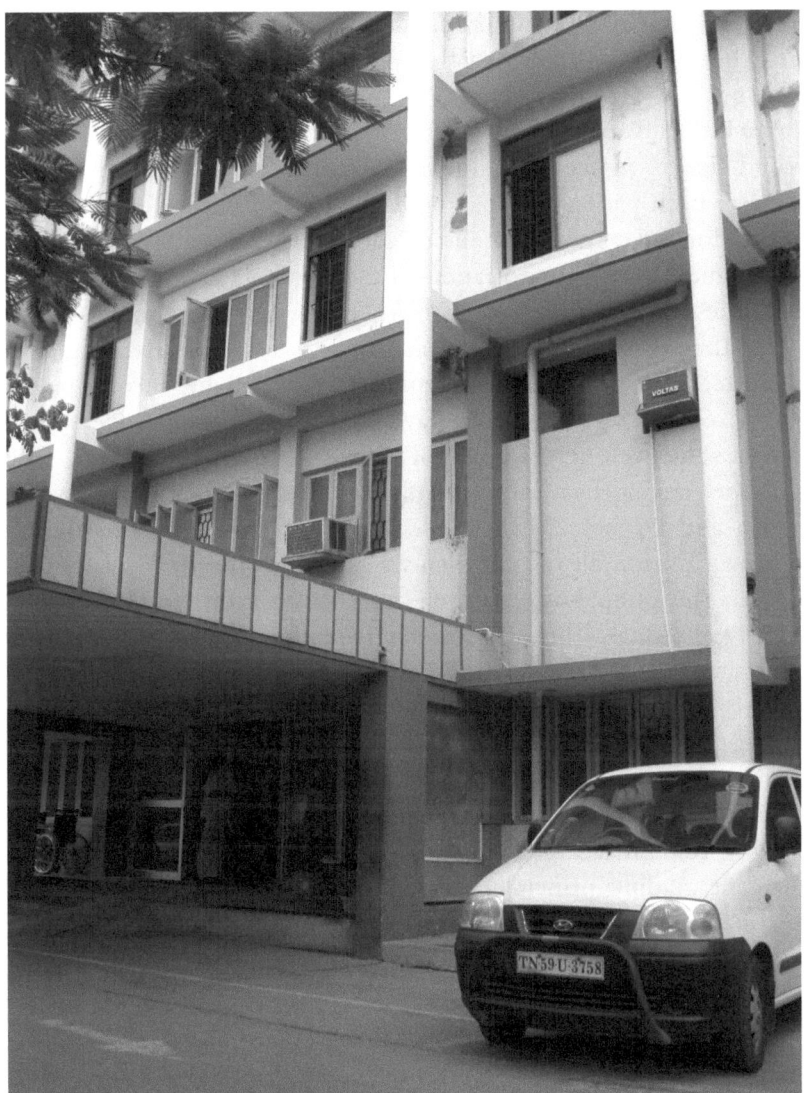

Fig. 3.1 Aravind Eye Hospital Outpatient Building (the first building on the central campus of Aravind Eye Care System in Madurai) which G. Srinivasan built floor-by-floor over five years as funds allowed (Photo by Logan D. A. Williams)

from the Indian government's national blindness control program and other donations cover all the costs for camp hospital patients (see Table 3.2).

Aravind calls each of the walk-in hospitals a "free hospital." At this second tier of service, the patient's fee is partially subsidized, but it is not free. Each patient will pay perhaps 700 Indian rupees ($10.34 US dollars) for the surgery alone and, additionally, he or she will have to pay for medicines, transportation to the hospital, and food at the hospital. The third tier of service is the executive tier where the patient can choose the size of his or her room, any extra beds for attending family members, a private room, or a room with A/C. Higher income patients in the executive service tier will pay 9000–15,000 Indian rupees for the cataract surgery alone, regardless of whether he or she is at an eye hospital in the Aravind Eye Care System, or at a corporate hospital's eye unit (Forgia and Nagpal 2012). While patients at Aravind cannot choose their own doctor, all the experienced surgeons on staff regularly rotate between the camp hospital, the "free" (or walk-in) hospital, and the executive hospital. This again exemplifies the ethos of sarvodaya. The numerous trainee surgeons only rotate between the camp hospital and the free hospital. Therefore, the executive hospital patients pay for the privilege of a surgical experience performed by the most skilled surgeons at Aravind.

Sri Aurobindo's spiritual teachings and Gandhian philosophies are partially responsible for Aravind's demonstration of sarvodaya as an emergent guiding principle (cognitive rule). Dr. Venkataswamy indicated in an interview that Gandhian philosophy influenced his medical practice (Venkataswamy 1992). He recalls attending a prayer meeting led by Gandhi as a child and having friendships with *Gandhiires* (followers of Gandhi) as an adult (Venkataswamy 1992). He also extensively studied Aurobindo's spiritual texts (Mehta and Shenoy 2011). Dr. Venkataswamy worked at Aravind Eye Hospital—Madurai every day, teaching, performing cataract surgery, and managing, until his illness and death. After his death in 2006, his picture joined the pictures of Sri Aurobindo and The Mother in the small shrines within each building across the various Aravind Eye Care System campuses. The leadership of Aravind continues along the path determined by Dr. Venkataswamy.

Table 3.2 Diverse revenue sources pay for expenses at the Aravind Eye Care System (India)

Revenues from sales (+)	Revenues from donations (+)	Fixed expenses (−)	Recurring expenses (−)
Ophthalmic consumable profits	Indian Government Remittances (World Bank in 1964); Government Sponsored Health-Insurance Scheme (i.e., Government of India or State of Tamil Nadu starting in 2007)		"Camp Hospital Tier" Patients no cost surgeries
"Executive Hospital Tier" Patient Fees; "Free or 'Walk-In' Hospital Tier" Deeply subsidized patient fees; Ophthalmic consumables sales	INGOs and individuals	Hospital equipment; Hospital vehicles; Land acquisition; Building construction	"Executive Hospital Tier" Surgeries; Staff Salaries Hospital consumables; "Walk-In Tier" Subsidized surgeries; Hospital staff training
	Government grants; Multinational company Local: businessmen, community leaders, religious organizations, etc.	Research laboratory equipment	Research projects
	Local Rotary Club	Building construction (Eye bank and its equipment)	Outreach eye camp
	Lions Clubs International Foundation	Building construction (one floor of LAICO in 1998)	

Sarvodaya is also demonstrated by creating different eye hospital levels suited for specific population densities and geographic areas. Since 2009, one of Dr. Govindappa Venkataswamy's niece's husband, Dr. Ravindran Ravilla, has led the Aravind Eye Care System. Aravind inaugurated its twelfth eye hospital campus in Madras (Chennai) in the state capital of Tamil Nadu, India on September 30, 2017 (Kumar 2014; Aravind E-News, October 2017). Each eye hospital (a tertiary eye care center) will eventually have ten or more affiliated vision centers (primary eye care centers). What Aravind calls vision centers are similar to stand-alone optical shops in the USA, with the addition of remote diagnosis by ophthalmologists through telemedicine. Dr. Venkataswamy encouraged early iterations of this idea before his death. Now, the Aravind Eye Care System has sixty-two vision centers across southern India.

Aravind demonstrates swadeshi and swaraj by maintaining autonomy in operations while partnering with national and international NGOs. The self-sufficiency and self-rule of the Robin Hood model of social entrepreneurship began with their self-funded physical and human infrastructure and continued through their autonomous operations. Aravind operates with economic independence thereby limiting the influence of NGOs in their organization while simultaneously encouraging close ties with these other NGOs.

There is evidence that, frequently, domestic NGOs in the global south find that linkages to external experts, agencies, and funders in the global north can be detrimental to their mission instead of enhancing their opportunities. An example is Shamba, a domestic NGO located in Kenya engaged in participatory agriculture research practices. This involved smallholder farmers selecting topics of scientific inquiry, and together with Shamba, participating, designing, and running experimental trials (Shrum 2000). Although this research was successful, Shamba found that too many linkages to other institutions and funders put pressure on their organization; eventually the participatory agricultural research followed the funding to a different split-off NGO (Shrum 2000). In contrast, community ophthalmology NGOs appear well able to establish and maintain the many national and international linkages required to fulfill their missions. They do this whether they are economically self-sufficient (Aravind, Loresho) or constantly searching for donations and investors (Tilganga, Sala Uno).

At the same time, Aravind also encourages knowledge exchange through its partnerships with global NGOs. Additionally, colleagues from the USA, the UK, and France encouraged their efforts, including Western colleagues from SEVA Foundation (see Chapter 2). Dr. Venkataswamy, his nephew-in-law Mr. Thulasiraj Ravilla, his youngest sister Dr. Natchiar, and his brother-in-law Dr. M Srinivasan have each served as board members of SEVA. Dr. Venkataswamy worked with SEVA Foundation and several other NGOs including Sightsavers International (HQ: UK) and the Lions Clubs International Foundation (HQ: USA).

As an international NGO, the Lions Clubs International Foundation is prominent in the autonomous global network to eradicate and control blindness because of its program to establish eye hospitals and eye clinics around the world. The Lions Clubs were established in 1917 in the USA. At an international convention in June 1925, the blind and deaf activist Helen Keller, styling herself as "opportunity ... a capricious lady," encouraged the Lions to "constitute yourselves Knights of the Blind in this crusade against darkness" by funding the then four-year-old American Foundation for the Blind (Keller 1925). She addressed her speech to Lions and Ladies; women could not become Lionesses until much later. Her story touched the Lions, and since that time Lions Clubs have become well known around the world for championing the blind and deaf.

The Lions Clubs came to India through the active efforts of an American military service member and Lion in 1956; his local Lions Club in Saxton, Pennsylvania sponsored the first two Lions Clubs in Bombay (Mumbai) and Delhi, India (Anonymous 1996). There are 3667 Lions Clubs across four Lions Districts (321, 322, 323, 324) and 42 sub-districts in India (Anonymous 1996).

Later, the Lions Clubs International Foundation (2011) created the Lions Clubs International Foundation SightFirst program in 1990. Lions Clubs International Foundation SightFirst claims responsibility for helping 30 million people to "have improved or restored vision" through "a focus on building comprehensive and economically viable eye-care systems" and by providing funds for "projects that deliver eye-care services, build or strengthen eye-care facilities, train professionals and build awareness about eye health in underserved communities" (Lions Clubs International Foundation 2011).

Many of the Indian Lions Clubs, approximately 600, have built eye hospitals or otherwise participated in the Lions Clubs International Foundation SightFirst program. Several of them have participated in trainings or consultations with the Lions Aravind Institute of Community Ophthalmology in order to improve their eye healthcare services.

Aravind's model of social entrepreneurship epitomizes self-sufficient, self-ruled eye hospital infrastructure that is good for India. Aravind uses a sliding scale fee structure to provide 66% of their patients with free or subsidized eye health care. The eye healthcare system serves approximately 2000 patients per day, and over 37 years of operation has conducted 4 million surgeries (Rosenberg 2013).

The Aravind Eye Care System is continuing to grow to provide eye health care for the millions of blind people inside and outside of India. To understand the rate of growth, contrast the 2.4 million outpatient visits and 285,967 surgeries (of which 66.3% were cataract surgeries) for the fiscal year April 2009 to March 2010, with the 3.5 million outpatient visits and 401,529 surgeries from April 2014 to March 2015 (see the Aravind Annual Activity Reports in Aravind Eye Care System 2010, 2015). Over these five years, Aravind doubled their number of hospital facilities providing primary or secondary level eye health care from five to ten. These numbers do not include: four Aravind-managed eye hospitals in northern India; or the new Aravind-managed eye hospital being developed for Nigeria in partnership with the Asian Nigerian foundation, Tulsi Chan Rai (Datta 2014; Mehta and Shenoy 2011).

Aravind is one of several prestigious eye units within India. The other three eye hospitals—L. V. Prasad Eye Institute in Hyderabad (which has a similar cost recovery model to Aravind); the Dr. R. P. Center for Ophthalmic Sciences in New Delhi (the eye unit within the renowned, government operated, All India Institute of Medical Sciences); and Sankara Nethralaya in Chennai (a completely charitable eye hospital)—have greater research output. According to the bibliometric analysis presented by P. Kirubanithi (senior librarian at Aravind Eye Care System in 2012), Aravind is the 4th best hospital in India judging by volume of peer-reviewed research publications, which places it relatively high in the clinical ophthalmology network within India. Aravind Eye Care System ophthalmologists publish in prestigious Western and European ophthalmology journals consistently and frequently; this also embeds them in the clinical ophthalmology network globally. Thulasiraj Ravilla became the first president of the WHO-IAPB Vision 2020 India program in 2004. The program set national goals for the eradication of blindness in India. Additionally, Aravind Eye Care System was the recipient of the inaugural Vision Award in 2007, from one of the largest biomedical science and humanitarian foundations in the world, the Antonio Champalimaud Foundation and also the 2010 Conrad N. Hilton Humanitarian Prize; both are worth more than 1 million US dollars (Mehta and Shenoy 2011).

The other three sites that I visited, the Tilganga Institute of Ophthalmology in Nepal, the Lions SightFirst Eye Hospital in Loresho, Nairobi, Kenya, and Sala Uno in Mexico City, Mexico, have each appropriated the Robin Hood model of social entrepreneurship from Aravind.

3.4   Sarvodaya Circumvents Kaplinsky's Dilemma

The Robin Hood model of social entrepreneurship in Global Health relies on a context-specific mix of funding pathways (public and civil society grants, public government subsidies, private cost recovery, consumable sales), and partnerships (local community embeddedness, institutionalized global friendships) and an overall ethos of sarvodaya. The work of community ophthalmologists primarily occurs in the global south, and the four units I have studied have similar Robin Hood models of social entrepreneurship for cataract surgery for the rural poor. All of these community ophthalmology units are interconnected within the subordinate network of community ophthalmology in the global scientific field of ophthalmology.

These community ophthalmology organizations have tried to up-scale their practices to fight avoidable blindness, resulting in slightly different Robin Hood models of social entrepreneurship. I argue that this increase in scale is a unique shift in the appropriate technology movement that represents an interesting solution to Kaplinsky's dilemma: Appropriate technology choices are produced and consumed on a large scale, where any "profits" from producing sighted individuals become reinvested in nonprofit charitable eye hospitals with a mission to address avoidable blindness. Therefore economies of scale are used. Instead of wealthy corporation owners and shareholders disenfranchising individuals in the long term through increased income inequality, local rural people are gaining sight cheaply which positively affects their long-term livelihood (and family welfare). Meanwhile, nonprofit NGOs operate with enough profit to facilitate long-term horizon infrastructure projects and this eventually results in more and better patient outcomes.

In contrast to market capitalism under neoliberal globalization, the social entrepreneurship practiced by these community ophthalmologists focuses on collective understandings of ownership when it comes to both the problem of, and the solutions for, diseases of avoidable blindness.

The Robin Hood model practiced by community ophthalmologists involves a sliding scale fee schedule with multiple tiers where the tier geared toward high-income patients generates a surplus that subsidizes eye health care for low-income patients. This effectively exempts the poorest patients from paying anything except for opportunity costs (household loss of income for able-bodied family member to escort blind family member, travel costs, etc.). It also results in enough surplus that eye hospitals can fulfill long-term infrastructure improvement and human resource training goals.

Long-term goals have involved further diversifying the service they provide across multiple levels of infrastructure: rurally based vision centers provide eye glasses, and urban-based tertiary eye hospitals provide a variety of clinical specialties; again this attempt to provide eye health care is focused on good for all, with access to care across rural and urban geographies. Thus by utilizing sarvodaya as a driving ethos, they have managed to circumvent Kaplinsky's dilemma. Propagating rural and semi-urban community-based eye centers for primary eye health care decentralizes power from urban areas in the global south.

Each community ophthalmology unit may have adapted its own, slightly different, model of social entrepreneurship; however, they typically credit the Aravind Eye Care System in India for devising the original model of social entrepreneurship. At Aravind, diverse revenue streams from public, private, and civil society sources allow them to provide eye healthcare services to many of the patients for free or deeply subsidized rates. In this Robin Hood model, government insurance remittances, direct government funding, private donations, and user fees serve as income. With multiple sources of income comes a greater degree of stability in each organization's finances. Moreover, they use surplus income to provide free or subsidized eye health services to low-income patients.

The multiple revenue stream of the Robin Hood model contrasts with the status quo financial model among many other ophthalmology units attempting public health work. The IAPB coordinates ophthalmology units and international NGOs that command annual budgets as small as $50,000 US dollars and as large as $18 million US dollars (Johns 1992). These community ophthalmology units are typically government eye clinics or domestic NGOs who depend upon government funding for anywhere between 5 and 80% of their total income (Johns 1992). They frequently have a mission to address blindness among impoverished populations, but not all of the necessary funds, equipment, or human resources.

The government insurance remittances or direct funding comes from the respective domestic governments of the community ophthalmology units. The donations may come from wealthy individuals, or from international NGOs, international agencies, and foundations such as Sightsavers International (HQ: UK), Orbis International (HQ: USA), Danish Agency for International Development (HQ: Denmark), or The Lions Clubs International Foundation (HQ: USA). The two South Asian ophthalmology units in India and Nepal have also partnered very closely with international NGOs such as the SEVA Foundation (HQ: USA), The Fred Hollows Foundation (HQ: AU), and the Himalayan Cataract Project (HQ: USA). Status and prestige, but few funds, come from being recognized by multilateral organizations such as the World Health Organization or the International Agency for the Prevention of Blindness. The dissemination of funds from international NGOs to domestic NGOs engaged in eye healthcare work serves as form of resource lodging (Harsh et al. 2010).

In Table 3.3, I have directly compared the percentage breakdown of paying versus subsidized (or non-paying) patients at Sala Uno, Loresho, Tilganga, and Aravind.

These community ophthalmology units in the global south engage in "production for and by the masses" (Kaplinsky 1990, 103). They use a combination of revenues from government insurance remittances, donations, sales of ophthalmic consumables, and patient fees to subsidize or provide free care for low-income patients. In India and Mexico, the governments provide remittances as part of an insurance scheme for patients in the informal economy without means to pay for surgery themselves. In Kenya and Nepal, the community ophthalmology organizations work hard to solicit donations to pay for such low-income patients in their eye camps and microsurgical eye camps. Some of the community ophthalmology units I have examined are more self-sufficient than others; for example, compare Aravind's and Loresho's ability to expand in size with Tilganga's and Sala Uno's constant quest for increased revenues in order to stay financially stable. The ability of each community ophthalmology unit to have surplus funds depends upon the suite of eye care services it offers, the density of patients it serves, and the relative expense of those services (depending upon the local context including, for example, existing government-supported infrastructure). In this Robin Hood model, any surplus becomes reinvested into creating human and physical infrastructure, such as more trained doctors and ophthalmic assistants, eye units within Aravind Eye Care System, or better technologies at Lions SightFirst Eye Hospital Loresho.

In the coming chapters of this book, I will describe how these community ophthalmology organizations have circulated science and technology globally. Using the aforementioned variety of funding pathways, and building upon partnerships with local businesses and foreign friends, they manage to circulate ophthalmic consumables and instruments and allied health professional trainees. This work in the global south falls under the

Table 3.3 Comparing percentages of paying versus subsidized (or non-paying) patients in the cost recovery models across four community ophthalmology units in 2012

	Paying patients (also called "Executive Hospital Tier" patients)	Subsidized patients ("Free Hospital" or "Walk-in Hospital Tier") and Non-paying patients ("Camp Hospital Tier")
	Choice of IOL; Choice of microsurgery (Phaco or SICS)	*Provided rigid PMMA IOL; Provided SICS*
Aravind (India)[a]	33%	66%[b]
	Separate accommodations; Paying patients choose amenities at cost (A/C or non A/C; private or shared, etc.)[a]	
Tilganga (Nepal)	66%	33%[b]
	Same accommodations as subsidized patients	
Loresho (Kenya)	25%	75%
	Separate accommodations	
Sala Uno (Mexico)	16%	84%[b]
	No inpatients yet	

[a]Regardless of tier, patients with complicating factors (e.g., high blood pressure, high intraocular pressure, high blood sugar) are given the safest surgery, manual SICS
[b]Government subsidies or INGOs pay for non-paying patients

radar (Kaplinsky 2011; Williams 2017), but would not have been possible without the radical financial innovation: the Robin Hood model. This radical financial innovation means that community ophthalmology professionals are embedded in their own appropriate technology niche in the civil society sector that is loosely linked to the existing Phaco-regime in the industrial sector (Williams 2017). As such, their work addresses a third concern with commercially embedded social enterprise organizations, that corporate sponsors indirectly influence the science created by the organization (Kleinman 1998). Since the community ophthalmology organizations I am describing in this book are more embedded in the civil society sector than the private industrial sector and also produce their own industrial products for consumption within their network, their work largely escapes this critique. This suggests the importance of fiscal autonomy for nonprofit organizations providing science and technology-based services.

While there are some points of commonality between the tenets of neoliberal globalization and South Asian philosophies of swadeshi, swaraj, and sarvodaya, the main point of contention between the two is their different answers to the question: what happens to the accumulated wealth in a technology production and diffusion process? Neoliberal globalization accrues wealth for the global elite, while South Asian philosophies of swadeshi, swaraj, and sarvodaya are interested in self-sufficient, community managed, local development (and thus locally shared wealth accumulation). This difference is at the heart of Kaplinsky's dilemma (1990).

One way of addressing Kaplinsky's dilemma would be shared ownership of any wealth produced through an appropriate technology innovation strategy. Piore and Sabel (1984) observed something like this at the employee-owned and employee-operated Spanish multinational company Mondragon. Similarly, Joshee (2012) commented that the British chemical company, Scott Bader, also operates as an (employee-owned) trusteeship. In these two examples, the local swaraj swadeshi elite-owned factory becomes a swaraj swadeshi factory cooperative (Bhatt 1982); the community members who worked there would split the dividends. In contrast, the Robin Hood model that the community ophthalmologists have chosen not only frequently employs local people, it also takes the accumulated wealth and reinvests it directly in service of the many community members who still have avoidable blindness—the prospective patients. Therefore, the Robin Hood model of social entrepreneurship is comparable, metaphorically, to a swaraj swadeshi factory splitting dividends between every person (employee and consumer) who crosses the physical plant's threshold.

3.5   Conclusion: Politics of Socio-Technical Systems and a Novel Financial Innovation

In this chapter, I have demonstrated that predominantly the third-sector (civil society) and additionally government and industry are involved in creating a new appropriate technology niche. Geels (2002) has already indicated in the multi-level perspective that the purpose of a stable socio-technical system is to configure the development of incremental innovations and new policies for technology development (including workforce development and labor policy). A newer insight is that while configuring incremental innovations is one way that socio-technical systems have politics; a second way that socio-technical systems have politics is by accumulating wealth and knowledge to a particular group of actors, while excluding other groups (Hård 1993). For community ophthalmology professionals, their purpose was to accumulate wealth and resources so they could redistribute some of it to users, while also remaining viable enough long term to challenge the incumbent regime. To do so, they had to link a variety of revenue streams together in new and contextually dependent combinations to create a finance model that was for the good of all. Simultaneously they developed a new appropriate technology niche. Aravind Eye Care System and Tilganga Institute of Technology are two prototypical examples of appropriate technology niches in peripheral countries within the world-system: India and Nepal.

This chapter has made it clear that the Robin Hood model is a model of social entrepreneurship. This novel finance innovation includes revenues from consumable sales, donations, and patients user fees. The patient revenue comes from a sliding scale fee schedule where the tier geared toward high-income patients subsidizes surgery for low-income patients. The Robin Hood model looks a little different at each eye hospital (see the Chapter 11 Appendix B). What the hospitals share in common is the ability to navigate between local and global financial institutions and domestic and foreign nonprofit partners, and to provide (a limited amount of) accountability to the communities in which they are embedded, without sacrificing autonomy. Each hospital has found a way to balance its commitments to patients, infrastructure, and partners. As appropriate technology niches and networks of production, they create two main products: (1) patients free of eye disease and, (2) infrastructure, both physical and human, to deal with the backlog of such patients. They are developing relationships with partners who contribute advice, time, funds, and expertise, without impinging upon the fiscal autonomy of the organizations. The Robin Hood model created at Aravind (or directly adopted or appropriated from Aravind) helps each eye hospital to navigate Kaplinsky's dilemma.

In the next chapter, I will elucidate how important it is for these social enterprise organizations to work with their local communities to fulfill their purpose of endogenous development of high-volume eye health care.

References

Alter, Sutia Kim. 2003. "Social Enterprise: A Typology of the Field Contextualized in Latin America." *Inter-American Development Bank.* https://publications.iadb.org/bitstream/handle/11319/2711/Social%20 Enterprise%3a%20A%20Typology%20of%20the%20Field%20 Contextualized%20in%20Latin%20America.pdf.

Anonymous. 1996. "History of Lionism in India." GVERI Resources Collection Box No. ORG-20. Govindappa Venkataswamy Eye Research Institute, Aravind Eye Care System, Madurai.

Aravind E-News. 2017. Aravind E-News, October. http://www.aravind.org/ default/aravindnewscontent/NI00000206.

Aravind Eye Care System. 2010. "Aravind Eye Care System Activity Report 2009–2010." *Annual Report.* Madurai, Tamil Nadu: Aravind Eye Care System. http://www.aravind.org/downloads/reports/AnnualReport910.pdf.

———. 2015. "Aravind Eye Care System Activity Report 2014–2015." *Annual Report.* Madurai, Tamil Nadu: Aravind Eye Care System. http:// www.aravind.org/content/aecsreport2015.html.

Arnold, David. 2000a. *Gandhi.* 1st ed. Harlow: Longman.

———. 2000b. *Science, Technology, and Medicine in Colonial India.* New York: Cambridge University Press.

Bandarage, Asoka. 2013. "The Buddha's Middle Path: Lessons for Sustainability and Global Well-Being." *Development* 56 (2): 232–40.

Bhatt, V. V. 1982. "Development Problem, Strategy, and Technology Choice: Sarvodaya and Socialist Approaches in India." *Economic Development and Cultural Change* 31 (1): 85.

Bowman, Andrew. 2011. "Mass Production or Production by the Masses? Tractors, Cooperatives, and the Politics of Rural Development in Post-Independence Zambia." *The Journal of African History* 52 (2): 201–21.

Cheru, Fantu. 1997. "The Silent Revolution and the Weapons of the Weak: Transformation and Innovation from Below." In *Innovation and Transformation in International Studies*, edited by James H. Mittelman and Stephen Gill, 153–69. New York: Cambridge University Press.

Coleman, Kate. 2011. "Proof of Sustainable Eye Care Systems in Africa, the Only Way to V2020." Unite For Sight 2011 Global Health & Innovation Conference, Yale University, New Haven, CT. Retrieved January 17, 2013. http://www.uniteforsight.org/conference/speaker-schedule-2011.

Datta, P. T. Jyothi. 2014. "Far-Sighted: Aravind Eye Care to Set up Hospital in Nigeria." *The Hindu Business Line*, January 20. http://www.thehindubusinessline.com/companies/farsighted-aravind-eye-care-to-set-up-hospital-in-nigeria/article5597886.ece.

Diwan, Romesh. 1987. "Mahatma Gandhi and the Economics of Non-Exploitation." *International Journal of Social Economics* 14(2): 39–52.

Forgia, Gerard La, and Somil Nagpal. 2012. *Government-Sponsored Health Insurance in India: Are You Covered?* The World Bank. Retrieved December 28, 2013. http://documents.worldbank.org/curated/en/2012/08/16653451/government-sponsored-health-insurance-india-covered.

Foucault, Michel. 2008. *The Birth of Biopolitics: Lectures at the College de France, 1978–1979*. Edited by Michel Senellart. Hampshire: Palgrave Macmillan.

Geels, Frank W. 2002. "Technological Transitions as Evolutionary Reconfiguration Processes: A Multi-level Perspective and a Case-Study." Research Policy, NELSON + WINTER + 20, 31 (8–9): 1257–74.

———. 2005a. "Conceptual Perspective on Systems Innovations and Technological Transitions." In *Technological Transitions and System Innovations: A Co-evolutionary and Socio-Technical Analysis*, 75–102. Cheltenham and Northampton, MA: Edward Elgar.

———. 2005b. "The Dynamics of Transitions in Socio-Technical Systems: A Multi-level Analysis of the Transition Pathway from Horse-Drawn Carriages to Automobiles (1860–1930)." *Technology Analysis & Strategic Management* 17 (4): 445–76.

———. 2005c. "Processes and Patterns in Transitions and System Innovations: Refining the Co-evolutionary Multi-level Perspective." *Technological Forecasting and Social Change*, Transitions towards Sustainability through System Innovation, 72 (6): 681–96.

———. 2007. "Analysing the Breakthrough of Rock 'n' Roll (1930–1970) Multi-regime Interaction and Reconfiguration in the Multi-level Perspective." *Technological Forecasting and Social Change* 74 (8): 1411–31.

Geels, Frank W., and Johan Schot. 2007. "Typology of Sociotechnical Transition Pathways." *Research Policy* 36 (3): 399–417.

Grosfoguel, Ramón, and Ana Margarita Cervantes-Rodríguez, eds. 2002. *The Modern/Colonial/Capitalist World-System in the Twentieth Century: Global Processes, Antisystemic Movements, and the Geopolitics of Knowledge.* Westport, CT: Greenwood Press.

Hård, Mikael. 1993. "Beyond Harmony and Consensus: A Social Conflict Approach to Technology." *Science, Technology & Human Values* 18 (4): 408–32.

Harsh, Matthew, Paul Mbatia, and Wesley Shrum. 2010. "Accountability and Inaction: NGOs and Resource Lodging in Development." *Development and Change* 41 (2): 253–78.

Harvey, David. 2005. *A Brief History of Neoliberalism.* New York: Oxford University Press.

Hess, David J. 2005. "Technology- and Product-oriented Movements: Approximating Social Movement Studies and Science and Technology Studies." *Science, Technology & Human Values* 30 (4): 515–35.

Hess, David J. 2016. *Undone Science: Social Movements, Mobilized Publics, and Industrial Transitions.* Cambridge, MA: The MIT Press.

Hwami, Munyaradzi. 2016. "Frantz Fanon and the Problematic of Decolonization: Perspectives on Zimbabwe." *African Identities* 14 (1): 19–37.

Jalali, Rita. 2008. "International Funding of NGOs in India: Bringing the State Back In." *Voluntas* 19 (2): 161–88.

Johns, Alan W. 1992. "The Role of International Non-governmental Organisations in Dealing with Cataract Blindness in Developing Countries." *Documenta Ophthalmologica* 81 (3): 345–48.

Joshee, Reva. 2012. "Challenging neoliberalism through Gandhian trusteeship." *Critical Studies in Education* 53 (1): 71–82.

Kaplinsky, Raphael. 1990. "The Institutional Framework of Appropriate Technology (AT) Development and Diffusion: Brick Manufacture in Three African Countries." In *The Economies of Small: Appropriate Technology in a Changing World*, 74–103. Rugby, Warwickshire: Practical Action Publishing.

———. 2011. "Schumacher Meets Schumpeter: Appropriate Technology below the Radar." *Research Policy* 40 (2): 193–203.

Keller, Helen. 1925. Helen Keller's Speech at 1925 International Convention. Cedar Point, Ohio: Lions Clubs International. Retrieved February 1, 2013. http://www.lionsclubs.org/EN/about-lions/mission-and-history/our-history/lions-history-hkspeech-print.php.

Kleinman, Daniel Lee. 1998. "Untangling Context: Understanding a University Laboratory in the Commercial World." *Science, Technology, & Human Values* 23 (3): 285–314.

Kumar, S. Vijay. 2014. "Aravind Eye Hospital Plans 700-Bed Facility in Chennai." *The Hindu*, February 2. http://www.thehindu.com/news/cities/chennai/aravind-eye-hospital-plans-700bed-facility-in-chennai/article5643435.ece.

Lingam, Lakshmi. 2013. "Development Theories and Community Development Practice: Trajectory of Changes." In *The Handbook of Community Practice*, edited by Marie Weil, Michael Reisch, and Mary Ohmer, 195–214. Thousand Oaks, CA: Sage.

Lions Clubs International Foundation. 2011. "LCIF Sight and Blindness Programs." Retrieved November 5, 2012. http://www.lcif.org/EN/our-programs/sight/index.php.

Mahadevan, Ashok. 2007. "Miracles by the Thousands." *Reader's Digest*, January, 3–9.

Manikutty, Sankaran, and Neharika Vohra. 2004. *Aravind Eye Care System: Giving Them the Most Precious Gift*. Ahmedabad: Indian Institute of Management.

Mehta, Pavithra K., and Suchitra Shenoy. 2011. *Infinite Vision: How Aravind Became the World's Greatest Business Case for Compassion*. San Francisco, CA: Berrett-Koehler Publishers.

Monroe-White, Thema. 2014. "Creating Public Value: An Examination of Technological Social Enterprise." In *Emerging Research Directions in Social Entrepreneurship*, edited by Larry Pate and Charles Wankel, 85–109. Advances in Business Ethics Research 5. Dordrecht: Springer.

Natchiar, G., and Tulika D. Kar. 2000. "Manual Small Incision Sutureless Cataract Surgery—An Alternative Technique to Instrumental Phacoemulsification." *Operative Techniques in Cataract and Refractive Surgery* 3 (4): 161–70.

Natchiar, G., A. L. Robin, R. D. Thulasiraj, and S. Krishnaswamy. 1994. "Attacking the Backlog of India's Curable Blind: The Aravind Eye Hospital Model." *Archives of Ophthalmology* 112 (7): 987–93.

Natchiar, G. N., R. D. Thulasiraj, A. D. Negrel, Shrikant Bangdiwala, Raheem Rahmathallah, N. Venkatesh Prajna, Leon B. Ellwein, and Carl Kupfer. 1998. "The Madurai Intraocular Lens Study I: A Randomized Clinical Trial Comparing Complications and Vision Outcomes of Intracapsular Cataract Extraction and Extracapsular Cataract Extraction with Posterior Chamber Intraocular Lens." *American Journal of Ophthalmology* 125 (1): 1–13.

Ninan, Anup S. 2009. "Gandhi's Technoscience: Sustainability and Technology as Themes of Politics." *Sustainable Development* 17 (3): 183–96.

Ojha, Arvind. 2013. "The Journey of Indian Civil Society: From the Gandhian Movement to Contemporary NGOs." Department of History, College of Humanities and Social Sciences, North Carolina State University, Raleigh, NC.

Ouaissa, Rachid. 2015. "Frantz Fanon: The Empowerment of the Periphery." *Middle East—Topics & Arguments* 5: 100–106.

Piore, Michael J., and Charles F. Sabel. 1984. *The Second Industrial Divide: Possibilities for Prosperity.* New York: Basic Books.

Rosenberg, Tina. 2013. "A Hospital Network with a Vision." *The New York Times Opinion Pages—Opinionator.* Retrieved April 16, 2013 http://opinionator.blogs.nytimes.com/2013/01/16/in-india-leading-a-hospital-franchise-with-vision/.

Rubin, Harriet. 2001. "The Perfect Vision of Dr. V." *Fast Company*, January 31. Retrieved May 1, 2009. http://www.fastcompany.com/42111/perfect-vision-dr-v.

Schumacher, Ernst F. 1973. *Small Is Beautiful: Economics as If People Mattered.* London: Blond & Briggs.

Seelos, Christian. 2014. "Theorising and Strategising with Models: Generative Models of Social Enterprises." *International Journal of Entrepreneurial Venturing* 6 (1): 6–21.

Seyfang, Gill, and Adrian Smith. 2007. "Grassroots Innovations for Sustainable Development: Towards a New Research and Policy Agenda." *Environmental Politics* 16(4):584–603.

Shrum, Wesley. 2000. "Science and Story in Development: The Emergence of Non-governmental Organizations in Agricultural Research." *Social Studies of Science* 30 (1): 95–124.

Smith, Adrian. 2002. "Transforming Technological Regimes for Sustainable Development: A Role for Appropriate Technology Niches?" SPRU Working Paper Series 86, University of Sussex, Brighton. https://www.researchgate.net/profile/Adrian_Smith15/publication/237978079_Transforming_technological_regimes_for_sustainable_development_A_role_of_alternative_energy_niches/links/54240a4a0cf238c6ea6e89d4.pdf.

———. 2007. "Translating Sustainabilities between Green Niches and Socio-Technical Regimes." *Technology Analysis & Strategic Management* 19 (4): 427–50.

Smith, Adrian, and Rob Raven. 2012. "What Is Protective Space? Reconsidering Niches in Transitions to Sustainability." *Research Policy*, Special Section on Sustainability Transitions 41 (6): 1025–36.

Tabin, Geoffrey. 2007. "The Cataract Blindness Challenge Innovations Case Discussion: Aravind Eye Care System." *Innovations: Technology, Governance, Globalization* 2 (4): 53–57.

TedIndia. 2009. Thulasiraj Ravilla: How Low-Cost Eye Care Can Be World-Class. | Video on TED.Com. India: TED Conferences LLC. Retrieved November 2, 2012. http://www.ted.com/talks/thulasiraj_ravilla_how_low_cost_eye_care_can_be_world_class.html.

Tidrick, Kathryn. 2006. *Gandhi: A Political and Spiritual Life*. London: I.B. Tauris.

Venkataswamy, Govindappa. 1992. "Spiritual Consciousness and Healing: An Interview with Govindappa Venkataswamy." By Missy Daniel. *Second Opinion* 18 (1): 68–81.

Virmani, Arundhati, and François Lépineux. 2016. "Aravind Eye Care System as Transformational Entrepreneurship: Spiritual Roots, Multi-dimensional Impact." *Philosophy of Management* 15 (1): 83–94.

Williams, Logan D. A. 2017. "Getting Undone Technology Done: Global Techno-Assemblage and the Value Chain of Invention." *Science, Technology and Society* 22 (1): 38–58.

Willoughby, Kelvin W. 1990. *Technology Choice: A Critique of the Appropriate Technology Movement*. Boulder, CO: Westview Press.

Ydstie, John. 2011. "India Eye Care Center Finds Middle Way to Capitalism." All Things Considered, NPR. http://www.npr.org/2011/11/29/142526263/india-eye-care-center-finds-middle-way-to-capitalism.

4

Witnessing Rural Blindness: Standardizing Benchmarks from Eye Camps

If we take [the] outreach program....we have innovated the whole planning process: How to plan the outreach program?; How to set targets?; What methods are to be followed?; What should be different parameters for different outreach programs?; What should be the benchmarks for each parameters?; How to monitor that?; How to make our resources much more optimally utilized?; How to make a judgment on outreach program whether it is productive or non-productive program? (Mr. R. Meenakshi Sundaram, MHM, Aravind Eye Care System 2012)

Patients moved like clockwork through the small eye camp run by ten staff persons from Aravind. The process by which a person became a patient was routine. The prospective patients first registered for the eye camp with an ophthalmic assistant or Sister. From there, the patients moved through each station where a Sister: provided the patient with a service or treatment, made notations onto his or her patient record, and sent him or her on to the next station.

At one station, there were two ophthalmologists performing patient examinations: one Tibetan two-year fellow sponsored by the SEVA Foundation and one Indian Aravind employee. They worked with an ophthalmic assistant in a classroom with chalkboard-lined walls that

© The Author(s) 2019
L. D. A. Williams, *Eradicating Blindness*,
https://doi.org/10.1007/978-981-13-1625-8_4

was decorated by children's art projects hung along wires across the ceiling. The children's art projects, occasionally stirred by the air flowing through the open doorways, were the only witnesses to the eye exams besides the occasional patient relative and visitors to Aravind like the group of management trainees I was with.

Across the dirt-packed courtyard of the school, a second room held three ophthalmic assistants who were performing refraction on patients, grinding and fitting lenses for eyeglasses, and selling glasses. Two more ophthalmic assistants checked visual acuity. An Aravind employee, Mr. Mohammed Gowth, explained that, in the modern eye screening camp we were visiting, the various stations mirror those of the outpatient clinic in the eye hospital (Williams 2012, May 9; Natchiar et al. 1994).

The outreach eye screening camps espoused by the Aravind Eye Care System are very successful in treating a high volume of patients. To illustrate this success R. Meenakshi Sundaram (senior manager of the Outreach Department), related the 2009–2010 statistics for the system's flagship hospital in Madurai (Williams 2012, March 19). From April 2009 to March 2010, outreach camp managers from the Aravind Eye Hospital, Madurai, held 362 regular comprehensive eye screening camps for approximately 108,000 patients (Williams 2012, March 19; Aravind Eye Care System 2010). For those patients whose cataracts require immediate surgery, 38% have on the spot transportation by minivan from the rural eye camp to the Aravind Eye Hospital, Madurai (Williams 2012, March 19). The rest receive an appointment and transportation (or in some cases just an appointment). The success of Aravind's eye screening camps comes, in part, from standardizing emergent practices into specific benchmarks.

In his presentation to a first-year business student team from the University of Michigan Ross School, R. Meenakshi Sundaram emphasized that benchmarks for the outreach camps had not been created at Aravind when they first started running camps, however, after creating the outreach camp benchmarks, Aravind has made them "quite scientific" over time (Williams 2012, March 19). What Aravind and other high-volume eye hospitals refer to as outreach is very important in feeding a high volume of patients to their tertiary eye care centers. At Aravind, the outreach camp benchmarks evolved over more than thirty years. During discussions at Monday meetings, the outreach camp managers gradually created specific benchmarks through an inductive process of moving between collated data on camp attendees and patient outcomes over many years. These benchmarks allowed them to plan for high volume and to gauge whether the tertiary eye care center affiliated with each camp would reach its planned patient intake.

In this chapter, I will primarily discuss the emergence of best practices among the Aravind Eye Care System and the Tilganga Institute of Ophthalmology for educating and recruiting rural patients with cataract disease and other eye blindness. I have arranged the remainder of this chapter as follows: Sect. 4.1 summarizes organizational theory on community embeddedness, the multi-level perspective conceptualization of rules, and a feminist science studies theory called strong objectivity. Next, Sect. 4.2 explains the modest witness from science and technology studies. It also highlight the ways that community ophthalmology professionals, acting as a collective of less modest witnesses, contested beliefs that persisted among poor, rural non-users in the incumbent socio-technical regime about blindness' inevitability with old age. Section 4.3 demonstrates the important role of community partners to gain rural patient's trust when working from urban eye hospitals. Section 4.4 showcases how economic necessity at Aravind resulted in the eye screening camps and transporting patients as a technical incremental innovation and an emergent practice that disputed the behavioral norms of rural ophthalmologists in India. Section 4.5 reveals that the geophysical, psychosocial, and socioeconomic context of Nepal requires microsurgical eye camps as an important practice at Tilganga to provide eye health care to rural poor patients. Section 4.6 argues that local context and global embeddedness influenced the Indian government's policy decision to ban eye surgical camps nationwide. The chapter conclusion, Sect. 4.7, suggests that community ophthalmology professionals are embedded in local and global communities and skillfully navigate these relationships in order to support their appropriate technology niches in India and Nepal.

4.1   Theory: Community Embeddedness, Rules, and Strong Objectivity

In this chapter, I argue that challengers are embedded in a local community, which helps them to incorporate more high-status actors into supporting the niche, to learn from their work, and to adjust their expectations and vision while further developing the emergent and incoherent rules of their autonomous network.

Unlike NGOs which depend solely upon donations to continue charitable work, these social enterprise organizations partnered with local stakeholders. With these partnerships came greater community embeddedness, where the NGOs "access and build local resources including the trust of community members...and also forming stable relations with powerful external stakeholders" (Seelos et al. 2011, 352); these NGOs have greater incentive to go beyond transferring basic essential medical services and technology (characterized by duplication and dependence) to develop new regionally tailored services and technology (characterized by adaptation and endogenous development). To do so, they first must focus on community ownership of eye health education and patient recruitment.

Creating eye camps as technology-practice simultaneously began stabilizing the network of community ophthalmologists. Emergent practices by community ophthalmology professionals included increasing local community involvement, recruiting patients, effectively using limited resources (technological, scientific, and human), and moving from handwritten data to locally produced clinical management software. Over time, these emergent practices became codified into standards; such standards are included in the appropriate technology niche's formal rules (Bakker et al. 2015, 157; Geels 2005). These emergent protocols codified their multiple, local, geo-political and geophysical contexts into benchmarks and standards for the entire network of community ophthalmology professionals.

In addition to formal rules, cognitive rules were active among the stabilizing network of community ophthalmology professionals. Community ophthalmology professionals utilized strong objectivity to advance a humanitarian agenda and medical science in order to reach the unreached (Harding 2015; Pokhrel 2003).

There is a theory in feminist standpoint epistemology called strong objectivity (Harding 1991, 1992, 2008), which talks about the relationship between individual identities, social structures, and research or design problem choice. Strong objectivity's starting assumption is that the structure of science as an institution contains built-in implicit worldviews, which then become part of the knowledge production process. These implicit worldviews in knowledge production processes support and affirm the status quo, including existing relationships of inequality in society.

Strong objectivity suggests that those within marginalized groups have greater epistemic authority to produce scientific knowledge than those within elite groups. This is because their peripheral social location allows them to understand the politically and socially contingent nature of knowledge production and be reflexive about it. In short, they have strong objectivity when making knowledge claims from below, and frequently (but not always) from their own homes.

Strong objectivity acknowledges and symmetrically evaluates the contingent nature of the knowledge production process. By acknowledging and evaluating this cultural and social relativism, strong objectivity is thus inherently maximally objective without falling into judgmental relativism (Harding 1991, 142; 2015). In contrast, weak objectivity does not attempt to evaluate the cultural and social relativism of science, but instead upholds science as value-neutral (Harding 1992, 2008, 2015).

Both strong objectivity and weak objectivity are detached and reflexive. However, unlike weak objectivity, strong objectivity does not make a pretense of neutrality. Instead, strong objectivity is not disinterested but involves humanitarian interest (Harding 1992, 2015). As such, the researcher is not neutral or disinterested (in the sense of the Mertonian norms; Merton 1973; Mulkay 1976) but does remain appropriately detached (Harding 1992). Being both interested and detached, the researcher follows all necessary formal procedures to justify high-quality results with a social justice bias to solve a problem of a marginalized group (Harding 1992, 2009, 2015).

Community ophthalmology professionals privilege the standpoint of the blind, rural poor. They utilize strong objectivity, which requires the researcher to empathize with the problems of a particular marginalized group.

4.2   The Less Modest Witness and Eye Health Education to Reach the Unreached

"Reaching the Unreached" is a popular phrase among community ophthalmologists and other public health professionals working in South Asia. The founders of the Aravind Eye Care System in India and Tilganga Institute of Ophthalmology in Nepal, Dr. Venkataswamy and Dr. Ruit, were originally from rural villages. For them and their employees, "reaching the unreached" means going to rural areas to provide eye health care to the poor. Through eye camps, community ophthalmology professionals have had the chance to experiment with different ways to provide eye health care far from the wealthy urban centers. The importance of physical distance does not equate to an emotional or intellectual disinterestedness. Instead, community ophthalmology professionals are a less modest witness collective: As a group, they have a humanitarian interest paired with a scientific detachment that allows them to collectively demonstrate strong objectivity.

Médecins Sans Frontières (Doctors without Borders) exemplifies a less modest witness collective; this organization engaged in using and creating technical expertise through reflexive advocacy to create "motivated truth" (Adams 1998; Redfield 2006). By using the term "witnessing," anthropologist Peter Redfield is referring to an earlier concept called the "modest witness." The modest witness points toward a scholarly conversation in science and technology studies about how the act of publically viewing and reacting to natural experiments, which emerged in Victorian England, has coalesced into community norms for scientists (Shapin 1985; Merton 1973; Mulkay 1976). A modest witness is not just a skeptical communal sharer of universal knowledge (Merton 1973; Mulkay 1976). Typically, a modest witness is disinterested and displays discrete experimentally based gains in knowledge (Shapin 1984). In contrast, the less modest witness collective actor described by Redfield (2005, 2006) is notable in its avowed humanitarian interest versus disinterest.

Before they could act as a less modest witness collective, community ophthalmology professionals had first to establish and maintain trust in three different communities: with patients who have had poor previous experiences with eye health care and also with local and global partners in the global field of international development upon whom they rely for logistical support and funds (see Chapter 3).

In the 1960s, many rural ophthalmologists were asking, how do you reach the unreached (Pokhrel 2003)? They were concerned about the rural patients that lived far away from eye hospitals available in urban centers. They needed to figure out how to bring these patients to the city for care, or alternatively, how to bring eye health care to the rural areas. The bottom line, however, is that these community ophthalmology professionals needed to turn rural villagers into eye healthcare consumers. Doing this involved both teaching eye health education and contesting local societal norms.

The majority (82%) of all persons with avoidable blindness are aged fifty years or older (Pascolini and Mariotti 2012). This is culturally inscribed in many places around the world where access to eye health care is minimal or nonexistent. For eye camps to work successfully, it is very important that prospective patients are aware that their eye disease is potentially treatable. Therefore, these professionals had to convince prospective patients that their eye health problems were not inevitable with old age, and this involved contesting societal norms. In his presentation at the Unite for Sight Global Health and Innovation conference, Dr. James A. Clarke (2011), a Ghanian national and co-founder of Crystal Eye Clinic in Accra, explained, "We have a saying: when you get old your hair turns white, your eyes turn white, and then you die." By white eyes, he was referring to the advanced stage white cataracts that are opaque to light. In a documentary about the Aravind Eye Care System, Dr. Larry Brilliant, muses, "You know in a way, blindness is a fatal disease in India. The life expectancy after blindness is two and a half or three years. If you can't feed yourself and your family, then there's a — there's a bad expression in India which is that a blind person is someone who is a mouth but no hands" (Krishnan 2004). Blind people are generally old and devastated by their inability to care for themselves or their families in a subsistence agriculture context. There have been several studies in Western industrialized nations that indicate many blind people have suicidal ideation (Williams 2008). What I learned from interviews with various outreach camp managers and other eye healthcare professionals in Mexico, Kenya, India, and Nepal is that many blind people are not aware that there is treatment for their eye problems. Especially, for cataract disease (which causes 50% of blindness), often a surgeon can easily correct their blindness and restore them to full sight.

Health education then becomes very important. Outreach camp managers are keen to convince different demographic populations that they should seek eye health care. As R. Meenakshi Sundaram explains (Williams 2012, March 19), disease priorities may depend upon age, and "50+ is a driven market." He explains that Indian eye camps typically segment disease by age along the following lines: At 50+ there is a chance for problems such as cataracts; 50+ also has a chance for glaucoma, retinal diseases, and diabetic retinopathy (the last only occurs in 5% of the cases); 40+ typically presents with presbyopia (therefore camps target workplaces to provide reading glasses); and children may have congenital problems (so camps target schools). However, in a typical eye screening camp, "after cataract, the next highest problem is refraction/glasses." Thus, eyeglasses can immediately correct the avoidable blindness in 40% of camp patients aged 16–49 (Williams 2012, March 19). This aligns with the 2010 statistics from the WHO, where cataracts cause 51% of avoidable blindness, and refractive errors cause 43% of visual impairment (including blindness; see Pascolini and Mariotti 2012).

Considering the wide variety of potential visual diseases and problems, teaching eye health education is important to make poor patients into health consumers. This occurs through various means. Unite for Sight publishes pamphlets in Hindi differentiated by gender to encourage recognition of eye health problems among rural

Indian families (Staples-Clark 2011). Similarly, the Aravind Eye Care System publishes a magazine called *Kannoli* once a month in Tamil on recognizing eye problems and controlling them (Aravind Eye Care System 2015).

In addition to educating patients and contesting societal norms, these medical professionals had to figure out how to access these primarily rural prospective patients at a distance.

4.3 Gaining Trust at a Distance Through Community Embeddedness

There are two levels of community embeddedness through which relationships of trust must operate: locally between the eye hospital and its community partners to operate rural eye camps and supralocally between the eye hospital and more distant governments, funders, and multilateral organizations.

Community involvement was an incremental innovation that community ophthalmology professionals at Aravind and Tilganga implemented to provide eye health care to rural poor patients. Community partners are arguably more visible in daily rural village life than in an urban eye hospital operating far away. Over time, this has meant that community partners have become increasingly important for an eye camp's success.

In one example, Tilganga partners with people from the local community for the outreach microsurgical eye camps (OMSECs). Gil (a pseudonym) is an Australian expatriate who has volunteered for many years at Tilganga. He believes it is the local organizers that make the OMSEC a success. Gil (unpublished interview, 2012) recalls the origins of the OMSECs, saying,

> They used to use a school; all the classrooms make [a] good operating theatre ward and things. They used local youth groups to organize it locally. They would tape all the flyers around the hills by foot and give them out to get people to come. [Also], they used to put ads on the radio in Nepal advertising it. That is how it used to happen.

The local community partners select the site and start advertising at least one month before the camp will occur. During Tilganga's OMSECs, the partners provide camp furniture and all of the food for the patients.

A second example also demonstrates the important work of community partners who advertise, sponsor, and set up the camp. On May 9, 2012, I joined a group of management and medical trainees from eye hospitals in Bangladesh and the state of West Bengal, India. Together we travelled in a minivan from the Aravind campus in Madurai to the village Batlagundu (near the Aravind Eye Hospital in Theni, Tamil Nadu) to gain insight into how the eye screening camp worked (Williams 2012, May 9). From one of the main (paved) roads in the village, we entered a dirt-packed courtyard surrounded by school buildings formed in a U-shape. Short ramps and small stairs led from this courtyard, up the high curb, and onto the first floors of the various buildings in traditional south Indian architecture. These ascents were easily navigable by those who were able-bodied but those who were blind required an escort. In assorted rooms on the first floor, there were different stations for the ophthalmic assistants to perform their assigned tasks (Williams 2012, May 9). As it was early in the day when we arrived (perhaps around 9:30 a.m.), the thirty or so prospective patients present did not meet my expectations for the hundreds of people that such eye screening camps are said to typically attract. However, the biggest surprise I sustained was the order of events for our visit, which started with representatives from Gramma Vidiyal, the local community partner, sharing some basic information about their philanthropic work (Williams 2012, May 9).

The representatives explained that, as a micro-credit institution, Gramma Vidiyal's mission focused on women's empowerment. Their philanthropic endeavors, in addition to eye camps, included sponsoring camps for: ear, nose, and throat; breast cancer; and cervical cancer. They expected to serve two hundred patients that day, and Gramma Vidiyal had spent 8000 INR to pay for three meals each for the Aravind Eye Care System staff, for advertising (audio and newspaper print), and for renting the venue (Williams 2012, May 9). From Gramma Vidiyal's self-description, I gathered that the local people trust the community partners to facilitate access to useful goods and services because of years of past experience with them.

In the above details, it becomes clear that community partners and outreach eye camps together act as a decentralized arm of the distant urban eye hospital. The local community partner provides the logistical support and funding, while the eye hospital provides the medical staff and ophthalmic consumables. Sir John Wilson credits the global gains in addressing avoidable blindness to the "leaders of rural ophthalmology in India, who were prepared to see their hospital not as a static centre of exclusive treatment but as a focal point of a rural programme with mobile teams achieving genuine community involvement" (Wilson 1988, 3). Thulasiraj Ravilla suggests in his TedIndia (2009) Talk that community involvement in outreach camps was an "early innovation" of the Aravind Eye Care System. Each of the urban eye hospitals in the Aravind Eye Care System is affiliated with a geographic region. Within each region, camps are organized and reorganized by Aravind outreach camp managers many times per week, most weeks per year. This means that across the system they are working with hundreds of such community partners, from micro-credit institutions to local businessmen, Christian clergy, Hindu gurus, or nonprofit service associations such as local Lions or Rotary clubs.

Community partners and previous patients informally recruit new patients through word of mouth. Informal recruitment of new patients is a key component of Aravind's eye screening camps (Mani 2013). R. Meenakshi Sundaram also discussed how previous patients act as "ambassadors" (Williams 2012, March 19). In the early twentieth century, rural Indians learned quickly about their family and friends' poor quality visual outcomes after the eye surgical camps conducted by the British Army (Elliot 1917). In contrast, now word of mouth spreads quickly within the rural area about high-quality visual outcomes after an eye screening camp and free surgery. After Aravind eye screening camps are promoted for several years in a particular rural location, many more patients start seeking out eye healthcare services.

The community outreach directors at Aravind, Loresho, and Tilganga pointed out that, once prospective rural patients have learned to trust them as eye healthcare providers, there is an interesting effect: The patients now come with the exact amount of funds required for cataract surgery. These eye health "consumers" are then sometimes surprised to learn: (1) Their blinding eye condition does not require cataract surgery; or (2) they need to lower their blood sugar before cataract surgery (Williams 2011, September 12). Over many years, the social norm that blindness is part of old age is disrupted in places where eye camps are regular and frequent. Patients have become aware that cataract surgery can be easily treated with high-quality outcomes. Now the eye hospitals have to tackle other types of patient education related to complicating factors like diabetes (Namperumalsamy et al. 2003; Official Website of the President 2018).

Eye hospitals must trust and work with community partners to exchange data and vice versa. Aravind and Tilganga work closely with partners to exchange data. Local community partners want the patient data; the eye hospital wants the logistics data (where was marketing performed, how much did the venue cost, and so forth). Both can use these data to make truth claims in their reports about the number of rural villagers turned into patients. Local community partners report to their executive boards and the broader community. No one reports to the villagers (who are presumably happy and sight-whole).

In addition to being a distant judge of outreach eye camps, community ophthalmology NGOs must inspire trust from distant judges such as the state, the WHO, and the IAPB. The "Robin Hood model" utilized by Aravind, Loresho, and Sala Uno relies on remittances from the government to pay for the low-income patients (see Chapter 3). Therefore, the government acts as a distant judge to evaluate the quality of eye hospitals' work. This distance is achieved by evaluating patient statistics far away from where eye hospitals perform patient care.

In addition to governments, distant judges of community ophthalmology NGOs include the WHO Prevention of Blindness Program and the IAPB. Eye hospitals around the world regularly collect data about population eye health through the Rapid Assessment of Avoidable Blindness (RAAB) survey and report results to national governments, the WHO Prevention of Blindness Program, and the IAPB RAAB open access data repository. Therefore, the small staff for the WHO

Prevention of Blindness Program in Geneva can then publish a new report every couple of years on the state of avoidable blindness worldwide. They also can determine whether and how the WHO's efforts to mediate and reduce blindness worldwide (operating through the IAPB and other nonprofit organizations) are effective (Foster and Resnikoff 2005; Pascolini and Mariotti 2012). Meanwhile, the WHO Prevention of Blindness Program and the IAPB have enough data to "design an epidemic" (Mahajan 2008)—their joint Vision 2020 program. Vision 2020 offers specific guidelines and benchmarks that voluntarily participating eye units (eye clinics or eye hospitals) must meet in order to reduce and eventually eliminate blindness.

Establishing trust is part of developing standards and demonstrating objectivity. The above examples further reveal why community ophthalmology professionals, as a less modest witness collective (Redfield 2005, 2006), must establish and maintain trust with the various communities to which they are connected. To engender trust among local community partners who are far away, their accounting practices should show not only the surgeries performed, but also the high-quality visual outcomes.

Historian of science Theodore Porter (1992) studies the history of accounting in order to better understand the importance of standards and objectivity. He suggests that such standards come into being, in order to take personal discretion (or judgment) away and to replace it with quantified discretion. Thus, to Porter (1992), standards' significance resides in their ability to create a distance between a centralized decision-maker and a decision at the periphery. One can still exert centralized power, but at a distance so it appears diffuse or decentralized (Porter 1992). This appearance of decentralization allows standard-makers to bolster their declining discipline-based authority with increased authority from disinterested mechanical objectivity (Timmermans and Berg 2003, 138–40). As Porter explains,

> The purposes of accounting and related forms of quantification are to be understood not mainly in terms of a logic of market capitalism, but of political values —usually some mix of justice, openness, and restraint on personal discretion. Their force depends on types of human communities, on forms of power. Objectivity is synonymous with public knowledge

in a deeper and more interesting sense than we have yet realized. (Porter 1992, 641)

Aravind's and Tilganga's reputation derives from the authority imbued in the data they publish in newsletters and annual reports on their high-quality patient outcomes. These published data act as "motivated truth" and openly exhibit these two institutions' collective "less modest" witnessing. Therefore, community ophthalmology professionals demonstrate strong objectivity based on a humanitarian interest in the standpoints of rural poor people that is additionally bolstered in its authority by detached mechanical data.

Eye hospitals working to control and eradicate blindness must be trusted in the scientific field and the field of international development. Having a good reputation makes each a desirable partner according to both the local community leaders (i.e., local religious leaders and businessmen) and foreign leaders in international development. Aravind's and Tilganga's international partners, such as Lions Clubs International Foundation, SEVA foundation, and The Fred Hollows Foundation, republish their facts and figures. Aravind Eye Care System and the Tilganga Institute of Ophthalmology face national and international scrutiny of their work's scientific merit (see Chapter 8). This is performed, at a distance, through the organized skepticism of journal article peer review (Merton 1973). The data from large community ophthalmology units help bolster the weaker disciplinary power community ophthalmology professionals have within the global field of ophthalmology in comparison with clinical ophthalmologists. This data's circulation also serves to unite the autonomous global network to eradicate and control blindness.

Although community partners are central to standards creation in community ophthalmology, such partnerships were not the only "early innovation" at Aravind and Tilganga. The eye camp itself had to emerge as a set of design and procedural practices that could become codified into standards and up-scaled to address the problem of avoidable blindness. Two different eye camp types have emerged from the autonomous global network within the intersecting global field of ophthalmology and the global field of international development. Both Aravind's screening eye camps and Tilganga's outreach microsurgical eye camps provide an immediate impact on patients' lives.

4.4 Codifying Benchmarks in Eye Screening Camps at Aravind

Standards have power to transform the world by transforming practices (Timmermans and Berg 1997, 2003; Timmermans and Epstein 2010).

> The protocols...by prescribing highly detailed sequences of action, they become the means through which facts can be produced and, at the same time, a crucial part of the networks through which the facts can be performed. (Timmermans and Berg 1997, 297)

Following this argument then, it is possible that the patient's local social world will be transformed by the procedural and design standards of the eye camp. By articulating and then acting on their desire to "reach the unreached," community ophthalmology professionals were inventing new eye camp protocols and changing the lives of rural blind people.

By trying to reach the unreached, community ophthalmologists are engaged in collective witnessing. The technical expertise of the camp is one way to enact a collective form of witnessing. A camp is a transient and unembellished space and "the knowledge it produces is always undeniably motivated and built out of facts assembled directly in the service of humane values" (Redfield 2006, 17). This knowledge is produced through a form of "collective advocacy" (Redfield 2005), where truth is undeniably motivated.

The eye camp's data about patients are produced directly in the service of a medical humanitarian movement: working to address the backlog of patients with avoidable blindness in poor rural areas of the world. Over time, the data from the eye camps have been standardized into benchmarks deployed to train outreach camp managers. Outreach camp managers can use the standardized benchmarks in order to make reliable and viable decisions at a distance from the eye hospitals with which they are affiliated.

On the one hand, eye camps are very common in the history of eye health care in South Asia. From the 1940s and onwards, there were eye camps in India and Pakistan (Wilson 1988). Historically, such medical service camps have been around in India for more than a hundred years (Elliot 1917; see Chapter 2). However, Dr. Venkataswamy brought the concept of eye camps down from northern India to southern India. Furthermore, eye screening camps were an early invention at Aravind that used fewer resources than surgical eye camps.

Aravind started out in the 1970s and 1980s by experimenting with outreach eye camps by always performing eye screenings and occasionally performing surgery on-site. Almost from the beginning, their eye camps only involved screenings and they advised patients to come to the hospital in Madurai for surgery (Aravind Eye Care System 1981, 11). The Aravind Eye Care System started performing eye screening camps only (without any surgeries) from necessity; they could not afford to mobilize the instruments to perform surgery in the field. Because of this, the Aravind Eye Care System encountered some mocking and controversy among their ophthalmology colleagues in India, as what they referred to as outreach camps in the 1970s and 1980s were really screening camps for eye diseases.

Instead of performing surgery in the field, Aravind community ophthalmology professionals would just perform the screening and either treat minor problems on-site, or ask the patient to come to the hospital in Madurai. When the patients never showed up, they started providing transportation to these patients on a specific date. Later, this evolved into providing same-day transportation to patients at the screening camp, to bring them to the hospital for surgery. Sir John Wilson (1987) writes in the *British Journal of Ophthalmology* that, "Last year over 900,000 cataract operations were performed in India. Most of these operations were in rural camps." Thus, in the late 1980s, other eye hospitals performing surgical eye camps at the time did not consider Aravind's screening camps to truly be outreach.

To better understand the reach of these earlier eye screening camps, the statistics from the 496 camps offered in 1985 show, that the Aravind Eye Care System performed 8324 surgeries on camp patients transported from the camp to the hospital and 3580 surgeries on camp patients within the camps (Aravind Eye Care System 1985, 5). In their annual report, they explained their rationale for this saying that, in their outreach eye camps, the cases of surgery occurred only at rural locations that were too remote to make transportation back to the hospital in Madurai feasible (Aravind Eye Care System 1985, 5). In addition to performing eye screening camps without surgery, Aravind also made another argument against the status quo of the time in 1980s India.

The second argument that the Aravind Eye Care System made, which was against the norms of the time in Indian rural ophthalmology, was that completely free camps decrease positive health-seeking behaviors. At Aravind's eye screening camps, they charge the patients a nominal fee to purchase eyeglasses to encourage positive health-seeking behaviors. Typically, patients receive a visual acuity check and refraction with a written prescription free of charge. These same patients can purchase eyeglasses at the subsidized price of $5 or $6 (Williams 2012, March 19). Of the approximately 108,000 patients diagnosed in eye screening camps by the Aravind Eye Hospital, Madurai, from 2009 to 2010, 19% had eyeglasses prescribed; 86% of those with prescriptions received eyeglasses at the camp (Williams 2012, March 19). Ophthalmologists diagnosed specialty eye diseases other than cataract in 6.8% of the eye camp patients; 37% of those were advised to come to the hospital in Madurai (Williams 2012, March 19). Out of those with specialty diagnoses, 79% traveled on their own recourse to the hospital for further evaluation and care (Williams 2012, March 19).

Aravind continued to differentiate their eye screening camps from the typical medical service camp practices of the period; they began to use ophthalmic assistants in the camps to decrease costs and increase patient volume. Aravind conserves the time of the most expensive resource in the eye camps, the ophthalmologist, in a similar manner to how it manages the patient flow in the eye hospital. Sisters (also called mid-level ophthalmic personnel, ophthalmic paramedics, or ophthalmic assistants) perform routinized tasks in the eye camp just as they do in the eye hospital.

The planning process for eye screening camps at Aravind has been routinized, and camp organizers must develop a prediction for each camp's expected size. They use three main indicators to develop their prediction: population density of the targeted geographic area; age segmentation of diseases of avoidable blindness in India; and any historical patterns for eye screening camps in the targeted area. Once they predict the camp size, they can determine the age (and thus the disease) breakdown by percentage can be determined in advance. R. Meenakshi Sundaram explains two such benchmarks as problems to be solved (Williams 2012, March 19),

> PROBLEM: Set target of 300 outpatients and 50 cataract [patients] but there were only 35 cataract [patients diagnosed]
> ANSWER: Therefore, the distribution of age [among the targeted number of outpatients] does not include the minimum [target]
> [THE BENCHMARK:] [A target] of 60% of [patients in the eye camp are] 50+ years-old patients
> PROBLEM: Target of 300 outpatients and 60% are 50+ years-old patients, but still only 35 cataract [patients diagnosed]
> ANSWER: The cataract surgery acceptance rate was less than [the target]; the [camp] patient counselor is accountable for the cataract surgery acceptance rate
> THE BENCHMARK: [A target] of 90% [of the eye camp patients diagnosed with cataract surgery will acquiesce to surgery].

Based on the camp organizer's prediction, there is a specific staffing pattern (Williams 2012, March 19; Natchiar et al. 1994). Each camp organizer has an affiliation with a specific hospital from which he or she draws their medical staff. Mr. Mohammed Gowth explains that the number of staff required multiplies according to the expected number of patients (Williams 2012, May 9). The smallest camps consist of approximately 200 people (and require nine or ten staff persons, including one refractionist and two doctors). A camp of 400 people would require three refractionists and three doctors, with one being more senior or a specialist (Williams 2012, May 9; Natchiar et al. 1994). The largest camp can get up to 1500 people (Williams 2012, May 9). Arguably, the camp's projected size matters less than the fulfillment of benchmarks for converting diagnosed patients into surgical patients. This conversion is necessary in order to address the backlog of rural poor patients with eye disease.

R. Meenakshi Sundaram (unpublished interview, 2012), comments, "If we are not meeting our productivity, then everything is underutilized. When we started facing these problems, then we started thinking how we could develop a structure to avoid this in the future... The parameters have been added one by one... The benchmarking was based on the experience." These emergent practices that started within eye camps and the Aravind Eye Hospital, Madurai, and that pre-exist much of the health management literature, eventually became institutionalized as checklists, benchmarks, and other documented processes and procedures (Prentice 2018). Later these handwritten records became sophisticated clinical management systems, i.e., the Clinic Score Card (Aravind Eye Care System 2010) and other management software produced and sold by the Aravind Eye Care System (see Chapter 7 to trace the likely software users).

The community ophthalmology professionals (including managers, ophthalmologists, and support staff) worked together to create benchmarks to directly address the need to scale up eye healthcare services to treat the high numbers of patients with avoidable blindness. Their pursuit of motivated truth created both targets and benchmarks from these desired outcomes and tabulated data. Motivated truth is seemingly universal although shaped in the crucible of local values and ideologies.

Over time, eye screening camps became known as a major innovation because they provide valuable eye healthcare services at a much smaller cost than surgical eye camps for a much larger number of prospective patients. The routines for eye screening camps have been shaped by an existing infrastructure of schools and paved roads within southern India. This is the unrecognized capital investment of governments in the philanthropic sector (McGoey 2014). Additionally, the population density within southern India—by region, by town, and by the distance between towns—has fed into the benchmarks created by Aravind Eye Care System.

Aravind was not the only eye hospital that was designing eye camps to transform the world. In contrast, in the contiguous nation of Nepal, the mountainous terrain and the many communities dotted along those ranges have shaped the eye camp design and benchmarks for Tilganga Institute of Ophthalmology.

4.5   Local Universality and Outreach Microsurgical Eye Camps at Tilganga

A few thousand miles north and more than three decades later in the country of Nepal, Tilganga determined that outreach microsurgical eye camps (OMSECs) are appropriate for the remote areas of the world with challenging terrain. The Tilganga Institute of Ophthalmology was focused on "unreached" people in remote areas of Nepal (which is divided into plains, hills, and mountainous districts). Tilganga argued the opposite of Aravind that outreach microsurgical eye camps are different from typical outreach eye camps because they provide surgical clinics. Community ophthalmology professionals at Tilganga argued that developed countries already have coverage for eye health care, while developing countries are trying to increase coverage. Increasing coverage generally means increasing the patient volume. The medical coordinator, Nabin K. Rai (2012), remembers Tilganga's origins and says that,

> Our work means, how to reach our service as far as possible; meaning as remote as possible a community. We were staying in the capital city but we were comparing our service here in the capital and there in the rural village and asking, 'how do we make the same class of treatment?'

This focus subsequently evolved into three kinds of outreach programs: (1) short-term outreach microsurgical eye camps (OMSEC); (2) one-day eye screening camps; and (3) community-based long-term program eye healthcare service delivery (a community branch of Tilganga). From 2008 to 2009, there were 8 OMSECs outside and 12 inside Nepal. In the 2009–2010 fiscal year, there were 19 camps planned in Nepal, India, China, and North Korea. The Tilganga Institute of Ophthalmology expected to conduct over 20 camps inside Nepal and 6–8 outside for the 2011–2012 fiscal year.

Dr. Ruit and his colleagues were obviously interested in extending eye health care from the urban core to the semi-urban and rural periphery in Nepal. Doing this in the Himalayan Mountains presents its own unique challenges. Access to these areas is only practical in the foothills;

moving surgical equipment much higher along infrequently traveled "hiking" paths is an improbable task. Thus, these OMSECs bring surgical care to the patients, but only after someone has carried these blind and low vision patients down from their remote mountain villages to the foothills (Mason 2010).

Tilganga brings its own medical supplies and also a kitchen staff and supplies for the staff's cook tent. They clean the school (or any other building with good windows and doors) and otherwise prepare it during the one or two days preceding the OMSEC in order to make it into a temporary hospital. An OMSEC usually occurs over three days. Day 1 is the screening; Day 2 surgery starts. Each patient receives postoperative instructions and any medicines needed. After four weeks, the patients come back to the same place for a follow-up outpatient examination.

The service that Tilganga provides to rural people is not just for Nepalese. They also perform OMSECs in other countries, including North Korea. Every year, just in Nepal, they perform approximately 30–35 one-day screenings and approximately 15 OMSECs. The outreach microsurgical eye camps provide an immediate impact. An ophthalmologist at Tilganga (2012) describes an OMSEC's impact in this way:

> I went to this camp in a place Rasuawah, it it's near the mountain near the Tibetan border… there was this one lady they brought her in the stretcher. A woman and a man carrying the stretcher. She had cataract in both eyes she was not able to see for two years. I operated on both eyes at the same time. The next day I realized … the woman on the stretcher was daughter-in-law and for 24 years had been a widow. The old lady … Mother in law [who helped carry the stretcher] saw the daughter-in-law was so happy, she was in tears. Daughter in law was crying, 'now I am happy I can support the family; I can go out in the field and work for my children.' I worked on 50 patients. This made me realize that I did something great there. This really impacted. A lot of stories like that. This made me realize that there are so many people like that lady who are waiting for me; that memory keeps in my mind; that gave me a big lesson. I want to go to camps outside Nepal; meet more people like that.

The outreach program manager at Tilganga, Khim B. Gurung, agrees that a key feature of an outreach microsurgical eye camp is the immediate impact (2012). This means that expectations become quickly fulfilled and that the patient (together with her local or foreign benefactor) will very likely be satisfied with the transaction: her visual outcome and its cost. The cost is free in terms of the surgery itself, but not in terms of the money raised by her family members to transport the patient down from further up the mountain into the camp located in the foothills. Most of the donors who have been supporting OMSECs for years want to continue; they are inspired and motivated to give more funds. There is something about the very visible work going on the ground, in giving the blindsight, which is incredibly appealing to donors.

Tilganga is proud of their outreach microsurgical eye camps, which they feel have uncompromising quality on a par with their hospital-based surgical services. OMSECs are uniquely Nepalese as Khim B. Gurung explains (2012),

> [In] India, they have poor acceptance of eye camp surgery from the provider side because they had faced problems such as surgical complications with their eye camps. They also have realized that it is due to poor quality of service. Therefore, they are very much against the eye camps. But ours, we don't compromise on the quality. So we set up the surgical table just like here in the hospital. Even though it's not exactly like here, but all the possible consequences of complications we try to remove or minimize them. So, the surgical eye camp set up looks like a temporary surgical theater. We sterilize the whole room, even the furniture. Most of the furniture for the surgical room, we bring from Tilganga.

As described in the above quote, Tilganga staff brings the surgical furniture from their hospital in Kathmandu or the closest satellite eye hospital. With such an accommodation to ensure surgical aseptic practice, Tilganga believes they have developed a good approach to reach the rural community through the microsurgical eye clinics and community eye centers.

The eye camps did not start out well-organized. Originally, the patients would fight with each other to get into the camp. Perhaps inspired by those school classrooms, the Tilganga staff would purchase children's exercise notebooks, tear out a page, tear the page into quarters, write the patient's name and age on each quarter, and give them to the (typically blind or low vision) patients to keep track of as a medical record. Over time, with experience and iteration, this evolved into a more formal system for tracking patients, tracking the eye examination data for each eye, etc. Like Aravind, Tilganga institutionalized emergent practices for maximum patient throughput in the camp. The eye camp's design standards and procedural standards emerged from their early practices.

Timmermans and Berg (1997) argue that "local universality" requires building standards on to pre-existing networks composed of heterogeneous actors both human and non-human. Therefore, the differences between eye camps in India and Nepal illustrate that the same global network to eradicate blindness enacts different meanings and protocols for "high quality" eye health care that is tied to local contexts. Thus, there is a "multiplicity of local universality" (Timmermans and Berg 1997, 287). These universal data have been shaped by the collective work of local community ophthalmology professionals, local and foreign nonprofit organizations, local businessmen, gurus, priests, and other community leaders.

Collectives within networks make standards (Timmermans and Berg 1997). While both institutions, Aravind and Tilganga, coexist as network builders in the same autonomous global network of community ophthalmology, they each are embedded in slightly different cultural contexts with differing governmental approaches to innovation and medicine. In order to transform the lives of rural patients, they developed new standards (design and procedural) for eye camps. These standards emerged from their practices over time.

Community ophthalmologists have a humanitarian interest in treating a high volume of patients. As community ophthalmology professionals collectively performed the actions they deemed necessary to address the large backlog of rural poor patients with cataract disease, they were both: (1) forming the autonomous global network to eradicate blindness within the field of ophthalmology and (2) creating the processes for which this network is known (high volume, affordable, accessible, and appropriate). The need for a high-volume patient throughput is seen over and over again as they assembled benchmarks and standards out of emergent practices to treat a backlog of patients with avoidable blindness.

4.6   Local Context and Global Debate Shapes Eye Camp Policy

Context matters in the formation of institutions such as laboratories and their emergent practices (Kleinman 1998; Scott 1991, 12–13). The question of how the historical geophysical context shapes the institutions and organizations that then create new practices and standards deserves more attention by scholars studying science, technology, and inequality (Hess et al. 2016; Kleinman 1998). Above, I have described how a shift in space (from India to Nepal) and in time (an advance of thirty years) has radically changed the "eye camp" as a technology-practice, within the same autonomous global network to eradicate blindness in the same region of the world. The distinct physical geographies and contexts of Aravind and Tilganga also include different government policy responses to poor quality patient outcomes in surgical eye camps.

The trouble was that, by the 1990s when Tilganga first started undertaking them in Nepal, surgical eye camps had already gained a poor reputation in India where they often produced poor quality results in terms of high complication rates and infection rates, and low patient return for follow-up services (Fletcher et al. 1999; Johnson 2000; Singh et al. 2000; Wilson 1988). The broader global field of ophthalmology discussed this concern in peer-reviewed literature (Johnson 2000; Singh et al. 2000). Singh et al. (2000), writing from the Liverpool School of Tropical Medicine in the UK, studied the cost-effectiveness of three practices for providing eye health services in Mysore, a city in the southern state of Karnataka, India. They evaluated government surgical eye camps, state medical colleges, and NGO eye screening camps with transportation to the affiliated hospitals for surgery. They pointed out that prior to their study, visual outcomes for eye camp patients had only measured outpatients who returned months later to the camp or to its affiliated hospital. Therefore, the authors argued, these former studies self-selected camp patients with good visual outcomes instead of camp patients who remained blind or low vision after surgery (see Singh et al. 2000). Patients with poor visual outcomes likely did not have the resources to have someone accompany them back to the hospital in order to complain about their poor outcomes after surgery in an eye surgical camp. Thus, it was likely that camp patients received poor visual outcomes more frequently than the previous peer-reviewed literature had reported (Singh et al. 2000).

This debate in the global field of ophthalmology precipitated official national policy to ban surgical eye camps in India. As Aravind started refining the eye screening camps, they were able to argue that the advantages of such camps included: decreased resource use, better surgical outcomes, and positive health-seeking behaviors. Singh et al. (2000) specifically mentioned the Aravind Eye Care System's eye screening camp as one that was cost-effective and potentially usable by the Indian government. Therefore, it appears that over twenty-six years (from 1976 to 2002), the emergent practices in Aravind's eye screening camps influenced Indian policy to make surgical eye camps illegal.

The Government of India indicated in its 2000 report, entitled *Major Schemes and Programmes,* that it wanted "[t]o shift from the eye camp approach to a fixed facility surgical approach... for better quality of post- operative vision in operated patients" (Ministry of Health and Family Welfare 2000, 21). In March 2002, Dr. Rao, the director of the L.V. Prasad Eye Institute in Hyderabad (in the southern state of Telangana), claimed that, "[t]here is a government mandate that prohibits surgery in makeshift facilities," (Ocular Surgery News Asia Pacific Edition 2002). Later, in the Annual Plan published on December 31, 2002, the Indian government indicated,

In order to improve the quality, [the] [District Blindness Control Societies] DBCS will ensure that:
Surgeries are conducted in dust free, sterile operation theatres;
(Planning Commission 2002, 211)

Banning eye surgical camps in India does not appear to have decreased the cataract surgical rate. On the contrary, a report from the *Indian Journal of Community Medicine* suggests that cataract surgical rates in India in 2008 continue to increase with better visual outcomes (Jose et al. 2010).

Aravind has been performing eye screening camps for over thirty years; it will likely never return to performing surgical eye camps. Thulasiraj Ravilla (unpublished interview, 2012) explains this probability in terms of the costs to mobilize all the equipment required for a surgical eye camp,

> [T]oday for you to operate on a patient they have to do a lot of pre-op. assessment now you have to find out exactly what power lens to insert, further need ultrasound equipment you require. Things like keratometer [to assess astigmatism or corneal dystrophy] and things like that. You require surgical microscope to put in the lens and then you would require slit lamp things like that…. So you require [a] lot of gadgets if you really want to do well because we thought that [without these instruments] you would have a very serious compromise on the outcomes. So mobilizing all this into the field … makes it even more difficult. Some of those microscopes, the high end ones, they are very expensive. Even the low end ones would cost about say 15,000-20,000 [US] dollars, you know, you kind of drop them or something then that's gone…. there are some exceptions like say in the hilly terrains of Nepal and also some parts in India where it is just impossible to mobilize patients… in those areas it still makes sense that you take whatever efforts should need to set up shop there… I mean it is more difficult but then [Tilganga still will] do it.

As Thulasiraj Ravilla explains in the quote above, the costs of mobilizing surgical equipment into the field for surgical eye camps are prohibitive, and the value to the patients is not high enough to make it a worthwhile practice to standardize in India for the plains regions. However, this position should be re-evaluated for accessing rural patients in the mountainous Himalayan regions of India and Nepal. Dr. Ruit (2012) acknowledged the difficulties he and his staff encountered in convincing colleagues that their outreach microsurgical eye camps provided excellent outcomes for their patients in the face of the intense scrutiny the design of such eye camps underwent in India and globally (Mason 2010).

The key similarity between Doctors Without Borders physicians and community ophthalmologists in India and Nepal is how their geo-political and geophysical context shapes their less modest witnessing and collective advocacy. This geo-political and geophysical context in terms of time and space impacts the emergence of targets and benchmarks for the design and procedures of eye camps as a technology-practice. The historically contingent formation of the autonomous global network to eradicate blindness plays a role, as does South Asia's culture and population density. The geographic difference in terrain between southern India and Nepal also shaped their respective approaches to eye camp design. Finally, the Indian government's embeddedness in the larger global biotechnology industry (Valdiya 2010; Williams 2017), and the global denouement of surgical eye camps meant that the emergent designs for eye camps in India and Nepal are quite different from each other.

4.7 Conclusion: The Emergent Standard of High Volume

Standardization occurred in community ophthalmology through a collective and less modest witnessing process involving extensive trial-and-error, and a geo-political and geophysical context that included terrain challenges and a high density of patients. Community ophthalmology professionals were able to use scarce resources to provide eye health care to many patients. This involved community embeddedness (Seelos et al. 2011): These social enterprise organizations relied on close ties to domestic and foreign partners in order to create and disseminate eye health education, routine procedures, targets, and benchmarks. Community embeddedness helped community ophthalmologists to engage those outside their network in the work of supporting a new niche.

In two appropriate technology niches (Aravind and Tilganga), a high volume of patients has become a formal rule. Through the crystallization of thirty years of practice, the need for a high-volume patient throughput has become integral to the "Robin Hood model." Community ophthalmologists have a humanitarian interest in treating large patient numbers. The inherent necessity of a high-volume patient throughput appears over and over again as they assemble benchmarks and standards out of emergent practices to treat a backlog of patients with avoidable blindness. Economic gain is not the driving motivation for community ophthalmology professionals as they assemble population-based benchmarks, health education strategies, routines for eye screening, and education materials. Instead, the work performed (and subsequent data produced) goes toward scaling-up treatment to "reach the unreached," a high density of rural poor patients, with high-quality visual outcomes.

In the USA, high-volume regional healthcare centers became more prevalent after economic and sociology studies in the late 1970s and early 1980s showed decreased rates of mortality (Luft et al. 1979) and better outcomes for surgical patients (Flood et al. 1984). In contrast, it becomes clear in this chapter that high-volume eye healthcare centers have emerged concurrently in India and Nepal specifically to address a high density of patients with diseases of avoidable blindness. Eye camps were a necessary solution to meet the problem of avoidable blindness on multiple fronts including: identifying and recruiting patients; facilitating population eye health surveys; educating prospective patients; treating patients; and bolstering the authority of community ophthalmology professionals. Now Aravind's eye screening camps and Tilganga's outreach microsurgical eye camps are prominently known among community ophthalmologists around the world.

Eye camps are key sites where technology choices violate the norm of and produce motivated truth through strong objectivity. The production of benchmarks for high patient throughput in eye camps is undeniably purposeful in violating the scientific norm of disinterestedness.

> [L]ocal institutions not only influence the success or the pace of a transition, but also the configuration of the emerging socio-technical system. We have found this with respect to the emerging standards. (Bakker et al. 2015, 163)

Humanitarian interest was involved in the design of the RAAB survey, the eye camp, and other work routinization and data collection protocols. Data can be useful in generating benchmarks to address the backlog of avoidable blindness. Once generated, these benchmarks can become formal rules in the appropriate technology niche.

Now instead of merely collecting data to describe patient outcomes, benchmarks are useful in predetermining patient throughput into the eye hospitals from the screening camps. In this way, patient outcomes are also predetermined, at least by volume of disease type. By matching up patient throughput patients to these codified benchmarks, community ophthalmology professionals have greater assurance of meeting the Vision 2020 goals for successfully reducing the backlog of persons with avoidable blindness. Thus, the collective of community ophthalmology professionals is "less modest" (Redfield 2005) in the sense that they produce detached "motivated truth" (Adams 1998; Redfield 2006) instead of detached disinterested knowledge. This pursuit of motivated truth informed the mission and vision for Aravind and Tilganga as organizations and appropriate technology niches.

In the next chapter, I will describe how they accomplished the adoption and endogenous development of an existing surgical technology that could best serve their patients if produced locally at a lower cost: the intraocular lens

References

Adams, Vincanne. 1998. *Doctors for Democracy: Health Professionals in the Nepal Revolution.* Cambridge: Cambridge University Press.

Aravind Eye Care System. 1981. "AEH So That You May Know About Us." *Annual Report.* Madurai: Aravind Eye Care System.

———. 1985. "Aravind Eye Care System Activity Report 1985." *Annual Report.* Madurai: Aravind Eye Care System.

———. 2010. "Evidence Based Management Practices." *Workshop Proceedings.* October Summit 2010. Madurai: Lions Aravind Institute of Community Ophthalmology. http://www.aravind.org/os2013/eb.htm.

———. 2015. "ARAVIND PUBLICATIONS." http://www.aravind.org/default/publicationscontent/publication.

Bakker, Sjoerd, Pieter Leguijt, and Harro van Lente. 2015. "Niche Accumulation and Standardization—The Case of Electric Vehicle Recharging Plugs." *Journal of Cleaner Production* 94 (May): 155–64.

Clarke, James A. 2011. "Reaching The Poorest of the Poor." Unite For Sight 2011 Global Health & Innovation Conference, Yale University, New Haven, CT. Retrieved January 17, 2013. http://www.uniteforsight.org/conference/speaker-schedule-2011.

Elliot, Robert H. 1917. *The Indian Operation of Couching for Cataract.* London: H. K. Lewis and Co. Ltd. The Foundation of the American Academy of Ophthalmology Museum of Vision & Ophthalmic Heritage. San Francisco, CA.

Fletcher, Astrid E., Martine Donoghue, John Devavaram, R. D. Thulasiraj, Susana Scott, Mona Abdalla, C. A. K. Shanmugham, and P. Bala Murugan. 1999. "Low Uptake of Eye Services in Rural India: A Challenge for Programs of Blindness Prevention." *Archives of Ophthalmology* 117 (10): 1393–99.

Flood, Anne B., W. Richard Scott, and Wayne Ewy. 1984. "Does Practice Make Perfect? Part I: The Relation Between Hospital Volume and Outcomes for Selected Diagnostic Categories." *Medical Care* 22 (2): 98–114.

Foster, Allen, and Serge Resnikoff. 2005. "The Impact of Vision 2020 on Global Blindness." *Eye* 19 (10): 1133–35.

Geels, Frank W. 2005. "Conceptual Perspective on Sytems Innovations and Technological Transitions." In *Technological Transitions and System Innovations: A Co-evolutionary and Socio-Technical Analysis*, 75–102. Cheltenham and Northampton, MA: Edward Elgar.

Harding, Sandra. 1991. *Whose Science? Whose Knowledge? Thinking from Women's Lives.* Ithaca, NY: Cornell University Press.

———. 1992. "After the Neutrality Ideal: Science, Politics, and 'Strong Objectivity.'" *Social Research* 59 (3): 567–87.

———. 2008. *Sciences from Below: Feminisms, Postcolonialities and Modernities.* Durham, NC: Duke University Press.

———. 2009. "Postcolonial and Feminist Philosophies of Science and Technology: Convergences and Dissonances." *Postcolonial Studies* 12 (4): 401–21.

———. 2015. *Objectivity and Diversity: Another Logic of Scientific Research.* University of Chicago Press.

Hess, David J., Sulfikar Amir, Scott Frickel, Daniel Lee Kleinman, Kelly Moore, and Logan D. A. Williams. 2016. "Structural Inequality and the Politics of Science and Technology." In The *Handbook of Science and Technology Studies*, edited by Clark Miller, Laurel Smith-Doerr, Ulrike Felt, and Rayvon Fouché, 4th ed. Society for Social Studies of Science. Cambridge, MA: The MIT Press.

Johnson, Gordon J. 2000. "Improving Outcome of Cataract Surgery in Developing Countries." *Lancet* 355 (9199): 158–59.

Jose, R., A. S. Rathore, and Sandeep Sachdeva. 2010. "Community Ophthalmology: Revisited." *Indian Journal of Community Medicine: Official Publication of Indian Association of Preventive & Social Medicine* 35 (2): 356–58.

Kleinman, Daniel Lee. 1998. "Untangling Context: Understanding a University Laboratory in the Commercial World." *Science, Technology, & Human Values* 23 (3): 285–314.

Krishnan, Pavithra. 2004. Infinite Vision: Dr. Govindappa Venkataswamy. Aravind Eye Care System.

Luft, Harold S., John P. Bunker, and Alain C. Enthoven. 1979. "Should Operations Be Regionalized?" *New England Journal of Medicine* 301 (25): 1364–69.

Mahajan, Manjari. 2008. "Designing Epidemics: Models, Policy-Making, and Global Foreknowledge in India's AIDS Epidemic." *Science and Public Policy* 35 (8): 585–96.

Mani, M. K. 2013. "Letter from Chennai." *The National Medical Journal of India, On the Frontline of Indian medicine* 26 (4): 241–42.

Mason, Margie. 2010. "Nepalese Doc Is God of Sight to Poor." *The San Diego Union-Tribune*, March 20. http://www.sandiegouniontribune.com/news/2010/mar/20/nepalese-doc-is-god-of-sight-to-poor/.

McGoey, Linsey. 2014. "The Philanthropic State: Market–State Hybrids in the Philanthrocapitalist Turn." *Third World Quarterly* 35 (1): 109–25.

Merton, Robert K. 1973. "The Normative Structure of Science." In *The Sociology of Science: Theoretical and Empirical Investigations*. Chicago: University of Chicago Press.

Ministry of Health and Family Welfare. 2000. "Major Schemes and Programmes." New Delhi: Government of India. http://mohfw.nic.in/WriteReadData/l892s/8565929279Major%20Schemes%20&%20Programmes.pdf.

Mulkay, Michael J. 1976. "Norms and Ideology in Science." *Social Science Information* 15 (4–5): 637–56.

Namperumalsamy, Perumalsamy, Praveen K. Nirmalan, and Kim Ramasamy. 2003. "Developing a Screening Program to Detect Sight-Threatening Diabetic Retinopathy in South India." *Diabetes Care* 26 (6): 1831–35.

Natchiar, G., A. L. Robin, R. D. Thulasiraj, and S. Krishnaswamy. 1994. "Attacking the Backlog of India's Curable Blind. The Aravind Eye Hospital Model." *Archives of Ophthalmology* 112 (7): 987–93.

Ocular Surgery News Asia Pacific Edition. 2002. "India's Government Tackles Challenges of Eye Care." *Ocular Surgery News Asia Pacific Edition*, March. http://www.healio.com/news/print/ocular-surgery-news-europe-asia-edition/%7B718ad951-a6e3-403d-9f92-9c34e8c06c72%7D/indias-government-tackles-challenges-of-eye-care.

Official Website of the President. 2018. "First Lady Applauds Lions Eye Hospital for Excellent Services—Presidency." Official Website of the President > Briefing Room > Latest News. February 26, 2018. http://www.president.go.ke/2018/02/26/first-lady-applauds-lions-eye-hospital-for-excellent-services/.

Pascolini, Donatella, and Silvio Paolo Mariotti. 2012. "Global Estimates of Visual Impairment: 2010." *British Journal of Ophthalmology* 96 (5): 614–18.

Planning Commission. 2002. "Annual Plan 2003–2004: Chapter 4 Human and Social Development." Annual Five Year Plans. New Delhi, India: Government of India. http://planningcommission.nic.in/plans/annualplan/ap0304pdf/ap0304_ch4.pdf.

Pokhrel, Ram Prasad. 2003. *Reaching the Unreached: Three Decades of Struggle in Nepal.* Kathmandu, Nepal: International Forum. Retrieved April 30, 2009. http://www.rppokhrel.com/index.php?pageid=pub.

Porter, Theodore M. 1992. "Quantification and the Accounting Ideal in Science." *Social Studies of Science* 22 (4): 633–51.

Prentice, Rachel. 2018. "How Surgery Became a Global Public Health Issue." *Technology in Society*, Technology and the Good Society, 52 (February): 17–23.

Redfield, Peter. 2005. "Doctors, Borders, and Life in Crisis." *Cultural Anthropology* 20: 328–61.

———. 2006. "A Less Modest Witness: Collective Advocacy and Motivated Truth in a Medical Humanitarian Movement." *American Ethnologist* 33: 3–26.

Scott, Pam. 1991. "Levers and Counterweights: A Laboratory That Failed to Raise the World." *Social Studies of Science* 21 (1): 7–35.

Seelos, Christian, Johanna Mair, Julie Battilana, and M. Tina Dacin. 2011. "The Embeddedness of Social Entrepreneurship: Understanding Variation across Local Communities." In *Communities and Organizations*, edited by Christopher Marquis, Michael Lounsbury, and Royston Greenwood, 333–63. Research in the Sociology of Organizations 33. Bingley: Emerald Group Publishing Limited.

Shapin, Steven. 1984. "Pump and Circumstance: Robert Boyle's Literary Technology." *Social Studies of Science* 14 (4): 481–520.

———. 1985. *Leviathan and the Air-Pump: Hobbes, Boyle, and the Experimental Life: Including a translation of Thomas Hobbes, Dialogus Physicus de Natura Aeris by Simon Schaffer*. Princeton, NJ: Princeton University Press.

Singh, Aj, Paul Garner, and Katherine Floyd. 2000. "Cost-Effectiveness of Public-Funded Options for Cataract Surgery in Mysore, India." *The Lancet* 355 (9199): 180–84.

Staples-Clark, Jennifer. 2011. "Innovation & Outcomes: Understanding and Maximizing Real Impact." Unite For Sight 2011 Global Health & Innovation Conference, Yale University, New Haven, CT. Retrieved January 17, 2013. http://www.uniteforsight.org/conference/speaker-schedule-2011.

TedIndia. 2009. Thulasiraj Ravilla: How Low-Cost Eye Care Can Be World-Class. | Video on TED.Com. India: TED Conferences LLC. Retrieved November 2, 2012. http://www.ted.com/talks/thulasiraj_ravilla_how_low_cost_eye_care_can_be_wowor_class.html.

Timmermans, Stefan, and Marc Berg. 1997. "Standardization in Action: Achieving Local Universality Through Medical Protocols." *Social Studies of Science* 27 (2): 273–305.

———. 2003. *The Gold Standard: The Challenge of Evidence-Based Medicine and Standardization in Health Care*. Temple University Press.

Timmermans, Stefan, and Steven Epstein. 2010. "A World of Standards but Not a Standard World: Toward a Sociology of Standards and Standardization." *Annual Review of Sociology* 36: 69–89.

Valdiya, Shailaja. 2010. "Neoliberal Reform and Biomedical Research in India: A Story of Globalization, Industrial Change, and Science." PhD, Rensselaer Polytechnic Institute, Department of Science and Technology Studies, Troy, NY.

Williams, Logan D. A. 2008. "Medical Technology Transfer for Sustainable Development: A Case Study of Intraocular Lens Replacement to Correct Cataracts." *Technology in Society* 30 (2):170–83.

————. 2011, September 12. Direct Observation Fieldnotes. Eye Camp. Presbyterian Church, Rironi, Kenya.

————. 2012, March 19. Direct Observation Fieldnotes. Weekly Outreach Camp Meeting, Aravind Eye Hospital–Madurai.

————. 2012, May 9. Fieldnotes. Outreach Camp Notes. Notebook No. 7 (April 2012).

————. 2017. "Getting Undone Technology Done: Global Techno-Assemblage and the Value Chain of Invention." *Science, Technology and Society* 22 (1): 38–58.

Wilson, John. 1988. "Preventing Blindness, A Retrospective." In *World Blindness and Its Prevention: Volume 3*, edited by the International Agency for the Prevention of Blindness and Carl Kupfer. New York: Oxford University Press.

5

A Laboratory of Our Own: Technology Diffusion from the Incumbent Regime

Definitely people always had some kind of reservation that … the lab, that it's a very sophisticated very high tech kind of thing, and whether that could be done in Nepal? That was the big picture that people had. Even after we did make the lens, and we did the testing and everything passed [still] people looked at the packaging where it said, 'Made in Nepal? Oh it can't be a good thing.'….But we said that we have made a good thing, we have made such a good thing! Why can't we write 'Made in Nepal'? … (Community Ophthalmologist at Tilganga 2012)

The Tilganga Fred Hollows Intraocular Lens Laboratory inhabits a corner of the bottom floor in the original building on Tilganga's campus in Kathmandu, Nepal. The laboratory "clean room" has a modern high-tech presence (Mody 2001, 2005). Such modern high technology is neither obvious nor expected in Kathmandu—one of the top twenty most polluted cities in Asia (on par with Beijing, China, and New Delhi, India). Kathmandu's air quality is six times worse than the recommended particulate matter count from the World Health Organization (Asian Development Bank and CAI-Asia 2006b). In addition to having poor air quality, many Nepalese denizens are poor, making a living through subsistence agriculture. Nepal is known

© The Author(s) 2019
L. D. A. Williams, *Eradicating Blindness*,
https://doi.org/10.1007/978-981-13-1625-8_5

for its tourism and textile industries. Its first and most famous modern biomedical manufacturing facility, the Tilganga Fred Hollows Intraocular Lens Laboratory, is largely unknown and un-lauded outside the global field of ophthalmology and the global field of international development.

As one community ophthalmologist at Tilganga (2012) says, "To come out of the Nepal situation [and establish Tilganga] was already difficult for us. To establish in this dust, in this pollution; to have a clean room environment as one little island—that was difficult...." The island metaphor used by this ophthalmologist highlights awareness about the Nepalese desire to be bikasi or "developed" (Pigg 1992) and the role that Tilganga Fred Hollows Intraocular Lens Laboratory plays in fulfilling this desire. The laboratory is one small area of pristine air in a country where the wealthier inhabitants wear air filtering masks and respiratory infections are among the top five diseases (Asian Development Bank and CAI-Asia 2006a). Additionally, the history of the laboratory's inception highlights the power relations underlying the circulation of science and technology between dominant modern industrialized nations such as the USA and Australia and subordinate modern, less economically developed countries such as Nepal that some (incorrectly) consider to be "backward" or underdeveloped. These power relations come into play when the incumbent regime, entrenched in the USA and the UK, attempts to control the autonomous global network emerging from South Asia.

This chapter will explain how intraocular lens laboratories (high-tech biotechnology manufacturing clean room facilities with all accompanying technology sub-systems) were created by Aravind and Tilganga in India and Nepal during the 1990s, contravening Western assumptions about where high technology is designed, developed, and mass produced. For the remainder of this chapter, the structure is as follows: Section 5.1 introduces theory about diffusion and adoption from science and technology studies and sociology of communication; additionally, it describes how the incumbent regime injects innovation into the early stage niche, and how this early stage niche is challenging developmentalism. Section 5.2 illuminates South Asian ophthalmologists' arguments for why the poor visual outcomes from ICCE

combined with aphakic glasses made that surgery + technology combination inappropriate for patients in the global south. This contrasts
with Sect. 5.3, which describes a WHO expert panel's argument for
why IOLs, as a novel biomedical prosthetic, were not appropriate
for patients in the global south. The third section also describes how
this argument was refuted by community ophthalmology professionals working in South Asia. Community ophthalmology professionals in India and Nepal transformed that rhetorical refutation into a
physical manifestation; in each country, they created their own nonprofit laboratory for manufacturing IOLs. Section 5.4 discusses how
Aravind worked closely with SEVA Foundation to create Aurolab in
India, despite being risk averse and being discouraged by their other
foreign NGO partners, as well as experts from the global north.
Section 5.5 demonstrates that Tilganga worked closely with a foreign
NGO partner and its government (The Fred Hollows Foundation
and the Australian government), to create the Tilganga Fred Hollows
Foundation Intraocular Lens Laboratory. Section 5.6 explains that the
result for both eye hospitals is high-tech, biomedical manufacturing
clean room facilities that add to their esteem. Finally, Sect. 5.7 concludes by suggesting that owning their own nonprofit manufacturing
laboratories fulfills their goal to sell low-cost high-quality IOLs while
establishing their technical sovereignty and supporting their anti-developmentalist sensibilities.

5.1   Theory: Diffusion and Adoption

In this chapter, I argue that challengers use diffusion to bring incremental innovations from the old socio-technical regime as a radical
innovation in the appropriate technology niche. Diffusion is "the process in which an innovation is communicated through certain chan-
nels over time among the members of a social system" (Rogers 2003
[1962]). In traditional development programs, diffusion moves technology from dominant industrialized nations to subordinate less economically developed countries (Cherlet 2014; Packard 1997; Seely
2003). This occurs through foreign direct investment by multinational

companies or by development aid programs by governments and multilateral nonprofit organizations. For the subordinate countries, this is a passive process of receiving technology and expertise through "turnkey technology transfer." In this process of diffusion, those countries with greater high-technology production capacity consider subordinate countries to be consumers of their superior knowledge and goods.

> Western society was presented to have superior knowledge—in an absolute manner—with respect to non-European societies ….the type of K[nowledge] & T[echnology] that a society possessed, such as its agricultural techniques, tools, or writing system, was a measure of the evolutionary stage it found itself in. (Cherlet 2014, 778)

This view confirms and accentuates the high power and status held by those countries that are already dominant economically and politically in the global field. On the surface, the creation of intraocular lens laboratories in South Asia might seem just such a story line.

> The novelties are produced on the basis of some existing knowledge and capabilities and geared to the problems of existing regimes. The interpretation of the functionality of novelties occurs on the basis of existing regimes. (Geels 2005, 83)

As suggested by the quote above, novel innovations in a niche do not arise from a blank slate. This suggests that some novel innovations in the appropriate technology niche may start through the adoption of an innovation from the incumbent regime. Culture, politics, and values travel with a technology and its sub-systems (De Castro 1997; Parthasarathy 2006, 352). As has been argued in Chapter 3, challengers in the appropriate technology niche are well aware that their economic ideology of socially and environmentally limited growth contrasts with the incumbent regime's unlimited growth ideology. These challengers find that, instead of the typical process of diffusion, their process involved the adoption of a technology and the simultaneous challenge of developmentalist culture and values.

5.2   South Asians Argue Aphakic Glasses Are Not Appropriate Technology

In 2000, the British ophthalmologist, Harold Ridley, was knighted by Queen Elizabeth II; this honor was largely due to his influence in the global field of ophthalmology (Apple 2006). Although he is not the inventor of ECCE, his viable intraocular lens design is largely credited as sparking the change in the preferential method of performing cataract surgery from ICCE to ECCE (Apple 2006; Metcalfe and James 2000; Metcalfe et al. 2005). He started this work in the 1940s, when he introduced a biologically inert and stiff plastic intraocular lens made from poly-methyl methacrylate (Perspex). Ridley conducted the first ECCE with IOL insertion on a female patient on November 29, 1949, at St. Thomas' Hospital in London (Apple 2006). Intraocular lenses made it possible to have good visual outcomes for patients when operating only on one cataractous eye, whereas aphakic glasses work best when operating on two eyes. Thus, the ECCE+IOL procedure increased surgeons' willingness to operate on only one cataractous eye (Cairns and Sommer 1984). This meant that they could operate on cataracts earlier (which was significant for the difficulty of the procedure; see Chapter 6). Unfortunately, until the 1990s, lenses in the USA and UK were of poor fabrication quality and still caused many postsurgical complications (Apple and Sims 1996). Fast forward to fiscal year 2015, Alcon, the industry leader in ophthalmic consumables and equipment, realized 1.1 billion US dollars in sales of intraocular lenses alone (Ball 2016).

Decades after Ridley's invention, the idea to manufacture intraocular lenses locally in the global south for implantation in poor patients by southern ophthalmologists turned out to be rather contentious. Developmentalist expectations and assumptions among domestic and foreign ophthalmologists meant Aravind and Tilganga faced opposition to making laboratories of their own.

When Dr. Sanduk Ruit participated in the Nepal National Blindness Survey as a young general medical practitioner 1979–1980 (see Chapter 2), he learned that more than 56% of patients that underwent ICCE did not possess aphakic glasses after surgery, which meant they were still functionally blind despite having undergone an invasive surgical procedure. Likewise, these aphakic patients contributed to the very high blindness incidence—50% (Marseille 1994, 153). A young Dr. Ruit was pondering these problems as he began his ophthalmology residency in 1981 at the All India Institute of Medical Sciences in New Delhi (AIIMS, New Delhi).

Fifteen hundred miles south of New Delhi, in Madurai, Dr. Venkataswamy learned about a newer surgical technique that involved the implantation of an intraocular lens. The newer surgical technology-practice, ECCE+IOL, involved an experimental prosthetic: the intraocular lens substituted for the body's natural lens inside the posterior chamber of the eye. In 1980, Dr. Venkataswamy watched an ophthalmologist and friend, Dr. Richard Litwin (from the US SEVA Foundation), perform ECCE+IOL on a carpenter in Tamil Nadu state in southern India (Litwin 1988; Marseille 1994). The impact on the carpenter's vision was immediate and profound (Mehta and Shenoy 2011; Marseille 1994). According to Suzanne Gilbert (unpublished interview, 2010), this was the impetus for Dr. Venkataswamy's decision that every cataractous patient at Aravind should have such surgery. Only a year later, in 1981, the U.S. Food and Drug Administration approved intraocular lenses (IOLs) as an "experimental device" (Marseille 1994, 149).

Dr. Ruit finished his ophthalmology residency in New Delhi, India, in 1984 and then returned to Nepal before completing fellowships in Europe and Australia that helped crystallize some of his ideas. Dr. Fred Hollows, a visiting Marxist New Zealand ophthalmologist (working in Australia), came to Nepal in 1985 for a short-term project with the World Health Organization (WHO) to look at trachoma. Dr. Hollows encouraged a young Dr. Ruit to dream. In recalling the visit, Dr. Ruit said, "[a]t the time Fred Hollows was a worldwide expert. I was young and started talking about my ideas with him and we found that we had common interests. He called his wife and stayed an extra 15 days. As he traveled across Nepal to perform his study I also had him look at cataract cases. Later we kept in touch by phone." In the mid-1980s, Dr. Ruit was attempting to create a private clinic with a small team of staff, some of whom also worked with him at the government run Nepal Eye Hospital. Meanwhile, Dr. Ruit visited Holland (the Netherlands) to perform cataract surgery with esteemed ophthalmologists and inventors of intraocular lenses: Dr. Jan Worst and his mentor Dr. Cornelius Binkhorst (Cimberle 2015). Perhaps his work with the co-founder of the Jan Worst Research Group and the designer of implantable lenses for ICCE helped Dr. Ruit to contemplate what technologies could be adopted as an "intermediate technology" for blind Nepalese people.

Afterward, at the invitation of Dr. Hollows, Dr. Ruit and his wife went to Australia and stayed for one year in 1986 (Ocular Surgery News Asia Pacific Edition 2010). While in Australia, Dr. Ruit realized that ECCE+IOL was becoming a common surgery. When he returned to Nepal, he started discussing with his colleagues how they could simplify the technique and execute it locally, "at the community level." Although Dr. Ruit had trained in ICCE+aphakic glasses at AIIMS, New Delhi, he instead wanted to use the newer more advanced ECCE+IOL technique for all of his patients.

In the late 1980s, intraocular lenses were a new and unproven technology innovation in the USA and UK. At this time, ophthalmologists in less economically developed countries were still implementing the proven standard for cataract surgery, ICCE, and then providing aphakic patients with "cokebottle" glasses. Middle- and high-income Indian patients were able to pay for ECCE+IOL surgery, while low-income Indian patients were still receiving ICCE+aphakic cokebottle glasses. At the Aravind Eye Care System, this tiered system was facilitated by Western consumerism and biomedical innovation. Multinational companies such as Alcon were constantly inventing new types of intraocular lenses; "[t]he 1980s were a time of rapid innovation in IOL design. Companies were happy to donate last year's lenses and take the tax deduction [sic]" (Marseille 1994, 168). Therefore, some clinical ophthalmologists (and some ophthalmic consumables companies such as Alcon) had old IOLs in excess supply. Intraocular lenses that originally would be priced well above the average Indian monthly income were donated by the companies to help poor patients. The Aravind Eye Care System in India used these donated IOLs for their middle- and high-income patients in the late 1980s (Marseille 1994, 168, 172). This method of acquiring IOLs for Indian patients worked well for a while. It is pragmatic for Aravind. The doctors can justify the high rates that they charge middle- and high-income patients as the costs of the latest and greatest high technology from the West. Consequently, they can use the extracted wealth to subsidize low-income patients while providing them with the current proven technology of ICCE+aphakic glasses.

Both Dr. Ruit, a Nepalese civil servant, and Dr. Venkataswamy, at Aravind Eye Care System, realized that aphakic cokebottle glasses, the standard that many Westerners considered "appropriate tech-nology" in the global south for post-cataract removal vision correc-tion, were insufficient. Cokebottle glasses did not allow for peripheral vision, and patients easily misplaced or broke them (Mahadevan 2007; Tielsch 1998). Elliott Marseille describes Indian patients' response to ICCE+aphakic cokebottle glasses. He explains that this surgical proce-dure did not excite patients because the visual outcomes were not very good:

> I expected to see joy and excitement in that room and was disappointed that these patients seemed so unmoved by the miracle of modern eye surgery. I chalked it up to the legendary equanimity of the Indian soul. I learned later that their nonchalance was perhaps not so philosophical: their new vision was nothing to be very excited about.
>
> …
>
> These aphakic lensless patients are far from blind but a long way from having normal vision. Their glasses enlarge images by one third. Patients must look directly through the center of the glasses to avoid disorient-ing distortion. In practice, they are afflicted by varying degrees of fish-eye effects, astigmatism, and farsightedness. One tell-tale sign of the aphake is the way he crosses a threshold. He steps high into empty space before bringing his foot down onto the step. (Marseille 1994, 152–53)

As described above, many patients with ICCE+aphakic glasses had poor vision quality. Mr. Nabin K. Rai (unpublished interview, 2012), the med-ical coordinator at the Tilganga Institute of Ophthalmology, explains that such visual field distortion and restriction makes aphakic glasses par-ticularly inappropriate for people located in the mountainous regions of Nepal that deal with "the hills and elevation changes…[to] work in the field" as subsistence agriculture laborers providing for their families.

Ophthalmologists knew that intraocular lenses provided better post-surgical vision outcomes than aphakic glasses. Consequently, ophthalmologists at Aravind and Tilganga identified the necessity of reducing the cost of intraocular lenses so that their use could be for everyone (instead of only wealthy patients). To reduce the cost, they planned to manufacture the lenses locally. As such, they took a stance in a debate that was beginning within the global field of ophthalmology about which surgical technology-practice was best for the global south: the proven ICCE+aphakic glasses versus the newer ECCE+IOL.

5.3 WHO Argues IOLs Are Not Appropriate Technology

The debate about which surgical technology-practice was best for less economically developed countries in the global south took place primarily through interactions at international meetings. To begin with, the WHO Interregional Meeting on the Management of Cataract within Primary Health Care Systems occurred in Denpasar, Indonesia, in 1986 (The International Agency for the Prevention of Blindness and Kupfer 1988). This meeting aimed to closely examine the issue of what types of cataract surgery to perform in eye units across the globe with a particular emphasis on eye units in less economically developed countries.

The meeting participants were from esteemed eye clinics, eye hospitals, and non-governmental organizations located in countries all over the world. For example, at the meeting, there was one delegate each for Bolivia, Saudi Arabia, Malawi, Fiji, Vietnam, India, Jordan, and Thailand, while Indonesia sent two delegates (The International Agency for the Prevention of Blindness and Kupfer 1988). One delegate came from each of the following international non-governmental organizations: Christoffel-Blindenmission (Germany); the International Agency for the Prevention of Blindness (UK); the International Eye Foundation (USA); and the Royal Commonwealth Society for the Blind (now called SightSavers International, UK). The remaining fifteen delegates included three from Helen Keller International Inc. (USA) and eight from the WHO Program for the Prevention of Blindness secretariat (Switzerland). These individual and NGO participants wrote recommendations for large-scale cataract surgery with the goal of increasing the country cataract surgical rates and decreasing the backlog of patients with avoidable blindness due to cataracts (The International Agency for the Prevention of Blindness and Kupfer 1988). Their recommendations were summed as follows:

> There is general agreement that the safety, speed, and simplicity of the intra-capsular extraction [ICCE] under local anesthesia make it attractive and economic for the present purpose. Changing to the microsurgical technique of extra-capsular extraction would be dependent upon additional surgical skills and the availability of operating microscopes. Furthermore, it would incur a major decrease in surgical output…The insertion of intraocular lenses would further complicate both the surgical procedure and the follow-up care. This would again reduce the number of cases operated upon and, in addition, increase the costs. (The International Agency for the Prevention of Blindness and Kupfer 1988, 161)

As shown in the excerpt above, the official expert advice from the WHO, published by the IAPB, was that ICCE and aphakic glasses were the best surgical technology-practice for patients in developing countries because it was faster, cheaper, less complicated, and safer for patients than the unproven ECCE+IOL. This advice was spread unofficially as well. Bala Krishnan (Ph.D.), manager of Aurolab, recalls that in the late 1980s (2012), "[Doctors in the U.S.] thought ICCE was the only way they can give at least something to the patient…That was some input that we got, some input from people in the ophthalmology area." Dr. Ruit remembers (2012) that Western ophthalmologists such as Dr. Carl Kupfer argued, "do not overlook the conventional ICCE; ECCE is untested. It is too early for developing countries to have this technology; instead, clinical trials are needed."

Despite this "expert advice" from a representative panel of ophthalmologists at the WHO meeting, after Dr. Ruit returned from his 1986 visit to Australia, he started using donated IOLs for surgical eye camp patients in Nepal. Once he returned to Nepal, Dr. Ruit talked to Gil about the infeasibility of aphakic glasses "with the really thick lens" as an appropriate solution for patients after removing cataracts. Together they went to speak with the first ambassador of Australia to Nepal, whom they convinced to visit an eye camp in 1989. As a result, Australia donated several IOLs (500 US dollars' worth), which Dr. Ruit used for surgical eye camps. In those early days of implanting IOLs in Nepalese cataract patients, Dr. Ruit (2012) recalls the importance of their connection to the Australian ambassador, Les Douglas, who "was captivated by the idea; he was also a great do-er [sic]. He kept us in touch with some of the local organizations". Additionally, Johns Hopkins University supplied Dr. Ruit with donated lenses. Dr. Ruit's colleague, Dr. Alan Robin, an ophthalmology professor at the university's Wilmer Eye Institute used to bring his residents to Nepal to learn at Dr. Ruit's surgical eye camps. Throughout his work implanting IOLs in patients that came to the surgical eye camps, Dr. Ruit began building up evidence and statistics about how he adapted the surgical techniques he learned in Australia to Nepalese conditions (Ruit et al. 1991a, b). Thus, in 1989, the work of Dr. Ruit and his colleagues using IOLs in developing countries was interesting to quite a few people, in particular the WHO and the IAPB executive board.

The IAPB organized an international meeting in Nepal at the Yak and Yeti hotel, a five-star hotel in Kathmandu. Dr. Venkataswamy from Aravind, along with representatives from another high-volume eye hospital from Hyderabad, India, and the Christoffel-Blindenmission each presented their cases of performing ICCE+aphakic glasses on their patients. Dr. Hollows and Dr. Ruit were the only group that was presenting about systematically using ECCE+IOLs on their patients in a developing country. Not only did they feel ostracized because of their work's novelty, but also because of Dr. Hollows' arguments with other ophthalmologists in attendance.

From all accounts, Dr. Fred Hollows was opinionated and forthright. He called out the eye hospitals that instituted unequal eye care (i.e., high-income patients with IOLs versus low-income patients without IOLs), as mirroring the disparity between eye care in the so-called first world and third world. Gil (unpublished interview, 2012) recalls the meeting in this way:

...I remember Ruit coming out, and he said something like "I wish that Fred wouldn't talk like that. He uses such bad language with all these people." ...Fred used to say every-body should have the same quality of surgery. The Indians used to say, "We use the [ICCE] for all the poor patients." [Fred's response would be], "Would you give your bloody mother those glasses?" "Oh that's different." They wouldn't do it unless the patients would pay for it. Ruit was showing them, it can be done with poor patients. The really poor patients would have it free; the eye camps are free.

In a book celebrating twenty years at the Fred Hollows Foundation, Dr. Ruit recalls prematurely leaving the meeting and heading with Dr. Hollows straight for the bar (the Fred Hollows Foundation 2012).

Perhaps this tense confrontation was more productive than it first appeared. Dr. Sommer saw Dr. Ruit perform surgery using ECCE with IOL in the mid-1980s at the Nepal Eye Hospital. The off-cycle 1989 IAPB four-day conference series held in Baltimore, Maryland, was framed around control of cataract blindness, including the application of appropriate technology (IAPB 2016). A year later, Australian Dr. Hugh Taylor and his faculty colleague at Johns Hopkins University, Dr. Alfred Sommer, published an editorial entitled, "Cataract Surgery: A Global Perspective." They wrote reflectively in the article's opening, commenting on the polarization of the debate about utilizing ECCE+IOL in the global south (Taylor and Sommer 1990, 797). After reiterating the WHO expert panel's opinion about problematic issues in terms of cost, training, and safety, they ended with a call to end developmentalist attitudes, saying, "No single approach will work everywhere, but we need to accept the legitimacy of alternative approaches and be imaginative and open minded about their appropriateness" (Taylor and Sommer 1990, 798).

Dr. Ruit and Dr. Hollows had successfully refuted the developmentalist duality of two surgical techniques for rich versus poor patients. As a next step, ophthalmologists and technologists in South Asia in the early 1990s then had to figure out how to develop their own clean room manufacturing facilities to create intraocular lenses. Unfortunately, they found that challenging assumptions (held by both domestic and foreign peers) about the capability of less economically developed countries to produce such high technology was an ongoing process. The radical idea blossomed independently in India and Nepal: These South Asian NGOs would manufacture their own IOLs locally. In India, Dr. Venkataswamy, along with his US colleagues from the SEVA Foundation, partnered to work on this project. Similarly, in Nepal, Dr. Ruit worked closely with the Fred Hollows Foundation as a partner to create the IOL laboratory.

5.4 Aurolab: An Early Example of "Make in India"

The cataract surgical rate in India from 1989 to 1990 was too low at 1342 per million (Murthy et al. 2008). An increase in the cataract surgical rate needed to occur in order to begin to address the backlog of patients living with blindness, as well as the many new patients who would develop cataract disease each year. Additionally, within Aravind, there was some concern because the IOL supply from generous Western donors was drying up. This occurred in large part because the US government's Medicare program's mandated ceiling on the poly-methyl methacrylate IOL price of 200 US dollars had decreased the margins of Western companies from IOL sales. Therefore, the Western multinational companies were more interested in selling old stock to previously unexplored user groups in their home markets, instead of donating these unused IOLs for poor patients in the global south.

Dr. Venkataswamy eventually decided that Aravind would make their own IOLs. Bala Krishnan, Dr. Venkataswamy's niece's husband, returned from the USA to India in 1990 in order to assist in this process. He recounts the immediate arguments against creating Aurolab:

> However, the doctors in the U.S. thought that this man wants to do something beyond his capability or he is going to waste a lot of money doing something that is not relevant...Because it cost so much and with limited resources they can do limited numbers. That was the thinking of a lot of ophthalmologists at that time.

Internationally esteemed Western ophthalmologists, the World Health Organization, and the World Bank (a major source of funding for national eye programs in less economically developed countries) insisted that the domestic production and implantation of lenses in developing countries were not viable because of the high production costs and the inability to monitor for postsurgical complications (Mehta and Shenoy 2011; Marseille 1994). The Indian government, in turn, thought that Aravind's plan would sabotage their national eye program (funded predominantly through the World Bank).

Dr. Venkataswamy, despite his original decision to make IOLs at Aravind, was risk averse. In particular, he found the initial required monetary investment daunting. Since starting his charitable trust in the 1970s, he had steered Aravind very strongly and narrowly with an emphasis on economic self-reliance and on providing eye health care only (not expanding to other types of health care or other missions). However, as Bala Krishnan recalls, after Dr. Venkataswamy decided Aravind would make IOLs, there was some internal debate. The senior leadership pointed out Aravind's inexperience in product manufacturing, especially the high standards required for a biocompatible implantable prosthetic that would not fray or degrade within the body. Aravind Eye Care System doctors were unsure how they would handle the risks of an untested Aravind-branded lens. These primarily Indian doctors worried about a potential future where they might be blamed for using faulty locally made products. Many Western friends of Aravind were discouraging, saying, "You are already doing a good job in ICCE. Why do you want to spoil your name by doing something risky?"

At a certain point, Dr. Venkataswamy bowed under the pressure of negative feedback from his international peers and the daunting task of finding funds to develop a manufacturing facility. He tried to backtrack on his decision that Aravind would move forward with the manufacturing unit. Unexpectedly, Dr. Venkataswamy's youngest sister, Dr. Natchiar, interceded with a forceful argument that the project moves forward, which neither her eldest brother nor other Aravind staff expected (Mehta and Shenoy 2011). Bala Krishnan remembers that, over time, the doctors at Aravind saw the implantable biomedical prosthetic's value and how the IOL provided better visual outcomes in comparison with aphakic glasses. Therefore, despite understanding the financial risks and patient safety concerns, the doctors at Aravind determined that the project should continue. Aravind doctors told Bala Krishnan that, with his recent mechanical engineering doctorate and industrial experience in the USA, "it is up to you to figure out how to do it, but if you ask us we want that." Dr. Venkataswamy and the senior leadership at Aravind compromised; they would mitigate and reduce their risk by seeking part of the start-up funds for the new manufacturing unit from external sources.

Aravind requested assistance from several international NGOs, a few whom were already partnering with them on other projects. However, they found that these NGOs were also risk averse. These international NGOs saw themselves as providing services, not getting into the expensive and risky business of manufacturing ophthalmic consumables. The exorbitant projected cost of retraining doctors throughout the global south in the new ECCE technique made the market seem nonexistent, and consequently, the idea to manufacture low-cost IOLs seemed reckless and improbable.

Even the SEVA Foundation, where Dr. Venkataswamy continued to serve as an executive board member, was initially risk averse. Early on in the aphakic glasses vs. IOLs debate, Dr. Brilliant remained noncommittal (Marseille 1994). Finally, SEVA assigned social entrepreneur David Green to help Bala Krishnan and Sriram D. Ravilla (who became the operations manager at Aurolab) start the new manufacturing unit. SEVA invested 250,000 US dollars and Aravind's investment added up to a cost of approximately 100,000 US dollars (in terms of infrastructure, sending the engineers abroad for training, and recruiting new staff).

Neither Bala Krishnan nor David Green knew anything about IOL manufacturing. Nor did Aravind have the capability to develop such a manufacturing unit on its own. Therefore, they started researching the companies already making lenses in an effort to determine which companies were willing to help with creating Aravind's local manufacturing unit. It is important to note there were few medical consumables manufacturing companies in India in the early 1990s, and Aurolab was one of the first in intraocular lens production. There were, however, some companies interested in entering drug development (Valdiya 2010). Therefore, there were not any local models of ophthalmic consumable manufacturing for Bala Krishnan and Sriram D. Ravilla to investigate in India. Instead, they needed to get a turnkey solution from the West. This took one or two years, as many places where they inquired were unwilling to help. Finally, they found a company in Florida called IOL International (Sandhu et al. 2005) and worked out how much it would cost for a turnkey technology transfer. Then, they had to arrange the necessary funding, which came from SEVA, SightSavers International, and Aravind (Ibrahim et al. 2006).

After securing the funding, the technology transfer occurred on a turnkey basis for the agreed upon price, and they got started. Bala Krishnan and Sriram D. Ravilla went for training in Florida in September 1991. They set up the IOL manufacturing unit on one floor of the Aravind Eye Hospital, Madurai (now known as the "old hospital" or the "outpatient block"). Aurolab's inauguration took place at the end of January 1992. Sriram remembers (2012), "Initially, when we went, we were there for three months and we brought the [Standard Operation Procedure] SOP from there." Upon their return, Bala and Sriram spent the time explaining the SOP to Aurolab staff, while waiting for their newly purchased equipment to arrive. It came in a large crate that arrived before the US engineers and technicians who provided six weeks of installation and training. Afterward, Aurolab staff created IOLs and sterilized them on their own.

Aurolab produced the very first lens in April 1992. In between fabricating the first lens and being ready to ship the lenses, they went through some rough patches. The trainers from the company in Florida returned after six months. An Aurolab staff person (2012) explains:

> You know when we work with a technology partner, what we try to do is…[we] learn as much as we can… We do a lot of preparation… Usually we run into problems during the actual process: always you have some doubts, something does not go as they taught you, or you figure out something is not going quite right. We used to depend too much on them; always asking them…That is when we decided that we should develop our own skills looking at problems, how to solve them when they come up.

This meant that at Aravind, the transfer of a turnkey process to manufacture ophthalmic consumables involved considerable problem solving. After that first rough patch, there was a formal arrangement in which IOL International would review the quality of 50,000 lenses by purchasing a few of those lenses from Aurolab in order to cover their costs. Once IOL International confirmed the quality, then Aurolab's baseline standard was determined by that batch of lenses' manufacturing process, which they later attempted to improve.

Aurolab was an endogenous manufacturing unit in India, and yet many technological products that they produced, and the manufacturing processes that they relied upon, were invented outside the country. This provided both advantages and disadvantages. The advantage was that, once import duties decreased due to central government policy changes, their costs were quite low because they were not investing a lot in research and development. These low costs were important because their mandate from Dr. Venkataswamy was to make inexpensive, high-quality products. The disadvantage was that they were always following instead of leading in the production of new products (Williams 2017). This may affect their level of distinction among other technology producers within the field of ophthalmology. However, it does not necessarily impact their mission of bringing low-cost, high-quality ophthalmic consumables to the unreached.

At Aravind, they were surprised to find that low-cost IOLs alone were insufficient to bring the new ECCE+IOL technique to Indian patients. Instead, the diffusion of ECCE+IOLs in India required shifts in local policy and practice. Bala Krishnan said about the early production years at Aurolab that, without doctors who were already trained in ECCE with intraocular lens insertion, the typical Indian hospital would not adopt the IOLs made at Aurolab. In addition to the spillover effects of the Cataract Blindness Control Project (which paid for the training of ophthalmologists in the new ECCE+IOL technique), the Government of India also removed the excise tax on imported ophthalmic technologies, which could be anywhere from 100 to 200% of the original equipment cost (Ocular Surgery News Asia Pacific Edition 2002; World Bank 2002). With a guaranteed subsidy per patient guaranteed by the government, many Indian eye hospitals invested in training for their ophthalmologists to learn ECCE+IOL (see Chapter 2; Mehta and Shenoy 2011). Therefore, in comparison with 1986, when cataract disease represented 80% of avoidable blindness in India, in 1999, cataract disease represented 55% of avoidable blindness in India (Planning Commission 2002).

When Aravind first became interested in creating an intraocular lens manufacturing unit, there was not very much competition. A few years after Aurolab started, older Indian pharmaceutical companies diversified their product lines to include ophthalmic products. New companies also emerged to make ophthalmic products. The 1996 edited volume *Appropriate Technology in Ophthalmology* lists four producers of intraocular lenses (Buisman et al. 1996 [1988]): Shah & Shah, Calcutta, West Bengal, India, selling 18 US dollar lenses; Florida Medical Manufacturing selling a "turnkey" package instead of lenses; Aurolab, Madurai, Tamil Nadu, India, selling 10 US dollar lenses for nonprofit use (the same lenses cost 15 US dollars for commercial use); and Appasamy Associates, Chennai, Tamil Nadu, India, selling 10 US dollar lenses. In 2012, there were upward of 200 companies in India that manufactured ophthalmic consumables; however, only approximately seven to eight companies in India manufactured IOLs at that time, including Appasamy Associates in Chennai and IAO Care in Gujarat. As such, Aurolab was an established endogenous technology manufacturer long before Prime Minister Modi's "Make in India" campaign started in 2014. Aurolab is a nonprofit manufacturing unit, and it is managed by a charitable trust that is similar in membership to the Govel trust which governs the rest of Aravind Eye Care System.

The groundwork for successful diffusion of the IOL laboratory from the USA to India was laid by the Indian innovation culture shaped by government bureaucracy (Prasad 2005) and supported by government regulation (Parthasarathy 2007; Valdiya 2010); these shaped norms, values, and policies. The case of Aurolab clearly shows this, where the Indian government: decreased excise taxes, funded the training of ophthalmologists, and subsidized surgeries for low-income patients. These policy changes resulted in a quick ramp up in the sales of Aurolab IOLs. The work of challenging developmentalism to create "a laboratory of our own" was hard in India, but even more difficult in Nepal.

5.5 "A Clean Room Environment as One Little Island" in Nepal

Dr. Hollows and Dr. Ruit had a universal humanitarian orientation toward marginalized people in Nepal that was reflected in their work to redistribute high-technology and high-quality medicine from the wealthy to the poor. At first, Dr. Fred Hollows thought the lenses donated from Australia would be implanted in patients in hospitals in Nepal. He was disconcerted but delighted to learn that Dr. Ruit was using them in surgical eye camps with good outcomes. However, in Nepal, Dr. Ruit ran into the same problem as Aravind when using donated intraocular lenses—an inconsistent and diminishing supply. Dr. Ruit (2012) recounts that time, saying, "Fred was very sharp, we also started talking about lenses and he said, 'why don't we start manufacturing lenses locally?' As you know, we need the blessing of friends in the West to do something in a country [like] Nepal." The fact that Dr. Hollows reinforced Dr. Ruit's desire to produce lenses locally was unsurprising to those who knew him. A volunteer with the Fred Hollows Foundation recalls (2012) that,

> Fred Hollows was, at one time, a member of the Communist Party of New Zealand. His philosophy was one of universal humanism. He believed that everyone deserves a good quality of life. And he was a real rebel in terms of the kinds of things he did. Small things, like taking equipment out of the hospital at which he was working and using it for overseas work without telling anyone. His philosophy was one of redistribution to the poor and self-empowerment; empowerment in terms of reducing things that were needless.

Dr. Hollows had become a popular figure in Australia during the late 1980s and early 1990s due to his work on health programs for indigenous Australians and eye health programs worldwide; meanwhile, he was dying from kidney cancer (the Fred Hollows Foundation 2012). Dr. Hollows started raising funds for Eritrea and Nepal. Ophthalmologists in Eritrea persevered to give the gift of sight during the war against Ethiopia by performing surgeries in caves while hiding from the fighting (the Fred Hollows Foundation 2012). Gil explains that "Fred was a rebel"; apparently, he was sympathetic to Eritrean freedom fighters, and this partly explains his decision to build a lens manufacturing facility in Eritrea and in Nepal. Nepalese community ophthalmology professionals remember Dr. Hollows as a visionary, someone who was "innovative" and "far-sighted."

When Dr. Ruit proposed that Nepal manufacture intraocular lenses locally, his superior, Dr. R. P. Pokhrel, waged a war against him in the government-operated hospital, Nepal Eye Hospital (Mahadevan 2007). At the time, Nepal Netra Jyoti Sangh (the Nepal Eye Society) was located in the Nepal Eye Hospital in Kathmandu under Dr. Pokhrel's domain. Dr. Pokhrel did not support Dr. Ruit's idea, instead trying to stop it. Dr. Sanduk Ruit (2012) explains the resistance he encountered in the Nepalese ophthalmic community, where his colleagues dismissed his ideas to bring a new surgical technology-practice to Nepal as being "too complicated... too expensive ... [and] not appropriate." Some of his colleagues went as far as petitioning the Nepalese Prime Minister to shut down his nascent project. Gil (2012) recalls, "Dr. Ruit said, 'We're not going to succeed under Nepal Eye Hospital. We have to break away and do it ourselves'," and furthermore concludes, "…. It must be very difficult breaking away from it. The Maoists had the same problem, you know—the Maoists because they wanted to make change. And they could see there was no way they were going to be able to change things so they had to start a war...Some of these things have to be violent unfortunately."

By Maoists, Gil is referring to the rural peasants in Nepal who joined with the Communist Party of Nepal that declared civil war in 1996, a cease fire in 2006, and an end to war with the new Federal Republic of Nepal's formation in 2008 (Pyakurel 2006; United Nations 2006). Social scientists generally recognize that unequal socioeconomic power distribution is a precursor for violence; the Maoists who fought in the civil war were able to come to power based on the disenfranchised, and therefore disillusioned, rural and poor people of Nepal whose monarchy was ignoring their needs. Similarly, because Dr. Ruit became disillusioned with some of his ophthalmology colleagues at the Nepal Eye Hospital and the Nepal Netra Jyoti Sangh, he was motivated to eventually leave the hospital; but first he had to build a new network of collaborators and well-wishers.

A small group of what Dr. Ruit describes (2012) as, "young up and coming entrepreneurs, friends, and legal people," sat down at the Toshita Restaurant in Lazimpat, Kathmandu, for the first Nepal Eye Program board of directors meeting in 1991. Dr. Ruit and Dr. Hollows also spoke with the Australian ambassador to Nepal about the possibility of starting an intraocular lens laboratory. Gil remembers (2012), "Then the ambassador contacted AUSAID, which is like USAID, to see about money. In those days, you did not have to do anything, you just rang up. This is back in 1991 or 1992."

Once the Nepal Eye Program NGO was started, Dr. Ruit and his team left the Nepal Eye Hospital. At first, the Nepal Eye Program was neither popular nor even accepted by other Nepalese ophthalmologists. Nabin K. Rai (2012) explains the conflict as one between two organizations with different approaches to achieving similar objectives,

> We learned much [from Nepal Netra Jyoti Sangh/Nepal Eye Hospital], you know. One thing we learned was that we should be open to new things; we should respect new ideas and new challenges. My opinion on that is, if Dr. Pokhrel … had agreed with the views of Dr. Ruit I think it would have been possible to establish the IOL lab under Nepal Netra Jyoti Sangh. But the objectives of Nepal Netra Jyoti Sangh were a little bit different. Not only the people are different, but there was a different vision/mission. So, manufacturing is a little different than services.

While Dr. Ruit could not convince Dr. Pokhrel that an IOL lens manufacturing facility was a viable idea in a country with such limited resources as Nepal, he did make his former supervisor an advisor for the first board of the Nepal Eye Program in 1991. This may be why Dr. Pokhrel (2003) writes in his autobiography about being confused that the lens manufacturing facility was separate from the Nepal Netra Jyoti Sangh. However, Dr. Pokhrel left the advisory board of the Nepal Eye Program in 1992.

Dr. Ruit and his colleagues marshalled support from local religious leaders and the Australian government to start Tilganga Eye Center's construction, which was to include in one building: the clinic, the operating theater, the eye bank, and the intraocular lens manufacturing facility. The funds to create the Tilganga Fred Hollows Intraocular Lens Laboratory came from the Australian government. The Fred Hollows Foundation established intraocular lens laboratories in Eritrea and Nepal according to the wishes of Dr. Fred Hollows after his death in 1993 (the Fred Hollows Foundation 2012). The Fred Hollows Foundation was particularly interested in building the eye bank and the IOL manufacturing facility, but not the clinical or surgical areas. Thus, similar to the development of Aurolab in India, close partnerships with international NGOs mark the development of the intraocular lens laboratory in Nepal.

A community ophthalmologist at Tilganga says that, over time, they established linkages with a lot of international NGOs, such as the Fred Hollows Foundation, the Himalayan Cataract Project, and Orbis International. Whereas originally those international NGOs were predominantly involved with Tilganga, in recent years they are working through Tilganga with other eye hospitals in Nepal, such as the Danghadi Place Geta Eye hospital, the Golchha Eye Hospitals, and the Janakpur Eye Hospital.

Tilganga brought in turnkey technology from outside of Nepal to create the new laboratory. Once they secured funding partners for the IOL manufacturing laboratory, in 1993, Dr. Ruit then hired a general manager, Mr. Rabindra Shrestha, to supervise the highly sophisticated facility's construction. In addition to his responsibility in setting up the IOL laboratory, the general manager of new Tilganga Fred Hollows Intraocular Lens Laboratory was also responsible for supervising construction of the building as well as for selecting equipment. The construction team at Tilganga worked in parallel with the technical team from Fred Hollows, which supplied all the equipment for the laboratory start-up. Contractors from New Zealand installed the air conditioning system for the clean room environment while the workmen who laid out the vinyl flooring came from Australia. At that time, the Fred Hollows technical director, Ray Avery, and his team set up the IOL factory facility, including the furniture and equipment. On June 7, 1994, they inaugurated the building with King Birendra Bir Bikram

Shah Dev. The marketing manager, Santosh Sharma (2012), says that the vision statement for FHIOL is to produce the highest quality IOLs at an affordable price for the poorest people.

After six or seven months of manufacturing three-piece lenses, Tilganga-FHIOL switched to single piece lens manufacturing to keep up with changes in the USA and the UK standard poly-methyl meth-acrylate IOL designs; the visual outcome for the single piece lens was better for the patients. The Fred Hollows Foundation was responsible for finding a supplier for the turnkey technology transfer of single piece lens production. They chose Lenstec (St. Petersburg, Florida) and paid for Rabindra Shrestha (the production manager), together with the engineering manager and the quality assurance manager, to go to the USA for training in 1995.

Once they returned to Nepal, they ordered equipment, which started coming in May 1995. By the following month, they had started trial production of the single piece lens. For the five days between equipment setup and production start, they worked very hard on adapting the SOPs for production, quality assurance, microbiology, administration, and engineering from what they had received from Lenstec. They changed the SOPs to fit their own requirements, making them more stringent.

Next, they sterilized the high-quality lenses and sent them for verification by NAMSA, a company in the USA that predominantly tests ophthalmic products for such things as water content, ethyl content, and so on; all of the lenses passed their tests by December 25, 1995. By January 1996, Tilganga-FHIOL had started commercial production. Dr. Ruit and his colleagues then reported on the results of using Tilganga-FHIOL lenses in Nepalese patients and advocated for high-volume ECCE+IOL (Ruit et al. 1999).

They continue to update their manufacturing facility with the latest equipment. Rabindra Shrestha says (2012), "We have backup support—we train our staff to maintain equipment and we do have spare parts [and] raw material always stocked. All of this is based on internal funds, including the newer purchases of milling machines, and DAC machines…Training is included in the equipment costs." A community ophthalmologist at Tilganga (2012) comments on the surprise of foreign (presumably Western doctors) visiting Tilganga, saying, "Another thing ...doctors who come here, they always think that in a place like Nepal it can't be true that it has everything; that makes them surprised to see lots of equipment and instruments." It appears that developmentalist ideology tells foreign doctors to expect a "lack" of proper instruments and consumables in a low-income country like Nepal, while within the field of ophthalmology, these same doctors expect that safe and efficacious ophthalmology requires certain types of instruments, consumables, and operating theater practices. This generates a double standard about expectations for clinics in high-income Western countries versus low-income non-Western countries. Therefore, the community ophthalmologists have to challenge developmentalism among their local and foreign peers in the global field of ophthalmology. Doing so involves navigating the tension between, on the one hand, providing a community with prestige by demonstrating mastery of the latest mainstream technologies (De Castro 1997, 194; Kressley 1981, 308) and, on the other hand, serving the community's interests through the cheapest and best suited technologies.

5.6   An IOL Laboratory Brings the Eye Hospital Prestige

Although Aurolab is not the sole ophthalmic consumables manufacturer in India, it does make Aravind distinctive among high-volume eye hospitals in India. When I asked Bala Krishnan (2012) whether Aurolab gives Aravind added prestige, he said, "A lot of other hospitals like Shankara Netralaya and L.V. Prasad are major eye hospitals in India; they have a lot of other [specialty] units but not [the] manufacturing part." Bala Krishnan continued explaining that it is a common practice for an Indian company to start a hospital mainly to support its employees and then to extend it as a social responsibility to their community. However, in Aravind, the situation was flipped. They started the hospital and then when they saw the costs were very high for consumables, they moved into manufacturing with a mandate to provide low-cost products.

Dr. Venkataswamy set a mandate for Aurolab to produce low-cost high-quality intraocular lenses, and this has steered the manufacturing unit. Sriram D. Ravilla explains, "We sell 7 to 8 percent [of the IOL global sales volume] so we should make 80 to 90 million U.S. dollars, but our IOL division made less than 10 million U.S. dollars. We priced it that way." The year 2002 marked ten years of operation, and by this time, Aurolab had started making approximately 15 million US dollars yearly; they use the profits of 3–4 million US dollars to fund their growth. However, in the future they may look for investors to fund their growth. Unlike other companies, they are not making a huge margin, and unlike public health organizations, they are not spending a lot of money on distributing and marketing.

Aurolab has a five-year plan, which they re-evaluate every year. They are interested in meeting growth targets and revenue targets. Companies acting as original equipment manufacturers of equipment and parts marketed under another company's brand name are common in other industries (i.e., electronic devices). Sriram D. Ravilla explains how Aurolab serves as an original equipment manufacturer for another company: "[W]e are selling something in U.S. our sutures…not in our brand but in another company's brand." These sutures, because of their guaranteed sales in the crowded and difficult to enter US market, are the only product for which Aurolab has been willing to pay the very expensive fees required for US FDA approval. Although they are proud of being competitive in the global market for ophthalmic consumables, the employees at Aurolab emphasize their mandate to decrease the cost of these consumables in order to better serve low-income patients.

In addition to growth and revenue targets, at Aurolab they are also interested in people targets. Sriram D. Ravilla (unpublished interview, 2012) pointed out, "We are not looking only at the revenue part ....We would also like to measure the number of people we touch, the number of people that have been reached by our products and how we can reach the unreached." This emphasis on people targets is what has driven them to quietly contest developmentalism in ophthalmology and to build their own intraocular lens manufacturing laboratory.

Just as Aurolab brings distinction to Aravind and India, Tilganga-FHIOL likewise brings prestige to Tilganga and Nepal. A staff member at Tilganga (unpublished interview, 2011) explains, "The FHIOL factory is prestigious for Tilganga and prestigious for Nepal. The cost for IOLs [was] reduced from a price of approximately 100 U.S. dollars; now it is 3-4 U.S. dollar[s]. This makes a big difference to people of Nepal." Similarly, Rabindra Shrestha (unpublished interview, 2012) explains,

[t]his lab is different from other labs… We manufacture in clean room environment and our quality is very strict. The prestige from the Fred Hollows brand is added to Tilganga. The Fred Hollows Foundation is from Australia. In people's minds, Tilganga-branded intraocular lenses and other ophthalmic consumables are affiliated with The Fred Hollows Foundation. In some instances, even though we manufacture the lenses here in Nepal, some people don't believe we make them in Nepal. The brand is important.

I confirmed this perception of Tilganga-FHIOL lenses being "made in Australia" while I was in India during a casual conversation with a community ophthalmology professional from Bangladesh who came to Aravind for training.

Of the money produced by Tilganga-FHIOL, some goes toward further developing the laboratory, and the rest goes toward Tilganga's cost recovery model. Tilganga-FHIOL reserves some intraocular lenses to provide free of charge for patients in outreach camps conducted in Nepal and abroad. It is the only IOL manufacturer in Nepal, and thus, it is responsible for one hundred percent of the IOLs produced in the country (Sharma 2004).

The Fred Hollows IOL Laboratory distinguishes Tilganga (run by Dr. Ruit's Nepal Eye Program) from the many other eye hospitals in Nepal (run by Dr. Pokhrel's Nepal Netra Jyoti Sangh). At Tilganga, they feel like they are breaking the curve by selling intraocular lenses with high quality at low cost (see Fig. 5.1 for a photograph of IOL technicians working at Tilganga).

Prices for rigid poly-methyl methacrylate lenses at Tilganga are as follows: the deeply subsidized domestic or international rate 2 US dollars; the subsidized domestic only rate 3–5 US dollars; and the

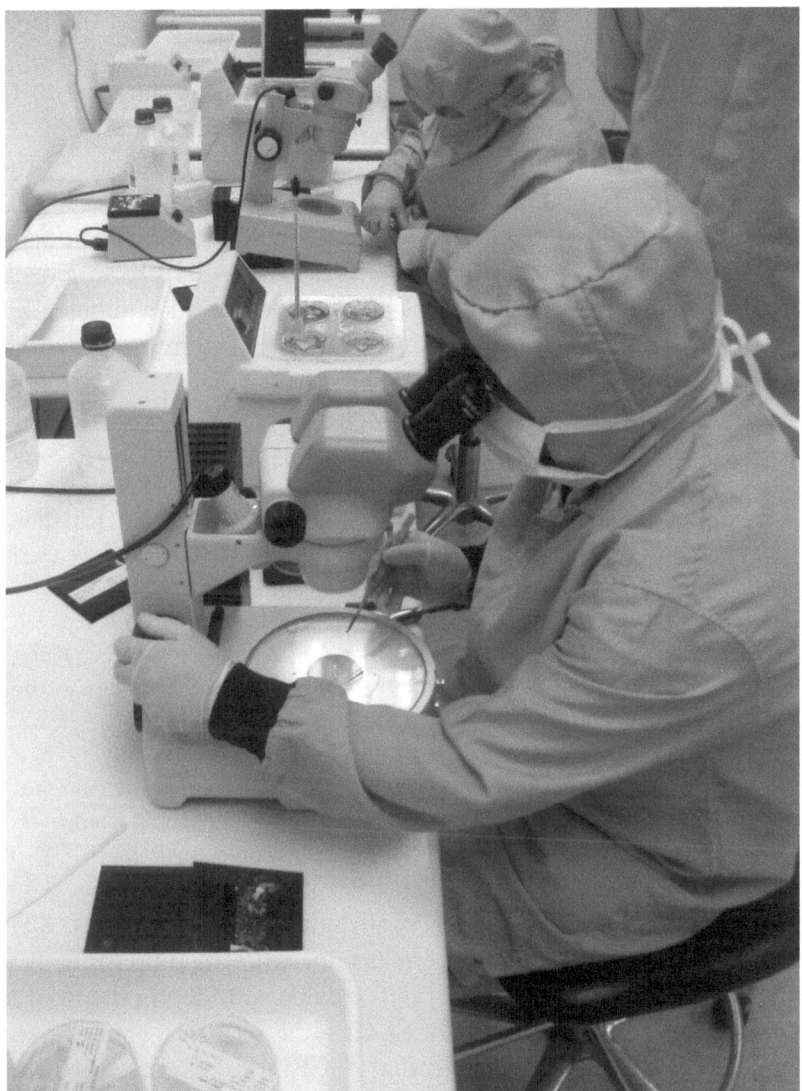

Fig. 5.1 Checking IOL surface quality under a microscope at Tilganga-FHIOL in Kathmandu, Nepal (Photo by Logan D. A. Williams)

international rate 4–4.5 US dollars. They supply the foldable lenses with injector and cartridge at a cost of 25 US dollars for industrialized countries like Australia and the UK (a comparable product is 200 US dollars from Alcon). At Tilganga, they are producing almost 350,000 lenses yearly, with about half of their market being domestic. They deeply subsidize 10,000 of the lenses they produce and additionally give away between 6000 and 8000 lenses for free. Nepal Netra Jyoti Sangh eventually became a major customer for Tilganga-FHIOL intraocular lenses. This large and consistent customer base made a key difference in the survival and thriving of Tilganga-FHIOL. A community ophthalmology professional at Tilganga (2012) recalls,

> First of all, before 1995 having IOL was the fashion. Fashion is a very glamorous thing. We used to say, "look the patient has a lens implant." Myself, this is a true story. Down at Nepal Eye Hospital (at that time there was no Tilganga) the lens would cost 100 U.S. dollars. And we used to say, "Oh that man is very rich," when he would come in the car, and have an intraocular lens and go. After [the] establishment of our lens lab from 1996, I remember 1995, July 21 or August 21, I remember being in [the] front of [the] building when we implanted the first lens in the patient and we did clinical trials. Then we started selling lenses for 5 U.S. dollars. Now everyone in this country has high quality surgery. Not only in Nepal but also in rural country [sic] like Afghanistan, Pakistan, Cambodia—they also have IOLs. We are sending our lenses from here. We made it possible for everybody not just rich people.

After there was widespread global availability of low-cost IOLs, WHO changed their expert opinion from denunciating to supporting IOLs for the global south. The WHO (1997), when considering the need for the widespread implementation of ECCE+IOL in Africa, could write in their 1997 workshop proceedings that ICCE+aphakic glasses had three problems. First, surgery had to be delayed until both eyes had developed cataract, as the glasses were not good for correcting only one eye with cataract. Second, if the glasses were lost, then the patients would again be functionally blind. The third problem was that, "Aphakic glasses can provide a good visual acuity, but at the expense of magnification, distortion, and restriction of the visual field" (WHO 1997).

As epidemiologist and Johns Hopkins University Professor, James Tielsch (Ph.D.), later wrote in 1998, the patient outcome with the combination of ICCE surgery and aphakic glasses was poor. Finally, Dr. Carl Kupfer changed his opinion; he published with senior medical officers from the Aravind Eye Care System in support of ECCE surgery with IOL implantation based on Aravind's results with Aurolab lenses in parts I, II, and IV of the four-part Madurai Intraocular Lens Study (Natchiar et al. 1998; Prajna et al. 1998, 2000).

A community ophthalmologist at Tilganga (2012) summarizes the economic logic of choosing ICCE+aphakic glasses or ECCE+IOL for addressing avoidable blindness at high volume. This ophthalmologist notes that both ICCE and ECCE have the same logistical requirements, including the need for suturing the wound and the need for other ophthalmic consumables besides suture. In the case of ECCE, the additional ophthalmic consumable is the IOL, and in the case of ICCE, it is aphakic glasses. In each case, one ophthalmic consumable visual aid must be purchased and transported to the surgical site. Those who argue that ICCE is best for Africa are arguing for a slightly lower price point, but much poorer vision (and no vision if the glasses break). Those who argue for the local production of aphakic glasses in Africa might instead start locally producing IOLs.

5.7 Conclusion: Catalyzing Anti-developmentalism and Technical Sovereignty

The global impact of Aurolab and Tilganga is clear from community ophthalmology professionals in the global south enjoying a greater degree of access to a variety of low-cost ophthalmic consumables, most especially intraocular lenses.

Adoption is not the correct word to describe the practices of South Asian technologists working in nonprofit eye hospitals on creating intraocular lens technology laboratories. The process of "turnkey technology transfer" primarily from the USA to South Asia (but also including Australia) went beyond passive acceptance or adoption of innovation from an incumbent regime. It involved the movement of an entire sub-system composed of: intraocular lens designs, production processes, manufacturing machines, even the flooring type affected the product quality. This sub-system was necessary in order to recreate intraocular lenses in the periphery instead of the world-system's center.

Although the technologies produced were incremental innovations, creating endogenous manufacturing facilities of high-tech biomedical prosthetics required a radical shift in thinking: an anti-developmentalist belief system. With the fiscal autonomy assured by their Robin Hood model, community ophthalmology professionals in the appropriate technology niche did not rely solely on traditional development aid but had diverse revenue streams. This fiscal autonomy meant they could incorporate anti-developmentalism as a belief system into the emerging, incoherent rules of their appropriate technology niche. This new rule allowed them to imagine and construct manufacturing laboratories of their own, with all necessary design, manufacturing and testing sub-systems. They did so through diffusion from the incumbent regime. This cognitive rule further established the appropriate technology niche for community ophthalmologists in the global south.

Thus, it becomes apparent that ophthalmologists and technologists in the global south invoke Schumacher's rhetoric of appropriate technology (small-scale and locally produced intermediate technology). Their previous work in eye camps leads them to begin to look for technological solutions to decrease costs and upscale the volume of cataract surgeries. Therefore, they are beginning to circumvent Kaplinsky's dilemma about the problem of scaling-up appropriate technology from small scale to large scale. As they do so, they find that they must go beyond Schumacher's definition of intermediate technology to what Willoughby calls "technology choice" (1990). They carefully consider the psychosocial and biophysical context of this choice, where the visual outcomes for patients are significantly better with ECCE and intraocular lenses than with ICCE and aphakic glasses. Moreover, they provide evidence of successful patient outcomes when changing from the old low-tech aphakic cokebottle glasses to the new high-tech intraocular lenses in less economically developed countries. Correspondingly, they argue that it is not any more difficult to manufacture intraocular lenses locally as it is to manufacture aphakic glasses locally.

Some science and technology programs are state-initiated for the purpose of establishing national sovereignty in the global field of science. Previous examples include nuclear sovereignty (Abraham 1998) and genomic sovereignty (Benjamin 2009). One conflicting example explained scientific sovereignty through the example of medication dispensing programs for trachoma which privileged multinational companies and technocratic decision-making over African state sovereignty (Samsky 2012). Above, I have described how ophthalmologists and engineers in nonprofit non-governmental organizations were asserting technical sovereignty through endogenous biomedical industry development in India and Nepal. These South Asian community ophthalmology professionals created their own laboratories to assert their right and establish their technical expertise to make medical technology choices while navigating local, regional, and global influences: they established technical sovereignty. The preexisting infrastructure of the existing biotechnology industry played a role at Aurolab in India (see Valdiya 2010). Meanwhile, the Nepalese community ophthalmology professionals had to import almost everything to Tilganga's Fred Hollows Intraocular Lens Laboratory as Nepal's first modern biomedical manufacturing facility. This demonstrates that national technical sovereignty is not just enacted through government–industry relationships; it can also be constituted through government–civil society relationships.

Throughout this book, I argue that diffusion from dominant to subordinate countries in the global field of science tells only part of the tale; additionally, other modes of science and technology circulation were involved. In the next chapter, I will explain how an additional mode of science and technology circulation called appropriation was utilized by South Asian ophthalmologists to create a radical new microsurgery technique, providing further benefits to low-income patients in the global south. The radical innovation of SICS was complimentary to the incremental innovation of IOLS and further propagated anti-developmentalist ethos in the community ophthalmology autonomous network.

References

Abraham, Itty. 1998. *Making of the Indian Atomic Bomb: Science, Secrecy and the Postcolonial State*. New York: Zed Books.

Apple, David J. 2006. *Sir Harold Ridley and His Fight for Sight: He Changed the World So That We May Better See It*. 1st ed. Thorofare, NJ: Slack Incorporated.

Apple, David J., and John Sims. 1996. "Harold Ridley and the Invention of the Intraocular Lens." *Survey of Ophthalmology* 40 (4): 279–292.

Asian Development Bank and the Clean Air Initiative for Asian Cities (CAI-Asia) Center. 2006a. Country Synthesis Report on Urban Air Quality Management: Nepal. Philippines: Asian Development Bank. Retrieved. http://www.adb.org/publications.

———. 2006b. Urban Air Quality Management: Summary of Country/City Synthesis Reports Across Asia. Philippines: Asian Development Bank. Retrieved. http://www.adb.org/publications.

Ball, Mike. 2016. "Alcon Division." Presented at the *Meet Novartis Management*, May 24–25.

Benjamin, Ruha. 2009. "A Lab of Their Own: Genomic Sovereignty as Postcolonial Science Policy." *Policy and Society* 28 (4): 341–55.

Buisman, Nico, Nico Dekker, Danny Haddad, and Peter Hardus. 1996. *Appropriate Technology in Ophthalmology*. Doorn, Netherlands: Intermediate Technology Information Ring.

Cairns, L., and A. Sommer. 1984. "Changing Indications for Cataract Surgery." *Transactions of the American Ophthalmological Society* 82: 166.

Cherlet, Jan. 2014. "Epistemic and Technological Determinism in Development Aid." *Science Technology Human Values* 39 (6): 773–94.

Cimberle, Michela. 2015. "Ophthalmic Community Grieves Jan Worst, Leader in IOL Innovation." *Ocular Surgery News*, September 29. http://www.healio.com/ophthalmology/refractive-surgery/news/online/%7B-d41d5119-16a3-4a32-9dad-af2be109f4ed%7D/ophthalmic-community-grieves-jan-worst-leader-in-iol-innovation.

De Castro, Leonardo D. 1997. "Transporting Values by Technology Transfer." *Bioethics* 11 (3–4): 193–205.

The Fred Hollows Foundation. 2012. *In Fred's Footsteps: 20 Years of Restoring Sight*. Sydney: The Fred Hollows Foundation.

Geels, Frank W. 2005. "Conceptual Perspective on Sytems Innovations and Technological Transitions." In *Technological Transitions and System*

Innovations: A Co-evolutionary and Socio-Technical Analysis, 75–102. Cheltenham and Northampton, MA: Edward Elgar.

IAPB. 2016. "IAPB History." IAPB History | International Agency for the Prevention of Blindness. http://www.iapb.org/about-iapb/iapb-history.

Ibrahim, Mahad, Aman Bhandari, Jaspal S. Sandhu, and P. Balakrishnan. 2006. "Making Sight Affordable (Part I): Aurolab Pioneers Production of Low-Cost Technology for Cataract Surgery." *Innovations: Technology, Governance, Globalization* 1 (3): 25–41.

The International Agency for the Prevention of Blindness, and Carl Kupfer, eds. 1988. *World Blindness and Its Prevention: Volume 3*. New York: Oxford University Press.

Kressley, K. M. 1981. "Diffusion of High Technology Medical Care and Cost Control—A Public Policy Dilemma." *Technology in Society* 3 (3): 305–22.

Litwin, Richard L. 1988. "Appropriate Elegance: Implanting New Ideas". In *SEVA a Decade of Stewardship*, edited by SEVA. GVERI Resources Collection Box No. ORG-14. Govindappa Venkataswamy Eye Research Institute, Aravind Eye Care System, Madurai.

Mahadevan, Ashok. 2007. "Miracles by the Thousands." *Reader's Digest*, January, 3–9.

Marseille, Elliot. 1994. "Intraocular Lenses, Blindness Control, and the Hiding Hand." In *Rethinking the Development Experience: Essays Provoked by the Work of Albert O. Hirschman*, edited by Lloyd Rodwin and Donald A. Schön, 147–75. Washington, DC: Brookings Institution; Cambridge, MA: Lincoln Institute of Land Policy.

Mehta, Pavithra K., and Suchitra Shenoy. 2011. *Infinite Vision: How Aravind Became the World's Greatest Business Case for Compassion*. San Francisco, CA: Berrett-Koehler Publishers.

Metcalfe, J. Stanley, and Andrew James. 2000. *Emergent Innovation Systems and the Delivery of Clinical Services: The Case of Intra-Ocular Lenses*. Manchester: Centre for Research on Innovation and Competition University of Manchester.

Metcalfe, J. Stanley, Andrew James, and Andrea Mina. 2005. "Emergent Innovation Systems and the Delivery of Clinical Services: The Case of Intra-Ocular Lenses." *Research Policy* 34 (9): 1283–304.

Mody, Cyrus C. M. 2001. "A Little Dirt Never Hurt Anyone: Knowledge-Making and Contamination in Materials Science." *Social Studies of Science* 31 (1): 7–36.

————. 2005. "The Sounds of Science: Listening to Laboratory Practice." *Science, Technology, & Human Values* 30 (2): 175–98.

Murthy, G. V. S., Sanjeev K. Gupta, Neena John, and Praveen Vashist. 2008. "Current Status of Cataract Blindness and Vision 2020: The Right to Sight Initiative in India." *Indian Journal of Ophthalmology* 56 (6): 489.

Natchiar, G. N., R. D. Thulasiraj, A. D. Negrel, Shrikant Bangdiwala, Raheem Rahmathallah, N. Venkatesh Prajna, Leon B. Ellwein, and Carl Kupfer. 1998. "The Madurai Intraocular Lens Study I: A Randomized Clinical Trial Comparing Complications and Vision Outcomes of Intracapsular Cataract Extraction and Extracapsular Cataract Extraction with Posterior Chamber Intraocular Lens." *American Journal of Ophthalmology* 125 (1): 1–13.

Ocular Surgery News Asia Pacific Edition. 2002. "India's Government Tackles Challenges of Eye Care." *Ocular Surgery News Asia Pacific Edition*, March. http://www.healio.com/news/print/ocular-surgery-news-europe-asia-edition/%7B718ad951-a6e3-403d-9f92-9c34e8c06c72%7D/indias-government-tackles-challenges-of-eye-care.

Ocular Surgery News Asia Pacific Edition. 2010. "Surgeon Brings Innovative Techniques to Ophthalmologists Worldwide." *Ocular Surgery News Asia Pacific Edition*. June. Retrieved April 29, 2013. http://www.healio.com/ophthalmology/news/print/ocular-surgery-news-asia-pacific-edition/{8EC07D3B-A963-4A73-A770-0B06574FF9A0}/Surgeon-brings-innovative-techniques-to-ophthalmologists-worldwide.

Packard, Randall M. 1997. "Visions of Postwar Health and Development and Their Impact on Public Health Interventions in the Developing World." In *International Development and the Social Sciences: Essays on the History and Politics of Knowledge*, edited by Frederick Cooper and Randall M. Packard. Berkeley and Los Angeles: University of California.

————. 2006. "Reconceptualizing Technology Transfer: The Challenge of Shaping an International System of Genetic Testing for Breast Cancer." In *Shaping Science and Technology Policy: The Next Generation of Research*, edited by D. H. Guston and D. R. Sarewitz, 333–58. Madison: University of Wisconsin Press.

Parthasarathy, Shobita. 2007. *Building Genetic Medicine: Breast Cancer, Technology, and the Comparative Politics of Health Care*. Inside Technology. Cambridge: MIT Press.

Pigg, Stacy L. 1992. "Inventing Social Categories Through Place: Social Representations and Development in Nepal." *Comparative Studies in Society and History* 34: 491–513.

Planning Commission. 2002. "Annual Plan 2003–04: Chapter 4 Human and Social Development." Annual Five Year Plans. New Delhi, India: Government of India. http://planningcommission.nic.in/plans/annualplan/ap0304pdf/ap0304_ch4.pdf.

Prajna, N. Venkatesh, K. S. Chandrakanth, R. Kim, V. Narendran, Selvi Selvakumar, G. Rohini, N. Manoharan, Shrikant I. Bangdiwala, Leon B. Ellwein, and Carl Kupfer. 1998. "The Madurai Intraocular Lens Study II: Clinical Outcomes." American Journal of Ophthalmology 125 (1): 14–25.

Prajna, N. Venkatesh, Léon B. Ellwein, S. Selvaraj, K. Manjula, and Carl Kupfer. 2000. "The Madurai Intraocular Lens Study IV: Posterior Capsule Opacification." American Journal of Ophthalmology 130 (3): 304–9.

Prasad, Amit. 2005. "Scientific Culture in the 'Other' Theater of 'Modern Science': An Analysis of the Culture of Magnetic Resonance Imaging Research in India." Social Studies of Science 35 (3): 463–89.

Pyakurel, Uddhab P. 2006. "Women in Armed Conflict: Lessons to Be Learnt from Telangana People's Struggle." Contributions to Nepali Studies 33 (2): 237–48.

Rogers, Everett M. 2003 [1962]. Diffusion of Innovations. 5th ed. New York: The Free Press.

Ruit, S., A. L. Robin, R. P. Pokhrel, A. Sharma, J. DeFaller, and P. T. Maguire. 1991a. "Long-Term Results of Extracapsular Cataract Extraction and Posterior Chamber Intraocular Lens Insertion in Nepal." Transactions of the American Ophthalmological Society 89: 59–76.

Ruit, S., A. L. Robin, R. P. Pokhrel, A. Sharma, and J. Defaller. 1991b. "Extracapsular Cataract-Extraction in Nepal—2-Year Outcome." Archives of Ophthalmology 109 (12): 1761–63.

Ruit, Sanduk, Geoffrey C. Tabin, Steven A. Nissman, Govinda Paudyal, and Rita Gurung. 1999. "Low-Cost High-Volume Extracapsular Cataract Extraction with Posterior Chamber Intraocular Lens Implantation in Nepal." Ophthalmology 106 (10): 1887–92.

Samsky, Ari. 2012. "Scientific Sovereignty: How International Drug Donation Programs Reshape Health, Disease, and the State." Cultural Anthropology 27 (2): 310–32.

Sandhu, Jaspal S., Aman Bhandari, Mahad Ibrahim, and P. Balakrishnan. 2005. "Appropriate Design of Medical Technologies for Emerging Regions: The Case of Aurolab, Paper No. IMECE2005-81291." In ASME Proceedings, Engineering/Technology Management, 213–18. Orlando, FA: The American Society of Mechanical Engineers Digital Collection. https://doi.org/10.1115/imece2005-81291.

Seely, Bruce Edsall. 2003. "Historical Patterns in the Scholarship of Technology Transfer." *Comparative Technology Transfer and Society* 1 (1): 7–48.

Sharma, Rupak D. 2004. "DDA Starts to Check Quality of Intraocular Lenses." *Ekantipur.Com—Nepal's No. 1 News Portal.* Retrieved March 20, 2009. http://www.kantipuronline.com/kolnews.php?&nid=25180.

Taylor, Hugh R., and Alfred Sommer. 1990. "Cataract Surgery: A Global Perspective." *Archives of Ophthalmology* 108 (6): 797–98.

Tielsch, James M. 1998. "Appropriate Technology for Cataract Surgery." *The Lancet* 352: 754–55.

United Nations. 2006. "Annan Welcomes Reinstatement of Parliament, Maoist Ceasefire." *UN News Service Section*, April 27. Retrieved April 29, 2013 http://www.un.org/apps/news/story.asp?NewsID=18273&Cr=Nepal&Cr1=#.UX265KLZ7_k.

Valdiya, Shailaja. 2010. "Neoliberal Reform and Biomedical Research in India: A Story of Globalization, Industrial Change, and Science." PhD, Rensselaer Polytechnic Institute, Department of Science and Technology Studies, Troy, NY.

Williams, Logan D. A. 2017. "Getting Undone Technology Done: Global Techno-Assemblage and the Value Chain of Invention." *Science, Technology and Society* 22 (1): 38–58.

Willoughby, Kelvin W. 1990. *Technology Choice: A Critique of the Appropriate Technology Movement.* Boulder, CO: Westview Press.

WHO. 1997. Cataract Surgery with Intraocular Lens Implantation in Africa. Geneva, Switzerland: WHO Programme for the Prevention of Blindness and Deafness. Retrieved http://whqlibdoc.who.int/hq/1998/WHO_PBL_98.70.pdf.

World Bank. 2002. "India—Cataract Blindness Control Project." 25232. Washington, DC: The World Bank. http://documents.worldbank.org/curated/en/238341468752788935/India-Cataract-Blindness-Control-Project.

6

The Hard Case of White Cataracts: Appropriation of Surgical Science

The essence that we all kept in our mind was equality. For example, we are always interested in developments in technology. Our role in Tilganga was to see how best this technology could be translated to the benefit of the community, thus making it more accessible and affordable. Furthermore modifications and simplifications are done so that the impact could reach hundreds and thousands. (Dr. Sanduk Ruit, unpublished interview, 2012)

In June 2009, I was in Nepal on pilot fieldwork to confirm or refute my tentative thesis: Science and technology disseminates from the global south outward. Tilganga Institute of Ophthalmology, situated in Nepal, seemed an unlikely place to confirm this thesis because of the country's small, poorly funded science and technology infrastructure (Singh and Bhuju 2001). Nepal represented a hard case, where, as sociologist Harry Collins (1982, 142 *Collins Emphasis*) explains,

to prove a general thesis you endeavour [sic] to prove it for the case where the thesis seems *least likely to hold*. The idea is that if you prove it for the case where it seems least likely to hold, it is fair to generalize to cases

© The Author(s) 2019
L. D. A. Williams, *Eradicating Blindness*,
https://doi.org/10.1007/978-981-13-1625-8_6

where it seems more likely to hold, whereas one has no warrant for generalizing in the other direction.

If I could prove a low-income country both produced and exported modern high-tech science and technology, then there was a chance I could make a more general case for innovation from below: Knowledge and artifacts developed by experts in the global south who are marginalized in the global field of science. Accordingly, I spent several hours in the operating theater at Tilganga to observe the new surgical technique for cataract surgery produced by Nepalese surgeon Dr. Sanduk Ruit. Dr. Ruit invented manual small incision cataract surgery (SICS); this surgical technique has helped to make Tilganga prominent among ophthalmology institutions in Asia.

In the operating theater, I stood to the medical resident's left, and she stood to the Nepalese surgeon's left. Together, the medical resident and I watched the Nepalese surgeon's microscope feed on the video monitor. The medical resident, who was from a US hospital and visiting Tilganga on a several month observership, explained everything I could see on the video monitor. The resident and I oscillated between gazing up at the monitor and looking down at the patients during their operations. Most patients had completely opaque cataractous lenses—white, with hard centers. However, I was confused because the surgeon used the expensive ultrasound phacoemulsification probe. I wondered, why did this surgeon use phacoemulsification instead of the inexpensive manual SICS technique? When I indicated my confusion, the resident pointed to another video monitor across the room where I could watch the renowned Dr. Ruit perform the inexpensive manual SICS technique.

Unmet surgical needs are 11% of the global burden of disease (Ozgediz and Riviello 2008). Nevertheless, surgery surgical facilities and training surgical personnel are neglected globally (Farmer and Kim 2008). South Asian community ophthalmology professionals have long been leaders in addressing this neglect. Hence, expert-users, such as these South Asian ophthalmologists, are adapting surgical techniques to meet their ideological and service provision goals. Therefore, Indian and Nepalese ophthalmologists appropriated cataract surgical sciences in the global field of science. While cataract surgery is one of the most frequently performed surgeries in the world (Minassian et al. 2000), judging by the WHO (2004) cataract surgical rates map, ophthalmologists most frequently perform cataract surgery on patients with early stage cataract in wealthy industrialized nations in the West or global north.

White cataracts are both a literal and figurative hard case for surgeons. They are physically more difficult to surgically remove than early stage cataracts. Above, I have described how white cataracts are an allegorical hard case for epistemic sovereignty (Healy 2003), that is, whose knowledge counts as science. Thus, South Asian ophthalmologists had at minimum two motivations behind appropriating surgical sciences from Israel and the USA. In this chapter, I will discuss the fact that their first motivation was to make these surgical techniques useful for treating the physically "hard" case of white mature cataracts, and the second motivation was to move from being consumers of science to producers of science (Eglash 2004).

I have organized the remainder of this chapter, as follows: First, Sect. 6.1 summarizes theory on appropriation in science and technology studies. Section 6.2 describes why white cataracts are a difficult technical problem for both patients and surgeons. It also introduces a second technical problem—the long recovery times patients suffered when undergoing a specific cataract technique, the gold standard in the 1960s, called ICCE; and illustrates how Dr. Kelman solved the second problem by introducing phacoemulsification in the USA in 1967, which was too costly for widespread use on low-income patients. Thirdly, Sect. 6.3 utilizes appropriation theory to explain how Dr. Ruit created SICS in Nepal to again solve the problem of long recovery time, but to benefit low-income patients. Next, Sect. 6.4 again uses appropriation theory to expound on how Dr. Vasavada modified phacoemulsification in India for the advanced stage cataracts that typically occur in low-income rural patients. Subsequently, Sect. 6.5 illustrates how ophthalmologists from Ghana, Kenya, Mexico, India, and Nepal are conversant in the economic and scientific reasons to choose SICS versus Phaco for cataract surgery. I suggest the novel finance model discussed in Chapter 3 will not function effectively unless the South Asian surgeons are skilled in both the incumbent Phaco technique and the radical SICS technique. Section 6.6, concludes by indicating SICS is a radical innovation produced by domestic experts who have previously been identified by Westerner experts as consumers of Western scientific knowledge. Their identity is beginning to shift as they become knowledge producers—creating surgical sciences such as SICS and phacoemulsification. Finally, as an afterword, Sect. 6.7 reflects on Chapters 2–6 and discuss the multiple, complimentary knowledge and artifacts that are coming together with a radical ideology to form an interlocking innovation. These interlocking innovations are unique to the outsiders challenging the incumbent regime.

6.1   Theory: Appropriation

In this chapter, I argue that challengers to the incumbent regime use appropriation inside the appropriate technology niches to create radical innovations. Since diffusion and appropriation are concurrent in the niches, interlocking innovations form from the newly linked, incremental, and radical innovations that are multiple, complimentary, and contain sub-systems.

Appropriation is the movement from solely consuming a science or technology to actively producing a science or technology through: re-interpretation, adaptation, or re-invention (Eglash 2004).

> Appropriation, however, can be a two-way street....people outside the centers of social power...have been able to use materials and knowledge from professional science for their own kinds of technological production. (Eglash 2004, 4–5)

Eglash (2004) explains, users acting closer to the consumption side of the spectrum are engaged in reinterpreting the semantic association of a science or technology, a change in meaning. Users engaged in adaptation are midway between consuming and producing science and technology to suit their needs; they are both reinterpreting and re-using science and technology. Finally, toward the production side of the spectrum, appropriation involves changing the structure of a science or technology in addition to reinterpreting its meaning or changing its use. At this final stage, users have become producers, where they are engaged in reinventing science and technology and maximizing their social power.

Appropriation is bilateral and unidirectional; science and technology transfers one-way from a dominant to a subordinate position in the field. However, by moving from simple consumption to production of scientific knowledge and technology, the subordinate position can increase its social power.

The problem sequence of addressing white cataracts within the global field of ophthalmology demonstrates appropriation. A large domestic population of patients with white cataracts was a global problem in the 1940s until foldable IOLs were invented in the late 1980s. Then, it became a problem unique to countries with scarce health infrastructure in the rural global south. Two surgeons in South Asia each created a solution to this problem. Dr. Ruit reinvented the new surgical technique of SICS, and later explained to *The Kathmandu Post* (2003), "we have successfully adapted the technology to local conditions without compromising on the quality and outcome." Meanwhile, Dr. Vasavada adapted phacoemulsification for use on white cataracts. The two ophthalmologists encountered other problems while reinventing SICS and adapting phacoemulsification that they had to solve to make their surgical techniques viable for their target population of patients. I will illustrate how the appropriation of SICS and phacoemulsification resulted in the economically viable cost recovery schema I previously described in Chapter 3.

6.2   Hard White Cataracts and Lengthy Patient Recovery Times

White cataracts are advanced stage (or mature) cataracts that cause complete blindness. In white cataracts, the natural lens' nucleus is often swollen (or hardened) at the center making it opaque to light with a white appearance.

[White cataracts] used to be [common]....The story was don't operate until they are nearly blind because the outcomes [when operating on early stage cataract] weren't nearly so good. And I was in training in the early 60s — early 50s and 60s when people waited. The farmers ...would come — had to be led in almost when they had white cataracts. But you don't see that so much [anymore]. (U.S. ophthalmologist and former President of the International Council of Ophthalmology, Dr. Bruce Spivey, unpublished interview, 2013)

Insufficient preventative eye care services mean there is often a time delay between cataract onset and opacified lens removal. This delay between onset and removal is more likely to occur to patients in LEDCs. In comparison, private health insurance and government medical care are more widely available for patients in wealthy industrialized nations. At present, patients in the global south are more likely to have white cataracts than patients in the global north (Chakrabarti and Singh 2000). Therefore, at the Lions Eye Hospital–Loresho, in Kenya, the chief medical officer, Dr. Fayez Khan (unpublished interview, 2011), is skeptical of how early cataractous patients in the USA, Europe, and Australia receive surgery; he deals with "real blind people" (a subtext he tries to prevent wealthy privileged people from undergoing surgery too early).

There are three types of white cataracts: intumescent, mature, and hypermature. Intumescent cataract is very soft having some swollen and opaque natural lens fibers (Chakrabarti and Singh 2000; Tabandeh et al. 1994). Mature cataracts occur after intumescence. The natural lens is completely opaque in mature cataracts. Opaque mature lenses sometimes hide a dense, hardened nucleus. A mature cataract may infrequently develop in a younger patient; typically, younger patients have a softer nucleus (Tabandeh et al. 1994). Hypermature cataracts occur after maturity when the natural lens fibers have liquefied or the anterior portion of the natural lens capsule is fibrous (Chakrabarti and Singh 2000).

Working on white cataracts was very common for Dr. Ruit in the late 1980s when he first started performing cataract surgeries. It was physically difficult for the surgeon. The surgeon's work was furthermore complicated by poor access to surgical equipment, including microscopes and surgical instruments. While the problems with the procedure were many, one in particular stood out to Dr. Ruit—the recovery time for patients was too long. Sir Wilson also described this common problem with cataract surgery in the Royal Commonwealth Society for the Blind surgical eye camps in India, Pakistan, and Bangladesh:

> If it is possible to have a 'bottleneck' connected to a 'backlog' then the bottleneck in most eye camps is the time patients remain in the camp after treatment. The operation takes about 10 minutes, the convalescence from seven to 13 days. (Wilson 1987)

Typically, in most eye camps, only one doctor was available to perform examinations and surgeries. Dr. Ruit would usually go alone or might occasionally bring a foreign colleague along to participate and observe. Ophthalmic assistants had to carry patients into the surgical building (or tent) and out again. The patients had to spend two to ten days recovering from the (typically) ICCE surgical procedure before they could walk upright. With such long recovery times, a surgical eye camp meant almost a two-week commitment, including travel, surgery, and patient recovery.

Family members tasked with feeding, bathing, and generally caring for patients in the camp found such an extensive convalescent time period prohibitive. These family members would lose the opportunity costs of daily work over that time period (Williams 2008). Ophthalmology professionals throughout India and Nepal typically worked in government hospitals and private clinics. They would volunteer their time to participate in eye camps (funded by the government or NGOs) to help reduce the rural cataract backlog. These ophthalmology professionals likely also found this extensive time commitment daunting.

One solution to reduce the extensive time commitment of patients, family members, and community volunteers, in addition to eye hospital staff, was to make the recovery process shorter. With a shorter recovery time, the inpatient procedure becomes an outpatient procedure and patients could quickly return home with sight. Making the surgery ambulatory had the added benefit of increasing surgical acceptance by persons with blindness.

Thirty years earlier, a US ophthalmologist named Dr. Charles D. Kelman also found this problem of making cataract surgery into an ambulatory procedure interesting. As the story goes, Dr. Kelman was reclining with his mouth open in his dentist's chair when it occurred to him to create an ultrasound probe to emulsify the natural lens inside its capsular bag (making the procedure an adaptation of ECCE). The first phacoemulsification trial on a human subject occurred in 1967 (Hillman 2017).

From the early 1970s onward, Dr. Kelman, Dr. Robert Sinskey, and other prominent ophthalmologists perfected and diffused phacoemulsification technology. Ophthalmologists found it difficult to master the new phacoemulsification technique for various reasons (e.g., lack of training, lack of interest, and the controversy it caused in US ophthalmology circles). Many US ophthalmologists simply continued to remove cataracts with intracapsular cataract extraction using a large incision. Nonetheless, some prestige comes with knowing how to perform the "latest" and "most advanced" form of surgery; problems may be viewed as a challenge. It became preferred over manual ICCE in the USA by the late 1980s (Hillman 2017). The development of the foldable IOL gave surgeons an incentive to use a smaller initial incision into the eye which eventually led to the preference for Phaco.

Originally, the phacoemulsification ultrasound probe could be used through a small corneal incision (3 mm). However, the ophthalmologist would then have to enlarge that same incision in order to put the hard stiff plastic intraocular lens (5–7 mm) into the eye. This stiff plastic IOL was fabricated from the same inexpensive material, Perspex, as used by the British ophthalmologist, Sir Harold Ridley, for the first IOL he implanted in 1949 (Apple and Sims 1996; see Chapter 5). Since then, the design and materials had been refined, creating a lightweight and more easily implanted lens (Jaffe 1996). However, the surgeon still had to enlarge the small corneal incision before placing the cheapest (and most popular) stiff plastic Perspex lens inside the eye.

With the foldable intraocular lens, came the advent of a small corneal incision that remained small throughout the entire surgery. In 1984, Dr. Thomas R. Mazzocco created a foldable intraocular lens from silicone, a plastic-like material much softer than Perspex (Boyle 2007). One could place this foldable lens into the eye through the small corneal incision without enlarging the incision. The ability to keep the small corneal incision small through the entire surgery is preferable because it has three desirable outcomes: (1) it requires fewer sutures to close; (2) it heals faster; and (3) it reduces the incidence of post-surgical myopic astigmatism. Post-surgical myopic astigmatism is a form of nearsightedness (where the patient sees well up close, but has trouble seeing distant objects). Post-surgical myopic astigmatism is caused by the corneal incision deforming the cornea. For the patient to have closer to 20/20 vision, he or she would need to pay for additional vision correction for better distance vision: either eyeglasses or Lasik™ refractive surgery.

Phacoemulsification clinical trials with the new foldable lens design started in 1986 (Boyle 2007). Dr. Charles Kelman presented a paper on small incision phacoemulsification in 1988, calling it SICS (Program for the LaserPhaco Symposium 1988, March 27). The smaller incision enabled the eye to heal faster, which meant patients could leave the hospital right away, thus converting what was previously an inpatient procedure into an outpatient procedure.

Patient interest in an ambulatory (or outpatient) procedure provided some pressure on US ophthalmologists to learn phacoemulsification. However, the phacoemulsification technique was difficult to master, and some surgeons were better at it than others. Also, in comparison with ECCE, it was very expensive to maintain the phacoemulsification equipment and invest the high capital costs for remedial surgical training. Nevertheless, by the early 1990s, ophthalmologists in the USA most frequently performed phacoemulsification (instead of manual ECCE) because it was an ambulatory procedure that involved a very small incision decreasing the recovery time for the patient.

Wealthy white-collar US patients receiving the surgery appreciated the new ambulatory procedure. In 1993, ophthalmology surgeries represented the most frequent (28%) ambulatory surgeries performed at the independent surgical centers throughout the USA which were rapidly increasing in number (Durant and Battaglia 1993, 84). By 1994, 80% of the cataract surgeries in the USA were ambulatory in comparison with 8% of the cataract surgeries in the UK (Chell et al. 1994). British patients who underwent ambulatory cataract surgery reported they would recommend it to others even though it was not yet a common procedure in the UK (Chell et al. 1994).

6.3   Inventing SICS in Nepal

Making the cataract surgery into an ambulatory procedure was an important innovation in global surgical technology-practice that involved adopting microsurgery. To do this in Nepal meant creating a new type of ECCE by appropriating mini-nuc to create SICS in 1994. Ophthalmologists in Nepal believe they performed the first ambulatory surgery in the developing world when they utilized SICS technique with IOL implantation in surgical eye camps in the Himalayas during the 1990s. They felt their novel SICS technique was very controversial in the global field of ophthalmology during the mid-1990s. Not only did ophthalmologists debate ambulatory surgery, but additionally Nepalese patients themselves resisted ambulatory surgery:

> We had to start. If we had to admit the patients, then the staff would double; the running costs would be another 30-40%; so we started that on our own to make it easier to run the whole show... We had resistance from the patients themselves as well. All their lives you have the surgery then they have to be in the hospital. Now Tilganga is saying, "go home and come back the next day... you will be fine"... Now the patients don't even ask; it's the norm. If the patient is admitted now, then they ask the doctor "why?" (Ophthalmologist at Tilganga Institute of Technology 2012)

By the 1990s, US governmental agencies were providing health remittances for cataract surgeries such as phacoemulsification with short recovery times because they were less costly than cataract surgeries such as ICCE and ECCE with longer recovery times (Metcalfe et al. 2005). Similarly, this Nepalese ophthalmologist (see above quote) was cognizant of the huge cost differential and, therefore, preferred to provide the less-expensive outpatient care. Over time, Nepal followed the West and ambulatory surgery became the new standard practice for patients with cataract disease. This was only possible because Dr. Ruit appropriated mini-nuc to create SICS for inexpensive ambulatory surgery for Nepalese patients with white cataracts.

Dr. Michael Blumenthal invented the mini-nuc technique in Israel in 1994. Mini-nuc was novel because it did not require expensive viscoelastic (an artificial, biologically non-reactive, soft plastic or silicone material) nor suture (thread for sewing wounds closed). Dr. Blumenthal's procedure uses a small sclera-corneal tunnel incision (5–6 mm) to enter the eye. The small sclera-corneal tunnel incision that Dr. Blumenthal uses takes a long time to learn, but when performed properly it does not require expensive suture for the self-sealing wound (Blumenthal 1994).

The continuous curvilinear capsulorhexis is the first incision into the natural lens capsule. Consequently, after the continuous curvilinear capsulorhexis incision, the surgeon next utilizes hydrodissection: he or she directs the intense water pressure to separate the natural lens into the epinucleus and nucleus inside the natural lens capsule. Then, the ophthalmologist removes these two parts from the natural lens capsule and (through the sclera-corneal tunnel) out of the eye (Blumenthal et al. 1992). This procedure must occur under positive intraocular pressure in order to keep the lens pieces from damaging the cornea as they are removed (Blumenthal et al. 1992).

Throughout the surgery, a re-usable device called the anterior chamber maintainer sustains positive intraocular pressure inside the eye. The anterior chamber maintainer provides positive intraocular pressure from a constant feed of balanced saline solution elevated above the patient's head. This is why the mini-nuc technique never requires expensive viscoelastic (Blumenthal et al. 1992; Blumenthal 1994).

Dr. Blumenthal shares the results of his new procedure in a letter to the Community Eye Health Journal (which is circulated around the world by the World Health Organization Vision 2020 program at no cost to the recipients). In this letter, he says,

[T]here exists another system which is suitable to any part of the world and any economic situation. I developed the mini-nuc technique. With a very small number of instruments one can achieve safe and very high standard cataract surgery, with or without an [intraocular lens]…There are the means to perform perfect cataract surgery around the globe safely, no viscoelastic material, no sutures, very cost effective. The only thing to be done is to learn how to do it! (Blumenthal 2002)

Certainly replacing expensive single-use ophthalmic consumables with re-usable instruments or new techniques made Blumenthal's mini-nuc technique more viable for low-income patients.

Creating SICS required innovative changes, including reinterpreting the name from Kelman's phacoemulsification and modifying Blumenthal's mini-nuc technique to make it quicker and even less expensive. Both Aravind and Tilganga needed to determine which microsurgical technique (extracapsular cataract extraction, mini-nuc, or phacoemulsification) would have good post-surgical outcomes and keep costs low. In his publication about his technique, Dr. Ruit defines the problem as such:

Innovations that reduce the cost, complexity and operating time, but without compromising ocular safety and vision outcome, are urgently needed in the surgical management of cataract in the developing world. The size of the back-log and new caseload of cataract blindness, and the limited human and material resources most countries have available to devote to the problem, mean that any such innovation can have a disproportionate benefit in the numbers of patients treated effectively. (Ruit et al. 2000)

Dr. Ruit (unpublished interview, 2012) recalls Dr. Blumenthal demonstrating his technique when visiting Tilganga. Upon Dr. Blumenthal's death in 2007, Dr. Ruit (with his US and Nepalese colleagues at the nonprofit Tilganga Institute of Ophthalmology) had already standardized and begun disseminating an adapted form of Blumenthal's technique (Ruit et al. 2000, 2007; Tabin and Newick 2008; Tabin et al. 2008). The South Asian ophthalmologists (and their Western colleagues) working at Tilganga call Ruit's adaptation of Blumenthal's mini-nuc technique "small incision cataract surgery" (Ruit et al. 2000, 2007; Tabin and Newick 2008; Tabin et al. 2008). Dr. Kelman had previously applied the term SICS to his small incision phacoemulsification with foldable IOL. In fact, when I spoke with three US ophthalmologists in 2010, they were unfamiliar with the South Asian SICS; they thought I meant phacoemulsification. However, community ophthalmology professionals have now reinterpreted the name SICS to mean a manual, non-phacoemulsification, sutureless, microsurgical ECCE technique (Chakrabarti and Singh 2000; Natchiar and Kar 2000; Ruit et al. 2000).

Ruit and his colleagues performed one primary modification in order to reinvent mini-nuc into SICS making it cheaper and faster. Their modification was to use air to keep the anterior chamber at the correct depth instead of relying upon saline from the anterior chamber maintainer (Ruit et al. 2000). In Ruit's SICS technique, once the surgeon successfully implants the intraocular lens, then he or she irrigates the anterior chamber of the eye with water to force the air out. With these modifications, SICS does not require: suture, viscoelastic, or an anterior chamber maintainer. It does require a higher degree of surgical skill to complete the surgery safely without those consumables and tool. Ruit also indicates his technique uses hydrodissection for early stage or immature cataract (similar to Blumenthal's mini-nuc technique). However, hydrodissection is not necessary for advanced stage or mature cataract (Ruit et al. 2000).

Dr. Ruit is recognized as the inventor of SICS and is the most well-known champion of the procedure in Asia. As one ophthalmologist at Tilganga explained,

> I can't tell you if we are the ones doing it first, but we are definitely continuing to modify it so it is easier to learn or more cost effective.... It will be easier, or, there are different things going on, like, if I do it this way, I [will] use less instruments going into the eye, you know, that sort of thing? .... They are very small things which make a large difference,

but at the same time if I say, this is one of the modifications that we do—then others will say, that is not a modification, that is just one thing you do. Training is the main way of dissemination. (Ophthalmologist at Tilganga Eye Center, July 2009)

So this Nepalese ophthalmologist does not know who first created or used the manual SICS in South Asia. However, since patenting surgical procedures varies with national laws, the scientific literature serves as the evidence necessary to resolve priority disputes and name the first inventor. In this scientific literature, Dr. Ruit claims the title of inventor (Ruit et al. 1991a, b, 2000).

Similar to Dr. Ruit, Dr. R. D. Ravindran was one of the first South Asians to perform M-SICS in the region. By his own account, Dr. Ravindran introduced microsurgery to his colleagues at Aravind after attending an ophthalmology meeting in Boston in 1991. While the exact timeline of this introduction is unknown, since the late 1990s, the Aravind Eye Care System has taught and utilized a scleral-corneal tunnel incision with an instrument, called an irrigating vectis, and the consumable, viscoelastic, for their version of M-SICS (see Natchiar and Kar 2000).

While the additional instrument and consumable make Aravind's M-SICS more expensive than Dr. Ruit's SICS, M-SICS is also very popular. The most likely reason for M-SICS' popularity is that more ophthalmologists have been trained in it. Alternatively, Aravind's M-SICS might be more popular because it is easier to perform than Dr. Ruit's SICS.

Some might argue SICS and M-SICS are not innovative as they involve removing a high technology (or a salable product, the phacoemulsification machine and attached ultrasound probe) and adding an increase in the surgeon's surgical skill. However, these ophthalmologist-inventors and their allies report significant modifications which make the technique more efficient: 5 minutes for SICS in comparison with 15 minutes for phacoemulsification (Chang 2005a, b; Ruit et al. 2000). Tilganga conducted an "expert clinical trial" with the prominent US phacoemulsification surgeon, Dr. David F. Chang (Ruit et al. 2007; Wormald 2007). They point to this expert clinical trial as evidence SICS and phacoemulsification are two comparable surgical techniques with equivalent outcomes.

To promote their SICS, Tilganga published in prestigious English-language journals as *Current Opinion in Ophthalmology* and the *American Journal of Ophthalmology* as part of their dissemination strategy (Latour 1987; Tabin et al. 2008). They also participate in regional and international conferences and train domestic and referred (foreign, from all over the world) ophthalmologists in their surgical techniques. Later—perhaps because of their high visibility in the global field of ophthalmology—Tilganga and their partner NGO, Himalayan Cataract Project, were asked to demonstrate financially viable, high-volume cataract surgery to the United Nations Millennium Villages Project in Africa (see Chapter 7). Dr. Sanduk Ruit demonstrated M-SICS in instructor sessions at six American Academy of Ophthalmology (2018) meetings from 2001 to 2006. Likewise, Dr. A. Haripriya, the chief of the cataract clinic at Aravind Eye Hospital, Madurai, demonstrated M-SICS in skills transfer sessions at the American Academy of Ophthalmology (2018) meetings in 2010, 2011, and 2012. These peer-reviewed short courses establish that the surgical techniques of SICS and M-SICS, reinvented by South Asians, helped these community ophthalmologists to accrue social power in the global field of international development and in the global field of ophthalmology.

6.4   Adapting Phacoemulsification in India

Around the same time Dr. Ruit worked on appropriating SICs, other ophthalmologists were pondering a third technical problem: Poor post-surgical outcomes made phacoemulsification inappropriate to use for advanced stage white cataracts (Wormald 2007).

Phacoemulsification's global popularity with ophthalmologists seems incongruous considering its poor suitability to remove white cataracts. Initially, the idea was phacoemulsification would make removing the hardened natural lens easier (Metcalfe et al. 2005). However, patients with hard white cataracts commonly experienced poor post-surgical outcomes in the form of capsular plaques. The hardened (or dense) nucleus is a poor candidate for phacoemulsification because, after emulsification, the hard lens pieces are more likely to damage the natural lens capsule's endothelium (Vasavada et al. 1998). A damaged endothelium often results in later capsular plaques, which block vision and necessitate further surgery (Vasavada et al. 1998). For this reason, until the late 1990s ophthalmologists have not favored phacoemulsification surgery over extracapsular cataract extraction for this advanced stage of cataract (Chakrabarti and Singh 2000; Jaffe 1996; Vasavada et al. 1998).

My explanation contradicts part of the problem sequence described by Metcalfe et al. (2005). These business scholars claim phacoemulsification was the trigger for further innovation in lens design and surgical procedure, in part because of its usefulness for "hard cataracts" (Metcalfe et al. 2005). In contrast, I suggest the following two important points, based on the medical science literature as well as interviews with US ophthalmologists. Firstly, that phacoemulsification was not universally accepted as "the right tool" for the job (Casper and Clarke 1998) before the late 1980s. In other words, phacoemulsification was not widely utilized to correct cataracts prior to the introduction of the foldable intraocular lens which turned it into an ambulatory surgical procedure. Secondly, phacoemulsification was not particularly useful for hard white cataracts because it caused a post-surgical complication in the eye again resulting in blindness for the patient.

This alternative explanation still matches the diffusion charts made by Metcalfe et al. (2005), which demonstrate the increased uptake of phacoemulsification by ophthalmologists in the US and the UK starting in the 1980s. Additionally, this alternative explanation provides rhetorical space for describing a second important contribution to modern medicine made by marginalized ophthalmologists in the field of ophthalmology: An Indian pediatric ophthalmologist appropriated the phacoemulsification technique in order to make it viable for white cataracts in India.

Dr. Abhay Vasavada started the Raghudeep Eye Clinic in 1984. It is a for-profit clinic located in the state of Gujarat in western India. Raghudeep Eye Clinic has a dedicated research center affiliated with the Indian Department of Science and Technology. Volunteers from the Raghudeep Eye Clinic provide free cataract surgeries at the local Red Cross Hospital. They perform all cataract surgeries by phacoemulsification. All lenses are the expensive, high-quality Alcon AcrySoft® brand. Dr. Vasavada has been working with AcrySoft® lenses for more than a decade; he won a "best paper for session" on this research at the 2000

American Society of Cataract and Refractive Surgery meeting. He also won awards at the American Society of Cataract and Refractive Surgery meetings in both 2007 and 2008. Dr. Vasavada's journal article (see Vasavada et al. 1998, 1) detailed the changes in both the phacoemulsification technique and the operation theater necessary for the successful removing white cataracts with good post-surgical outcomes.

One adaptation was adding an endoilluminator, a tiny cylindrical light typically used to illuminate the inside of blood vessels, to the operation theater. Removing a white cataract with phacoemulsification is difficult. The opacity of white cataracts creates poor visibility conditions for a surgeon operating within a patient's eye. Changes were necessary in the operating theater to adapt it to performing phacoemulsification on white cataracts. Dimming the lighting in the operating theater and using an endoilluminator relieves the poor visibility for the surgeon operating upon eyes with white cataract (Vasavada et al. 1998; Chakrabarti and Singh 2000).

A second adaptation was adding a consumable, viscoelastic, to the technique. The intumescent (extremely swollen) cataractous lens is difficult to remove due to the increased intracapsular pressure. The increase in intracapsular pressure makes the continuous curvilinear capsulorhexis incision more challenging. Vasavada and his colleagues describe the necessary changes in the continuous curvilinear capsulorhexis incision required to adapt phacoemulsification for white cataracts (Vasavada et al. 1998).

While utilizing the ultrasound probe, the anterior chamber pressure should be carefully maintained to prevent natural lens material leaking from the natural lens capsule. If natural lens material leaks out, then viscoelastic is needed to fill the natural lens capsule and maintain anterior chamber depth so the ultrasound probe can continue to emulsify the lens without damaging the natural lens capsule endothelium (Vasavada et al. 1998; Chakrabarti and Singh 2000). Vasavada's phacoemulsification technique successfully demonstrated using viscoelastic to reduce the chances of post-capsular plaques after operating on white cataracts. After the ultrasound probe has completed breaking the lens, the surgeon suctions out the lens pieces and places the soft foldable intraocular lens into the natural lens capsule. Finally, a single suture (and occasionally no suture) seals the 3 mm corneal incision into the eye.

The Raghudeep clinic continued to report their successes in innovative surgical science at the American Society of Cataract and Refractive Surgery meeting in 2009. Dr. Vasavada gave the prestigious Binkhorst Lecture, which he entitled, "Pediatric Cataract: The Compelling Quest," for the 2011 American Society of Cataract and Refractive Surgery meeting. This invitation from the American Society of Cataract and Refractive Surgery reveals Dr. Vasavada's increased stature in the global field of ophthalmology primarily results from his pediatric ophthalmology work, not his incremental adaptation of phacoemulsification.

In summary, a South Asian ophthalmologist appropriated the phacoemulsification surgical technique for treating advanced stage cataract disease. His suggested changes include small modifications to the surgical technique itself (in the form of new tools from cardiovascular surgeries, a slight change in incision style, and the standardized use of viscoelastic) and to the operating theater (in the changes in lighting and magnification). With these adaptations in the technique and the theater,

> [w]hite cataract has ceased to be a contraindication to phacoemulsification ... [h]owever... [i]f there is difficulty at any stage (hard nucleus, repeated nucleus prolapse into anterior chamber), we recommend timely conversion to the manual nonphacoemulsification sutureless technique, which preserves most of the benefits of small incision cataract surgery [(also called phacoemulsification)]. (Chakrabarti and Singh 2000)

Due to Vasavada's inventive efforts, phacoemulsification can safely be used in the hard case of white cataracts with the qualification: If there is a problem during surgery, then the ophthalmologist should immediately convert to the manual SICS technique. The similarities between phacoemulsification and SICS are obvious: Each surgery is now technically appropriate for the hard case of white cataracts, and both solve the technical problem of long patient recovery times by utilizing the IOL as a complimentary technology. Community ophthalmologists choose to SICS versus Phaco for a variety of reasons.

6.5   Cost Recovery Requires SICS and Phaco

As demonstrated by their coverage at the Asia-Pacific Academy of Ophthalmology,

> In a head-to-head comparison of phaco and SICS, with the techniques performed respectively by [U.S. ophthalmologist] David Chang, M.D., and Dr. Ruit to treat 180 "typical cases"—patients with hyper-mature cataracts in Nepal—SICS was comparable in terms of safety. It also showed a distinct advantage in terms not only of cost, but also of ease, time, and visual outcomes in these cases. About 70% of the Nepalese patients who underwent phaco in Dr. Chang's hands achieved 20/60 or better vision; more than 90% achieved 20/60 or better after SICS with Dr. Ruit, (Anonymous 2010)

ophthalmologists in the autonomous global network to eradicate blindness discuss both the economic imperative and the scientific evidence for SICS. They really believe in its efficacy for resource-constrained settings. Reinventing SICS and adapting phacoemulsification for white cataract have put South Asian ophthalmologists in an enviable position: They are proficient in both surgical techniques and, therefore, are cognizant of the advantages and disadvantages of each. Community ophthalmologists believe both techniques are necessary for their social entrepreneurship model.

The scientific reasons for using SICS include the fact that SICS is safer for patients with white cataracts or complicating medical conditions. When I interviewed Dr. James Clarke (Crystal Eye Clinic, Ghana) at the Unite for Sight Global Health and Innovation Conference at Yale University in April 2011, he told me he preferred SICS because it did not require expensive sutures, was cheaper than Phaco, and also because, "SICS is a newer technology that has come in, it gives much better results at less cost .... The cataracts we see—they are very dense. We are not sure how well that Phaco will perform." Similarly, Dr. Sanduk Ruit (2012) asked, "[h]ow to make Phaco a safer technology? Put it in the heads of Western ophthalmologists that Phaco cannot be applicable to all cataracts in developing countries... Without question that there are a lot of cataracts in small developing countries that you cannot use Phaco and SICS is superior." In the 2007 expert clinical trial, Dr. Ruit and his colleagues found they had lower complication rates when they used SICS on white cataracts as compared to expert Asian-American Phaco surgeon Dr. Chang who used Phaco on similar white cataracts in Nepalese patients (Ruit et al. 2007). A clinical trial by Indians at a hospital in Pune, Maharashtra, India, also found SICS is better than Phaco for white cataracts (Gogate et al. 2005, 2007).

In Mexico, Dr. Juan Pablo Olivares (unpublished interview, 2012) discusses whether SICS or Phaco is better for hard white cataracts:

> I think that for very hard mature or hypermature cataracts that SICS is a better technique when done by a properly trained surgeon. Why? Because there aren't differences in visual acuity results as well as complication rates and the main advantage is that we spare the endothelial damage to the endothelial cells by not using Phaco; not using the ultrasound really helps with that. Hypermature or really hard cataracts are mostly seen in very old patients so the endothelial damage is already there; that would be my preferred technique for hard brown. [Dr. Ruit's SICS] technique was first described using an anterior chamber maintainer (using simcoe cannula to irrigate the anterior chamber constantly) and it is more difficult to perform. That technique has more complication rates than what Aravind does [for M-SICS]. With viscoelastic, even though it is more expensive the cost benefit to the patient is very good.

In the last week of September 2012, Dr. Olivares made a presentation at a congress for medical doctors based on the results at Sala Uno. When he or his team utilized M-SICS or Phaco both resulted in good outcomes for the patients and the same complication risk were the same. SICS/M-SICS has better one-day and one-week postoperative vision compared to Phaco (Ruit et al. 2007). As I previously pointed out, if there are any problems with Phaco, the surgeon must convert to ECCE or SICS.

Economic reasons for using SICS on white cataracts include its speed: At five minutes, SICS is faster than the fastest Phaco surgeon who typically takes fifteen minutes (Chang 2005a, b). It is also cheaper, as it is one-tenth to one-eighth the cost of Phaco (Chang 2005a, b).

Being fast and cheap is excellent for addressing the backlog of patients who are blind due to cataract, but the fact that the technique is manual and does not require electricity (unlike typical phacoemulsification probes) is a definite advantage for low-income countries with poor electricity infrastructure. In addition to the economic and scientific reasons, there is the social justice reason, which has close ties to the high-volume practices discussed in prior chapters. Dr. R. D. Ravindran (2012) suggests SICS is best for resource-constrained settings in order to address the backlog of individuals with cataract. Yet, the cost recovery from user fees would be incomplete without utilizing both SICS and phacoemulsification. The eyes of patients for whom surgeons choose SICS versus phacoemulsification differ for both scientific and economic reasons.

Ophthalmologists commonly utilize phacoemulsification for immature cataractous lenses diagnosed in patients with early access to medical care; such patients are typically located in urban industrialized areas. While phacoemulsification has a transnational definition of "high technology" that assumes modern Western scientific knowledge is the best and most important, it was demonstrated as inappropriate for advanced stage white cataracts, which are typically more prevalent in less economically developed countries. However, ophthalmologists in South Asia have engaged in a process of adaptation on a transnational stage to develop special techniques and changes in the operating theater. These special techniques and changes facilitate successfully applying phacoemulsification to the hard case of white cataracts while further validating its standing as "high tech." However, there are two reasons why the surgeon might convert from phacoemulsification to extracapsular cataract extraction (or SICS). The conversion is necessary if there are complications during phacoemulsification, or the patient has contraindications for phacoemulsification, such as high intraocular pressure, high blood pressure, or high blood sugar.

The scientific reason why one might prefer phacoemulsification is that, with its smaller incision, there is no astigmatism, thus there is no need for distance glasses (Dr. R. D. Ravindran, unpublished interview, 2012). The chief medical officer of Sala Uno in Mexico, Dr. Juan Pablo (unpublished interview, 2012), explains it this way:

I would also say that I would prefer Phaco for other types of cataract, for younger patients. [SICS is not as good as Phaco] [b]ecause of the astigmatism with a bigger incision. Younger patients in their forties are people who are still working; their expectation about the results is totally different than an 80-year-old person who is at home or watching TV or who does not have a very agitated style of living.

Dr. Khan (unpublished interview, 2011) in Kenya and Dr. Ravindran (unpublished interview, 2012) at Aravind make similar statements about the need for Phaco to satisfy white-collar or wealthy patients with their higher expectations for their post-surgical visual outcomes. Dr. Ruit (unpublished interview, 2012) agrees, saying that "Phaco is like a very committed fashion; there are a lot of MNCs interested there. It is a fantastic procedure." Depending upon a patient's social context and his or her surgeon's proficiency in SICS versus Phaco, patients who undergo Phaco surgery are less likely to require distance glasses and therefore may be more fashionable. Scientifically, Phaco may be better for patients who might have other eye diseases. An ophthalmologist at Tilganga Institute of Ophthalmology (unpublished interview, 2012) prefers Phaco personally saying, "If you have to do other surgeries in the future, such as glaucoma, it's a better surgery."

Decreasing the phacoemulsification equipment costs will make the technique more viable for the global south. Professionals at Aravind and Tilganga plan to continue to produce technology locally to make phacoemulsification machines less expensive. For example, Aurolab already produces their low-cost Pegasus phacoemulsification machine—but only for sale in India (Williams 2012, July 21). In 2011, Tilganga announced its plans to make a low-cost, battery-operated Phaco machine for use in their outreach microsurgical eye camps in Nepal.

Using Phaco is important for cost recovery in community ophthalmology. Aravind's model of social entrepreneurship requires the performance of phacoemulsification as distinctive because it is the "Western technique." Ophthalmologists can therefore justify charging the wealthier patients higher prices for the latest Western surgical technique and for the use of the expensive phacoemulsification ultrasound machine—the latest Western surgical technology. This conspicuous consumption enables the sliding scale fee system where high-income patients subsidize services for non-paying and low-income patients.

An economic reason for NGOs and government hospitals to continue using Phaco in resource-constrained settings is to keep high-income patients who might otherwise go to the private sector, which would reduce or eliminate the sliding scale fee schedule in the Robin Hood model of cost recovery. At this chapter's beginning, I discussed my confusion while completing 1.5 months of fieldwork at Tilganga in 2009. I wondered, why were they doing Phaco if they had reinvented SICS? Before returning to Tilganga in 2011, I posed this question to the ophthalmologists I interviewed at the Lions Eye Hospital, Loresho in Kenya. They answered that offering Phaco procedures is necessary to be competitive with other eye hospitals and clinics; in order to keep their rich patients, they had to offer the "laser surgery." Laser surgery is the vernacular term some South Asian and Kenyan patients use for phacoemulsification, which involves an ultrasound probe. It should not be confused with the term LaserPhaco which involves a laser probe invented by African American ophthalmologist Dr. Patricia E. Bath (Davidson 2005; Program for the LaserPhaco Symposium 1988, March 27).

In 2003, Loresho ophthalmologists were among the first Kenyan doctors to offer phacoemulsification. Dr. Khan (unpublished interview, 2011) remembers that,

> [b]efore we started offering phacoemulsification to treat cataract disease, there were only two other hospitals performing this Western technique [in Kenya]. High-income patients used to come to Loresho and ask, 'are you doing the laser surgery?' When the answer was no, they would go somewhere else to have their cataracts treated. Phacoemulsification was a necessity for survival; we were losing high-income patients to the private sector.

These high-income patients were necessary for their user fees to enable them to subsidize low-income patients. Now, Loresho claims to perform the most Phaco surgeries, corneal grafts, and SICS in Kenya.

Cost recovery requires conspicuous consumption resulting in fees from the rich subsidizing the poor. I saw a straightforward example of this when sitting in the waiting room of Dr. Jyotee Trivedy's executive clinic at Loresho in Kenya. In her clinic, a female nurse (or perhaps a counselor) was trying to convince a family to purchase phacoemulsification cataract surgery with Alcon lenses for their older male relative, because "it is the best Western surgery." Dr. Ruit (2012) explains that with "Phaco/SICS there is a cost differential. There is a lot of demand from the affluent community for Phaco. If you want to serve poor people you have to serve the rich people." When my mother visited the optical shop at Loresho, she commented with surprise that there was no perceptible cost difference between the cost of eyeglasses from Kenya and those from the USA (2011). While this cost recovery is very positive because it provides free surgery for the poor, it has a negative aspect: After moving away from a double standard of ICCE/ECCE at the global level for low-income countries/high-income countries, it appears to advocate a new double standard of SICS/Phaco at the local level for poor/rich patients.

Eye hospitals in LEDCs focus on the cost-effectiveness of SICS; this is why they want to disseminate it further. Nonprofit organizations in India and Nepal have developed SICS and focused on its cost-effectiveness. As a result, many South Asian ophthalmologists are experts in both SICS and phacoemulsification—knowledge held by very few Western ophthalmologists. The equivalent efficacy with faster speed and lower cost makes SICS more viable than phacoemulsification for any nation-state trying to reduce the cost of cataract surgery (Anonymous 2010; Blumenthal 2002; Ruit et al. 2007; Wormald 2007).

6.6   Conclusion: SICS Is a Radical Innovation from Below

Community ophthalmologists have problematized the developmentalist (and exceptionalist) understanding that Western industrialized countries create sophisticated high technology and disseminate it to less economically developed countries. Community ophthalmologists are producing high-tech surgical science from a peripheral location in the world-system: South Asia. With its higher density of patients with advanced stage white cataract, South Asia was a propitious location to advance cataract surgical practice in order to make the surgical science viable for the physically hard case of white cataracts. Therefore, the re-invention of SICS by Nepalese ophthalmologist Dr. Ruit and the adaptation of phacoemulsification by Indian ophthalmologist Dr. Vasavada together serve as a physical and figurative hard case (Collins 1982, 142). Each example of appropriation demonstrates domestic experts who are citizens of a less economically developed country can produce sophisticated science that is novel and contextually appropriate. This production of advanced modern science and technology in the global south is a necessary step before it can be circulated. Therefore, these examples serve as further evidentiary foundation for conceptualizing innovation from below.

Scientific and technical experts in the global south were interested in distributional justice and epistemic sovereignty; their interests influenced them to produce innovation from below. Firstly, community ophthalmologists were interested in distributional justice, that is, who benefits from the science. Through reinterpreting, adapting, and reinventing ambulatory SICS, these Indian and Nepalese ophthalmologists configured the patient-users (Woolgar 1991) of sophisticated high technology; they reinterpreted patient-users from the urban white-collar rich professional to the poor rural subsistence agriculture worker.

Secondly, community ophthalmologists were interested in epistemic sovereignty (Healy 2003). They wanted to assert themselves as credible, inventive experts without relying upon knowledge and surgical practices from the West. After reinventing mini-nuc to create SICS, both Dr. Sanduk Ruit and Dr. R. D. Ravindran have suggested SICS (M-SICS) is best for less economically developed countries (Ruit et al. 2007; Anonymous 2010). South Asian community ophthalmologists are using the radical innovation of SICS to challenge the necessity and suitability of "the master's tools" (Lorde 2003 [1983]) in the global field of ophthalmology, i.e., Western science and technology. This is on a global scale where local experts in resource-poor areas of the global south challenged the knowledge hierarchies separating them from foreign experts in wealthy industrialized countries of the global north (Nieusma 2007). Southern ophthalmologists reconfigured (Eglash 2004; Woolgar 1991) themselves by shifting their identities from expert-users to expert-producers of sophisticated surgical science.

Innovative users can produce advanced modern science and technology. While South Asian ophthalmologists upheld phacoemulsification as the gold standard for performing cataract surgery globally, they also became producers of scientific knowledge and high technology. They did so by proving SICS: has equivalent outcomes to Phaco, is safer than Phaco (for eyes with white cataracts or for patients with other complicating factors such as high blood pressure), and is better suited to the high-volume radical finance Robin Hood model to treat the backlog of patients needing cataract surgery.

In this chapter, I have demonstrated how medical scientists in LEDCs contributed to global modern science and technology in the field of ophthalmology. Utilizing scant resources, they have re-created two highly technical forms of surgery through "appropriation," where they have moved along the spectrum of "users" from consumption to production (Eglash 2004).

6.7   Afterword: Interlocking Innovations

[T]he way it is done is multiple. You know, it is done through training, it is done through consulting process, (pause) giving of products, giving applications for software. You know, IOL … that's a big part …. So I think it's happened in multiple ways. (Thulasiraj Ravilla, MBA, Aravind Eye Care System, unpublished interview, 2012)

The hard case of white cataracts provides a stopping point for reflection about how outsiders challenge an incumbent socio-technical regime, and the relationships between science and technology innovations developed in appropriate technology niches. Community ophthalmology professionals are challengers to the incumbent Phaco-regime; they created SICS as a radical innovation and adapted Phaco for white cataract as an incremental innovation. These two surgical innovations could have been competitors in a technology substitution transition pathway. Instead of being solely competing surgical innovations, they additionally are useful in the global south as complimentary innovations in appropriate technology niches.

Making surgical science both high quality and low cost is not enough; the entire process of eye health care should be inexpensive. For cataract surgery, this necessitates low-cost surgical science and technology consumables. Producing low-cost IOLs in the Global South has had a global impact providing IOLs very inexpensively to the world. By 2012, at Tilganga, the Fred Hollows Intraocular Lens Laboratory (FHIOL) was producing high-quality intraocular lenses certified by the European Union. It was also providing 80% of the lenses used in Nepal and selling lenses in Africa, Asia, and Australia. From 1994 to 2012, Tilganga-FHIOL produced 2 million lenses that they exported to forty countries (The Fred Hollows Foundation 2012).

Likewise, in 2012 Aravind's manufacturing unit claimed 7% of the intraocular lens sales worldwide (this measure is by volume, not by income); earlier they had claimed 10% in 2005 (Oregon Public Broadcasting 2005). Aravind Eye Care System reinvests all revenues (Rubin 2001). Having initiated the local production of low-cost, high-quality ophthalmic consumables in less economically developed countries, it is now the leader among three manufacturers in India that produce more than 1 million intraocular lenses a year (Aravind et al. 2008).

This demonstrates both Aravind and Tilganga together have gone past the 5% of the market indicating an innovation is ready to breakthrough from niche to regime (Geels and Schot 2007, 405; Rogers 2003). They have made both ophthalmic surgical science and technology consumables less expensive globally. However, the ancillary costs for energy, personnel, and technology maintenance exceed the cost of new medical technology (Kressley 1981, 312–13). This is the nature of a socio-technical system: Instruments are connected to the regime's other elements including ideology, flexible specialized labor, energy infrastructure, facility infrastructure, and expert labor. Inexpensive surgical science and cheap technology were both necessary, but the two alone were not sufficient. The result of South Asian community ophthalmology organizations using these radical and incremental innovations concurrently is that these fully developed innovations became linked together into interlocking innovations.

The socio-technical system transition (pathway no. 4) dealignment and realignment involve the co-evolution of multiple, complimentary, and sub-system innovations which, when linked together, make wider application possible (Geels 2005, 91, 97–99; Geels and Schot 2007). Typically, in dealignment and realignment, breakthroughs from the niche to the regime occur with multiple linked innovations, not just one singular artifact (Geels 2005, 98). This is because the multiple innovations relate to each other through positive feedback (Geels 2005, 97). Geels explores three ways positive feedback occurs among multiple linked innovations. I will add a fourth positive feedback mechanism to more robustly develop the concept of interlocking innovations.

The first way multiple innovations relate to each other through positive feedback occurs through cross-sectoral clustering. For example, changes in material science and the speed and frequency of communication, i.e., steel and the telegraph, influenced the technological transition in Europe from the sailing ship to the steamship (Geels 2005, 98). In this case, community ophthalmology professionals have, within the civil society sector, created innovations adapting from and participating in international development, industrial manufacturing, and hospital services sectors.

An additional mechanism by which multiple innovations provide each other with positive feedback is complimentary utility. Complimentary utility means a technology benefits from the presence of another linked technology. This benefit comes in at least two forms: (1) the newer linked technology creates a product or process that directly enhances the functionality of an existing or incremental technology; (2) an existing or incremental technology's design and widespread adoption in the niche constrains the newer linked technology's design in some manner. It becomes evident the complimentary utility of multiple linked innovations is related to rules of the socio-technical niche.

Above, I have demonstrated that, in the incumbent regime, Phaco could not become an ambulatory procedure until foldable IOLs were introduced; this demonstrates complimentary utility where the design of an incremental technology, the foldable IOL, constrained phacoemulsification's utility. Furthermore, I have illustrated that, in the appropriate technology niches, SICS was enhanced by the adaptation of Phaco for white cataracts (providing both to patients helped Aravind and Tilganga continue using the Robin Hood model of cost recovery).

SICS, a new scientific innovation, thus became "the right tool for the job" of addressing the backlog of advanced stage cataract disease, but not in isolation. SICS has complimentary utility with intraocular lenses, a technological innovation, to restore sight to patients with advanced cataract disease. These intraocular lenses are produced through highly labor intensive and labor specialized processes at low wages at Aurolab and living wages at Tilganga-FHIOL.

Likewise, SICS had complimentary utility with high patient volume with its checklisted processes, standards, and benchmarks to routinize a high patient throughput and increase surgical volume in eye hospitals and eye camps (Prentice 2018). High volume constrained both SICS and Phaco. Without high patient volume, the eye unit could not fulfill the first cognitive rule that is deeply entrenched in the autonomous global network: to eradicate and control blindness. Subsequently, high volume became a formal rule in community ophthalmology organizations such as Aravind, Tilganga, Loresho, and Sala Uno.

A third way that interlocking innovations contain positive feedback is through a sub-system innovation. Incremental innovations have accumulated over time and are hierarchically organized to form a sub-system that altogether improves overall performance (Geels 2005, 99). One example of a sub-system might be the clean laboratory for manufacturing biomedical prosthetics. Such clean room infrastructure typically includes special uniforms and protocols to reduce air particulate counts, vent hoods, computer numerically controlled lathes, other machines, magnifying glasses, microscopes, linoleum flooring, and positive pressure air ventilation systems. The users, processes, scientific knowledge, and technological artifacts which compose a "clean room" sub-system are quite complex with their own interdependencies (Mody 2005). This sub-system innovation was pivotal to endogenous production of intraocular lenses at low cost, which again supports the guiding principle of eradicating and controlling blindness.

A shared ideology is the fourth way that interlocking innovations contain positive feedback between multiple, linked, complimentary, and sub-system innovations. The radical ideology which helped shape the appropriate technology niches subsequently has influenced the formation of the interlocking innovations. This radical ideology can be represented by Gandhi's concept of sarvodaya or good for all (see Chapter 3). This ideology serves as a foundational building block upon which the many other innovations have been built. For instance, it is incorporated into the problem-sequence for surgical science (see above) and the development of management standards and health services benchmarks in eye camps (see Chapter 4). Therefore, this ideology serves as an early and important cognitive rule in the appropriate technology niche that influences the formation of the interlocking innovations and is carried along with them wherever they travel.

This was a practical building block for appropriate technology activists challenging the incumbent regime. Since their economic ideology strongly differed from the incumbent regime's practices and approaches, this economic ideology served as a point of commonality between persons of different cultures and geo-political origins interested in eradicating blindness. The financial innovation that emerged from this radical economic ideology was also important since the appropriate technology niches themselves were not attractive to the typical investors in the incumbent regime who might otherwise support technology niches.

By extending Geels' work, I define interlocking innovations as the multiple, complimentary, and sub-system innovations providing each other with positive feedback through a shared ideology. In this example, community ophthalmology professionals, working within their appropriate technology niches, have created interlocking innovations which are: a novel constellation of context-appropriate processes (or products) in science, technology, and management connected to each other by a shared economic ideology and other guiding mission (or cognitive rule).

The complimentary utility between the multiple innovations comprising an interlocking innovation means one innovation cannot breakthrough from niche to regime without the others (Geels 2005, 98). Innovations are first produced inside niches as separate, singular knowledge and artifacts. Once these multiple complimentary and sub-system innovations are linked and black boxed, they then circulate outside the niches. Altogether, these scientific, technological, financial, and organizational innovations, shared ideology, and rules are necessary to scale-up sophisticated surgical practices to address the eye healthcare needs of the rural poor at a low cost.

In Chapter 7, I discuss how Aravind and Tilganga train other community ophthalmology professionals in their interlocking innovations. The multiple and complimentary innovations created by Aravind and Tilganga are packaged and sold to other eye units. Selling low-cost interlocking innovations provides additional revenue and helps fulfill the larger mission of eradicating and controlling blindness. Domestic NGOs addressing avoidable blindness inside and outside of South Asia send their employees for training in both the surgical techniques and the management practices. Such training can enable them to then create cost recovery models similar to those of Aravind and Tilganga.

References

American Academy of Ophthalmology. 2018. "Meeting Archive." https:// secure.aao.org/aao/meeting-archive.

Anonymous. 2010. "APACRS Eye World Asia-Pacific Meeting Reporter: Reporting Live from the 25th APAO Congress Beijing, September 16–20, 2010." *Eye World Magazine*, September 20. Retrieved August 21, 2011. http://www.apacrs.org/edm/APAO/mr/web_09202010.htm.

Apple, David J., and John Sims. 1996. "Harold Ridley and the invention of the intraocular lens." *Survey of Ophthalmology* 40 (4): 279–292.

Aravind, Srinivasan, Aravind Haripriya, and B. Syeda Sumara Taranum. 2008. "Cataract Surgery and Intraocular Lens Manufacturing in India." *Current Opinion in Ophthalmology* 19 (1): 60–65.

Blumenthal, Michael. 1994. "Manual ECCE, The Present State of the Art." *Klinische Monatsblatter fur Augenheilkunde* 205 (5): 266–70.

———. 2002. "Cataract Surgery." *Community Eye Health* 15 (42): 26–27.

Blumenthal, Michael, Isaac Ashkenazi, Ehud Assia, and Michael Cahane. 1992. "Small-Incision Manual Extracapsular Cataract Extraction Using Selective Hydrodissection." *Ophthalmic Surgery* 23 (10): 699.

Boyle, Erin L. 2007. "Foldable IOLs Ushered in New Cataract and Refractive Paradigm." *Ocular Surgery News U.S. Edition*, June 1. http://www.healio.com/ophthalmology/cataract-surgery/news/print/ocular-surgery-news/%7B98997a7f-36ca-4ad0-b64c-4d5389834bff%7D/foldable-iols-ushered-in-new-cataract-and-refractive-paradigm.

Casper, M. J., and A. E. Clarke. 1998. "Making the Pap Smear into the 'Right Tool' for the Job: Cervical Cancer Screening in the USA, Circa 1940–95." *Social Studies of Science* 28 (2): 255–90.

Chakrabarti, Arup, and Seema Singh. 2000. "Phacoemulsification in Eyes with White Cataract." *Journal of Cataract & Refractive Surgery* 26 (7): 1041–47.

Chang, David F. 2005a. "Tackling The Greatest Challenge In Cataract Surgery." *British Journal Of Ophthalmology* 89 (9): 1073–1077.

Chang, David. 2005b. "A 5-Minute, $15 Cure for Blindness: Tackling Cataract Blindness in the Developing World." *Cataract & Refractive Surgery Today*, October, 49–51.

Chell, P. B., P. Shah, and A. R. Fielder. 1994. "Ambulatory Cataract Surgery: The Patients' Perceptions." *Ambulatory Surgery* 2 (3): 162–65.

Collins, Harry M. 1982. "Special Relativism—The Natural Attitude." *Social Studies of Science* 12 (1): 139–43.

Davidson, Martha. 2005. "The Right to Sight: Patricia Bath." Lemelson Center Invention Features: Patricia Bath. Retrieved November 20, 2010. http://invention.smithsonian.org/centerpieces/ilives/bath/bath.html.

Durant, G. D., and C. J. Battaglia. 1993. "The Growth of Ambulatory Surgery Centres in the United States." *Ambulatory Surgery* 1 (2): 83–88.

Eglash, Ron. 2004. "Appropriating Technology: An Introduction." In *Appropriating Technology: Vernacular Science and Social Power*, edited by R. Eglash, J. L. Croissant, G. Di Chiro, and R. Fouche, vii–xxi. Minneapolis: University of Minnesota Press.

Farmer, Paul, and Jim Kim. 2008. "Surgery and Global Health: A View from Beyond the OR." *World Journal of Surgery* 32: 533–36.

The Fred Hollows Foundation. 2012. *In Fred's Footsteps: 20 Years of Restoring Sight.* Sydney: The Fred Hollows Foundation.

Geels, Frank W. 2005. "Conceptual Perspective on Systems Innovations and Technological Transitions." In *Technological Transitions and System Innovations: A Co-evolutionary and Socio-Technical Analysis*, 75–102. Cheltenham and Northampton, MA: Edward Elgar.

Geels, Frank W., and Johan Schot. 2007. "Typology of Sociotechnical Transition Pathways." *Research Policy* 36 (3): 399–417.

Gogate, Parikshit, Madan Deshpande, and Praveen K. Nirmalan. 2007. "Why Do Phacoemulsification? Manual Small-Incision Cataract Surgery Is Almost as Effective, But Less Expensive." *Ophthalmology* 114 (5): 965–68.

Gogate, Parikshit M., Sucheta R. Kulkarni, S. Krishnaiah, Rahul D. Deshpande, Shilpa A. Joshi, Anand Palimkar, and Madan D. Deshpande.

2005. "Safety and Efficacy of Phacoemulsification Compared with Manual Small-Incision Cataract Surgery by a Randomized Controlled Clinical Trial: Six-Week Results." *Ophthalmology* 112 (5): 869–74.

Healy, S. 2003. "Epistemological Pluralism and the 'Politics of Choice.'" *Futures* 35 (7): 689–701.

Hillman, Liz. 2017. "Phaco Turns 50." *Eyeworld*, April. https://www.eyeworld. org/phaco-turns-50.

Jaffe, Norman S. 1996. "History of Cataract Surgery." *Ophthalmology* (Rochester, MN) 103 (8): 5–16.

Kressley, K. M. 1981. "Diffusion of High Technology Medical Care and Cost Control—Public Policy Dilemma." *Technology in Society* 3 (3):305–22.

Latour, Bruno. 1987. *Science in Action: How to Follow Scientists and Engineers Through Society.* Cambridge, MA: Harvard University Press.

Lorde, Audre. 2003. "The Master's Tools Will Never Dismantle the Master's House." In *Feminist Postcolonial Theory: A Reader*, edited by Reina Lewis and Sara Mills, 25–28. New York: Routledge.

Metcalfe, J. Stanley, Andrew James, and Andrea Mina. 2005. "Emergent Innovation Systems and the Delivery of Clinical Services: The Case of Intra-Ocular Lenses." *Research Policy* 34 (9): 1283–1304.

Minassian, Darwin C., Angela Reidy, P. Desai, S. Farrow, G. Vafidis, and A. Minassian. 2000. "The Deficit in Cataract Surgery in England and Wales and the Escalating Problem of Visual Impairment: Epidemiological Modelling of the Population Dynamics of Cataract." *British Journal of Ophthalmology* 84 (1): 4–8.

Mody, Cyrus C. M. 2005. "The Sounds of Science: Listening to Laboratory Practice." *Science, Technology, & Human Values* 30 (2): 175–98.

Natchiar, G., and Tulika D. Kar. 2000. "Manual Small Incision Sutureless Cataract Surgery—An Alternative Technique to Instrumental Phacoemulsification." *Operative Techniques in Cataract and Refractive Surgery* 3 (4): 161–70.

Nieusma, Dean. 2007. "Challenging Knowledge Hierarchies: Working Toward Sustainable Development in Sri Lanka's Energy Sector." *Sustainability: Science Practice and Policy* 3: 32–44.

Oregon Public Broadcasting. 2005. *The New Heroes: Their Bottom Line Is Lives.* Oregon Public Broadcasting. Retrieved March 1, 2010. http://www.pbs. org/opb/thenewheroes/.

Ozgediz, Doruk, and Robert Riviello. 2008. "The 'Other' Neglected Diseases in Global Public Health: Surgical Conditions in Sub-Saharan Africa." *PLOS Med* 5: e121.

Prentice, Rachel. 2018. "How Surgery Became a Global Public Health Issue." *Technology in Society*, Technology and the Good Society 52 (February): 17–23.

Program for the LaserPhaco Symposium. 1988. Patricia Bath Oral History Collection No. 753 Box No. 2. Lemelson Center/Archives Center, National Museum of American History, Smithsonian Institutes, Washington, DC, March 27.

Rogers, Everett M. 2003 [1962]. *Diffusion of Innovations*. 5th ed. New York: The Free Press.

Rubin, Harriet. 2001. "The Perfect Vision of Dr. V." *Fast Company*, January 31. Retrieved May 1, 2009. http://www.fastcompany.com/42111/perfect-vision-dr-v.

Ruit, Sanduk. 2003. "Dr Ruit: 'I Had a Puzzle to Solve' Interview of Dr. Ruit by Puran P Bista." *The Kathmandu Post*, December 29, sec. Editorial. http://www.ekantipur.com/the-kathmandu-post/2010/02/16/Business/Tomatoes-at-Rs-1-per-kg/5230/.

Ruit, Sanduk, Alan L. Robin, Ram Prasad Pokhrel, Anil Sharma, Joseph DeFaller, and Paul T. Maguire. 1991a. "Long-Term Results of Extracapsular Cataract Extraction and Posterior Chamber Intraocular Lens Insertion in Nepal." *Transactions of the American Ophthalmological Society* 89: 59–76.

Ruit, Sanduk, Alan L. Robin, Ram Prasad Pokhrel, Anil Sharma, and Joseph DeFaller. 1991b. "Extracapsular Cataract Extraction in Nepal: 2-Year Outcome." *Archives of Ophthalmology* 109 (12): 1761–1763.

Ruit, Sanduk, G. Paudyal, Reeta Gurung, Geoffrey Tabin, D. Moran, and G. Brian. 2000. "An Innovation in Developing World Cataract Surgery: Sutureless Extracapsular Cataract Extraction with Intraocular Lens Implantation." *Clinical and Experimental Ophthalmology* 28 (4): 274–79.

Ruit, Sanduk, Geoffrey Tabin, David Chang, Leena Bajracharya, Daniel C. Kline, William Richheimer, Mohan Shrestha, and Govinda Paudyal. 2007. "A Prospective Randomized Clinical Trial of Phacoemulsification vs Manual Sutureless Small-Incision Extracapsular Cataract Surgery in Nepal." *American Journal of Ophthalmology* 143 (1): 32–38. e2.

Singh, Ramesh M., and Dinesh R. Bhuju. 2001. "Development of Science and Technology in Nepal." *Science Technology and Society* 6 (1): 159–78.

Tabandeh, Homayoun, Graham M. Thompson, and Peter Heyworth. 1994. "Lens Hardness in Mature Cataracts." *Eye* 8: 453–55.

Tabin, Geoffrey, and Emily R. Newick. 2008. "Eye Care for the Millennium Villages." *Cataract & Refractive Surgery Today*, April. Retrieved February 27, 2010. http://bmctoday.net/crstoday/2008/04/article.asp?f=CRST0408_05.php.

Tabin, Geoffrey, Michael Chen, and Ladan Espandar. 2008. "Cataract Surgery for the Developing World." *Current Opinion in Ophthalmology* 19 (1): 55–59.

Vasavada, A., Raminder Singh, and Jagruti Desai. 1998. "Phacoemulsification of White Mature Cataracts." *Journal of Cataract and Refractive Surgery* 24 (2): 270–77.

WHO. 2004. "Global Cataract Surgical Rates in 2004." Retrieved February 1, 2007. http://www.who.int/blindness/data_maps/CSR_WORLD_2004.jpg.

Williams, Logan D. A. 2008. "Medical Technology Transfer for Sustainable Development: A Case Study of Intraocular Lens Replacement to Correct Cataracts." *Technology in Society* 30 (2): 170–83.

———. 2012, July 21. Direct Observation Fieldnotes. Vision 2020 India Conference. Govindappa Venkataswamy Eye Research Institute, Madurai, India.

Wilson, John. 1987. "Clearing the cataract backlog." *British Journal of Ophthalmology* 71 (2): 158–160.

Woolgar, Steve. 1991. "Configuring the User: The Case of Usability Trials." In *A Sociology of Monsters: Essays on Power, Technology, and Domination*, edited by John Law, 58–97. New York: Routledge.

Wormald, Richard P. 2007. "Phacoemulsification vs Small-Incision Manual Cataract Surgery: An Expert Trial." *American Journal of Ophthalmology* 143 (1): 143–44.

7

Training the New Cadre: Translation of Interlocking Innovations

LAICO uses the systems, right? They share what's happening in the hospital with the other hospitals, so they would gradually get to know what's happening .... they will have to be able to package it when they share it with someone else... to reach a packaging stage it takes time, that's why I said gradually. (Dr. S. Aravind, MBA, Aravind Eye Care System, unpublished interview, 2012)

One morning Suzanne Gilbert started her training session with some startling statistics highlighting the uneven patient access to trained medical personnel around the world (Williams 2012, July 17). She noted that patients in sub-Saharan African countries are at a great disadvantage compared to patients from industrialized countries in the Americas, when it comes to accessing medical services due to the "lack" of trained personnel. However, Suzanne's solution, as the director for SEVA Foundation's Center for Innovation in Eye Care, did not involve importing medical personnel from Western industrialized countries to provide short-term training to medical personnel, or short-term medical services to African patients. Instead, she focused on a multi-component system building process (Herzlinger 2010). That day, as an instructor at

© The Author(s) 2019
L. D. A. Williams, *Eradicating Blindness*,
https://doi.org/10.1007/978-981-13-1625-8_7

Eye Excel, she was focused on one component of the system building process: "teaching the trainers."

A sharp increase in human and physical infrastructure is necessary to address the backlog of avoidable blindness around the world and especially in less economically developed countries. The Eye Excel course at the Lions Aravind Institute of Community Ophthalmology (LAICO) is one infrastructure-building activity practiced by the Aravind Eye Care System. In addition to her primary job with SEVA Foundation, Suzanne is an Eye Excel instructor at LAICO a few weeks per year. The purpose of the Eye Excel course is to allow individual eye hospitals or eye units within a general hospital, to develop training programs. Instructors at Aravind's Eye Excel course are making the argument that training programs offer the opportunity both to increase trained medical personnel and to increase patient access to high-quality eye health care. They are attempting to counter the general perception among small resource-poor eye units that training programs are both a drain on existing resources and decrease the quality of care for individual patients. Considering the limited human and physical infrastructure to address the backlog of avoidable blindness, these training initiatives are filling an important role. This training involves translating the Robin Hood model, along with the other innovations in surgical technology-practice, operating theater management, etc., from South Asia outwards.

This chapter's purpose is to illuminate how interlocking innovations began to move from the niche to a new regime. The remainder of this chapter is organized as follows: First, Sect. 7.1, outlines the theory on translation in science and technology studies and niche accumulation in the multi-level perspective of socio-technical transitions and their areas of synergy. Section 7.2 sheds light on the decision of Aravind senior management to create a semi-periphery of calculation, a dedicated training center for eye health services, and the importance of recognition by the WHO. Next, Sect. 7.3 provides some startling observations about the subsequent south–south circulation of experts. Subsequently, Sect. 7.4 describes the short courses available at Aravind and Tilganga that transform expert professionals from the global south into systems thinkers. Section 7.5 explains how Aravind and Tilganga perpetuate their similar interlocking innovations and a systems thinking discourse as they reproduce their models of eye health care in other countries in the global south (such as a government hospital eye unit in Malawi). Finally, Sect. 7.6 concludes by summarizing how translation, which involves extraction, alignment, and transformation, accumulates niches, and operates through the unilateral imposition of power.

7.1 Theory: Translation and Niche Accumulation

In this chapter, I argue that the interlocking innovations developed by community ophthalmology professionals are translated, that is, they circulate globally, thereby developing a larger and larger market. This is called the niche accumulation in transition studies (Geels 2005a).

Translation, or the bidirectional, unilateral movement of knowledges and technologies, has several definitions. In business, science, and engineering, it is the route by which innovations move from the laboratory bench to the commercial market. Historical studies of science and technology translation have shown how colonial expeditions and botanical gardens enabled indigenous knowledges (e.g., plants, rocks, paths, waterways, and animals) to flow from the colonial periphery back toward the empire's center (Basalla 1967; Harding 2008; Hess 1995). These local indigenous knowledges served as a natural resource for experts in the West to create new scientific knowledge (e.g., botany, biology, cartography, geology, and zoology). This new scientific knowledge starts as Western and assumes universal significance (Englander 2014; O'Connell 1993).

Sociologists, geographers, and historians use the concept of immutable mobiles to describe how re-configured knowledges flow from centers of calculation outwards (Jöns 2011; Latour 1987; Raj 2006). Immutable mobiles are physically manifested ideas, knowledges, and processes; they are portable, unchanging, and can be easily aggregated to further scientific knowledge production (Jöns 2011 citing Latour 1987). A "standardized package" (Fujimura 1987) is a specific form of immutable mobile that involves routinized data collection processes and technology-practices for more doable scientific research. When two social worlds are closely interrelated with each other (e.g., two laboratories working on slightly different research problems in their respective sub-fields of biology, or, two culturally and geographically differentiated eye hospitals in an autonomous global network), then standardized packages move easily between them (Fujimura 1987). Standardized packages are unique because they help stabilize a particular scientific sub-field around shared vocabulary, shared instruments, and shared data collection processes (Fujimura 1988).

During translation, science and technology moves bidirectionally. This is demonstrated by the first direction, when indigenous knowledge moves from the periphery to the center of calculation, and the second direction, when immutable mobiles (such as maps) move from the center of calculation outwards (Latour 1987, 229). This bidirectionality is also seen as extracted experimental data, commonly used chemical or biological materials, and finalized experimental records, i.e., standardized packages, move between laboratories and peer-reviewed journals.

This movement occurs in a world-system with asymmetric power relationships between countries. Translation offers an illustration of this asymmetric relationship. In one example, social scientists in the periphery strategically translate scholarly knowledge produced in the center to enhance their status and prestige at home (Medina 2014). In Medina's (2014) example, as knowledge moves between nations and between contexts, its ascribed status changes, but the power of the center remains stable. In a second example, the intent of Western development workers was to listen to the Nepalese midwives and shamans as well as to train them: a bidirectional flow of Western and local knowledges. Instead, local knowledge was devalued and, in its place, modern Western obstetrics medical knowledge was prized: a unilateral imposition of Western knowledges on local people (see Pigg 1995). However, as Harding (2008, 42–43) notes,

> Latour seems completely unaware that [translation] … is also an account of how Western sciences and empires are inextricably interlinked, how they co-constitute each other, and in disastrous ways for those 'left on the outside' of the West's sciences and societies.

Therefore, Latour's (1987) theory of translation might be usefully amended to explore how, "structures, interests, actors, and identities are constructed historically, but at any given time, these phenomena have an established character, and this configuration has effects" (Kleinman 1998, 290).

I amend Latour's translation conceptually and empirically. I argue that uneven power relationships are central to translation as a mode of science and technology circulation that extracts, aligns, and transforms. When describing the translation of a new scientific practice from a laboratory outwards, Latour (1983, 151) wrote that,

> Pasteur cannot just hand out a few flasks of vaccine to farmers and say: 'OK, it works in my lab, get by with that.' If he were to do that, it would not work. The vaccination can work only on the condition that the farm chosen .... be in some crucial respects transformed according to the prescriptions of Pasteur's laboratory.

Expanding on this premise suggests that, in order for a standardized package to move from a center of calculation outwards, the dominant actor must carefully package extracted data for dissemination. The dominant actor must also select the new intended location and then extract necessary information about this location. It is then essential that the dominant actor prepares, stages, and modifies the new location in order to most closely mimic the center of calculation (alignment and transformation). Therefore, any act of extension operates through extraction, alignment, and transformation where those who are dominant enact a unilateral power relationship over those who are subordinate. Below, I offer a novel empirical example of how translation starts from locations in the semi-periphery of calculation in the world-system and impacts other locations in both the semi-periphery and periphery. In order to do this, I demonstrate the synergies between translation as a mode of science and technology circulation, and niche accumulation as a mechanism of innovation breakthrough from niche level to regime level in the multi-level perspective.

Niche accumulation occurs when a particular innovation, beginning with the niche where it was initially developed, gradually aggregates markets. If the innovation is applied in novel ways, it enters new technical markets. Likewise, when the innovation is utilized by more users, it absorbs new demographics such as: age, gender, ethnic background, income level, education level, location, attitudes, values, interests, hobbies, and firm size (Geels 2005c, 691).

Niche accumulation is not just the gathering of technology domains and users. The constitutive elements of a niche, that is, expectations and vision, social network, and knowledge derived from learning and reflection, are also accumulated; this forms a socio-cognitive aggregation (Bakker et al. 2015, 155 citing Geels and Raven 2006). Thus, niche accumulation has user, technical, and socio-cognitive dimensions.

To generate technological momentum, niche accumulation is required (Bakker et al. 2015, 155 citing Geels and Schot 2007; Hughes 1987). A socio-technical system with momentum has economies of scope and scale (Hughes 1987). Economies of scope and scale first develop during niche accumulation as challengers to the incumbent regime modify an innovation to be relevant and useful in an increasing variety of technical and user markets.

There are several similarities between niche accumulation and translation: enrolling allies, aggregating knowledge and mistakes, aligning worlds, and creating supralocal standards. Part of niche accumulation is accruing enthusiastic niche innovation adopters (Geels 2005b, 452; 2005c, 694; Latour 1987). This is similar to enrolling allies in translation. Linkages between actors (e.g., NGOs or firms, individuals, and government agencies) are important for: disseminating knowledge and artifacts, collaborating over shared interests, and circulating financial resources. These actors share emergent: cognitive rules (e.g., guiding principles, ideologies, and expectations) and normative rules (e.g., values).

In the case of community ophthalmology professionals, Dr. Venkataswamy had an overt interest in putting principles of rationality and efficiency into practice, even attending the McDonald's Hamburger University in Oak Brook, Illinois, USA in 1974 (Rubin 2001). Fordist assembly lines and Taylorist scientific management became popular in the USA in the early twentieth century (Nye 2013). Sociologist George Ritzer's (1996) McDonaldization thesis is useful to understand how these principles have gained global notoriety. Ritzer (1996, 292) explains that the "fast-food restaurant has combined the principles of the bureaucracy with those of other rationalized precursors (for example, the assembly line, scientific management) to create a particularly powerful model of the rationalization process." The popularity of rationality and efficiency as management principles in service industries means that Dr. Venkataswamy can confidently state,

> See, McDonald's concept is simple. They feel they can train people all over the world, irrespective of different religions, cultures, all those things, to produce a product in the same way and deliver it in the same manner in hundreds of places.... Supposing I'm able to produce eye care, techniques, methods, all in the same way, and make it available in every corner of the world. The problem of blindness is gone. (Dr. Venkataswamy speaking in *Infinite Vision* Krishnan 2004)

By focusing on rationality and efficiency, community ophthalmologists can link their appropriate technology niches to broader visions of a global world, with businesses that are productive, efficient, and have international reach (Krishnan 2004; Marseille 1994, 151; Mehta and Shenoy 2011; Rubin 2001). Therefore, while actors from the incumbent regime may not necessarily understand or agree with the radical economic ideology inherent to the appropriate technology niche, they are enthusiastic for the familiar elements of this globally shared vision, that is, increased productivity, and high efficiency. Inspiring such "cultural enthusiasm" in users advocating for specific policies and outcomes is part of successful technology breakthrough (Geels 2005b, 452; 2005c, 694).

Like translation, niche accumulation aggregates knowledge and mistakes from experiments with innovations. Learning occurs through parallel experimentation by a single actor (firm, individual, NGO, government agency), sequential experimentation by a single actor, or vicarious experimentation where multiple actors compare the results of parallel or sequential experiments (Raven 2007, 2393–95). Socio-cognitive accumulation includes gaining knowledge and mistakes from the various experiments (Bakker et al. 2015, 156).

Niche accumulation requires alignment between these actors' contexts within the niche, or between separate niches: especially in cases of widespread geophysical and psychosocial differentiation between actors sharing knowledge. This is true when the actors are engaged in already similar niches (such as Aravind and Tilganga), or in very different niches (e.g., Aravind and Loresho). The alignment process requires a lot of work (Raven 2007, 2395). Therefore, niche accumulation is not only aggregating the knowledge and mistakes from one laboratory or niche, it involves creating a knowledge-sharing platform (Raven 2007, 2395). This platform likewise serves to concentrate resources that are otherwise divided across the various niches (Raven 2007, 2395).

Niche accumulation results in the creation of supralocal technical standards. When local experimental outcomes or technical designs are amassed and embraced by many relevant actors, then the result is a technical standard (Bakker et al. 2015, 155–56). Standards involve abstracting robust supralocal knowledge from packaged, generalized aggregated local knowledge (Bakker et al. 2015, 155–56). During niche accumulation, actors create such standardized packages as part of aligning within and across niches. Likewise, translation involves an imposition of power over space where a set of internationally circulating standards, "constructs an invisible network … by establishing the authority of a particular representative, circulating it, and assuring that comparisons are made to it" (O'Connell 1993, 164–65).

Previous theories of translation or the multi-level perspective have not sufficiently elaborated the necessity of extraction, the early authority of one or more actor, and the recognition of that actor's authority as part of alignment and transformation among accumulated niches. In this chapter, I will do so by recounting how challengers to the incumbent regime disseminate their interlocking innovations through their own semi-periphery of calculation.

7.2   Creating a Semi-periphery of Calculation: North–South Recognition

LAICO's origin as a knowledge-sharing platform is rooted in challengers to the incumbent regime recognizing the fact that their interlocking innovations work well in southern India or central Nepal does not mean that these innovations would transfer easily. Indeed, it was recognizing the difficulty of implementing Dr. V's vision to eradicate needless blindness globally, that made the need for a consulting and training organization most evident.

Apparently, Dr. Venkataswamy met with the senior leadership at Aravind in 1990; they were looking for an opportunity for Aravind more consistently contribute their knowledge to the international ophthalmology community (Williams 2012, April 5). Around the same time, the Lions Clubs International Foundation (LCIF) created the SightFirst program and wanted to increase the productivity of existing Lions eye hospitals in India before investing in more. When the LCIF approached Aravind about training staff from Lions eye hospitals in India, Aravind asked them for $1.15 million US dollars to build the Lions Aravind Institute of Community Ophthalmology (Williams 2012, April 5; see Fig. 7.1).

Dr. Venkataswamy intended LAICO to be an internationally esteemed ophthalmology research, training, and consultation center. In the same Infinite Vision video (Krishnan 2004), Suzanne Gilbert fondly remembers Dr. V's first visit to the University of Michigan in 1978, three years after she had earned her Master's degree in Public Health with a concentration on Maternal and Child Health and Health Education (Krishnan 2004).

When Dr. Venkataswamy spoke to her about having a training facility similar to the one at the University of Michigan Medical School, she was charmed but skeptical; she recounts her earlier skepticism with a laugh because eighteen years later LAICO existed (Krishnan 2004).

Aravind used their own income, funds from old partners, and funds from their new partner, the Lions Clubs International Foundation, to develop the Lions Aravind Institute of Community Ophthalmology. The organization relied on close partnerships with international NGOs to partially fund the new training center's construction. LAICO was designed to have quite extensive infrastructure, with 50,000 square feet which included: the second and third floor offices, the first floor classrooms, the ground floor offices, dining hall, and a small conference room with air-conditioning and teleconferencing audio/visual setup that seats approximately twenty people. LAICO also had a basement level with a medium-sized lecture hall (approximately 150

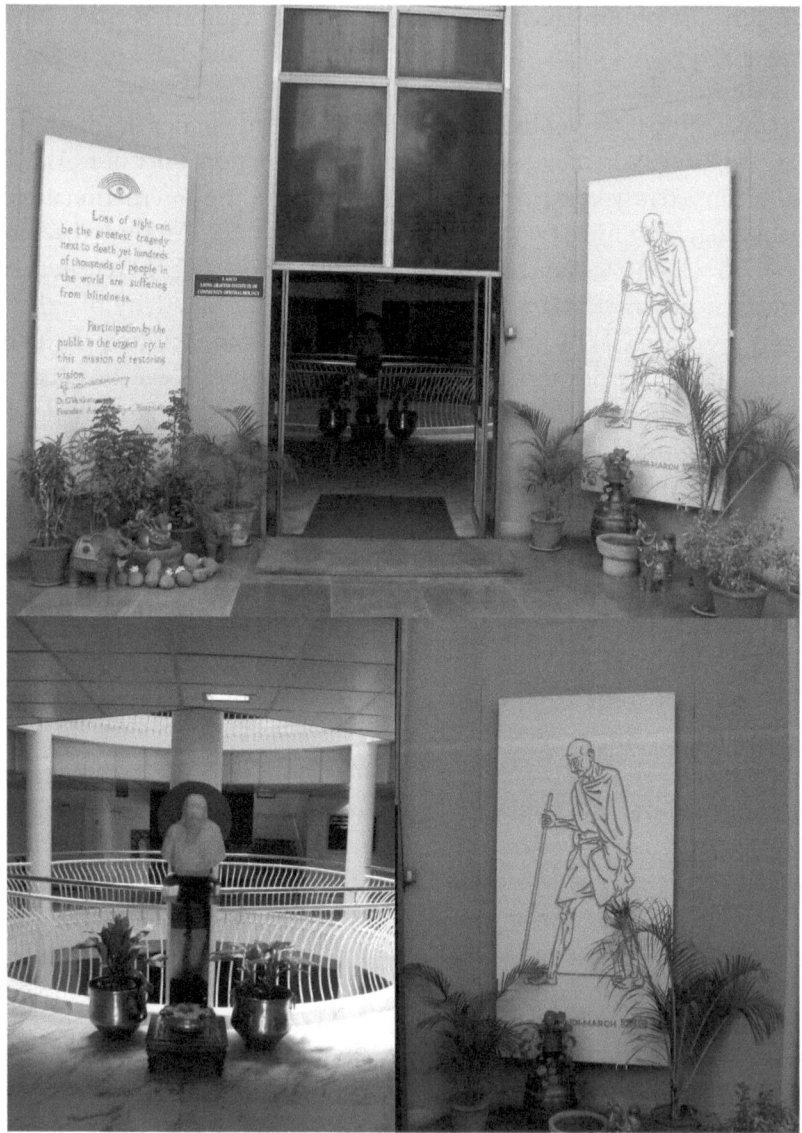

Fig. 7.1 Entrance to the Lions Aravind Institute for Community Ophthalmology which shows a drawing of Gandhi to the right of the doorway and a bust of Sri Aurobindo centered between the open doors (Photo by Logan D. A. Williams)

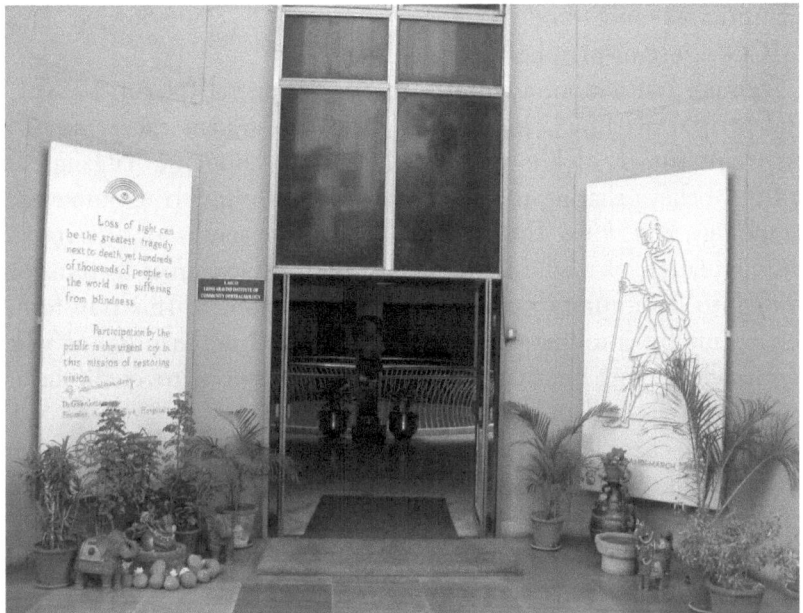

Fig. 7.1 (continued)

seats and audio/visual setup). The funds donated by the Lions Club International Foundation SightFirst program paid only for the 8000 square foot first floor which has four classrooms each varied in size from 30 seats to 65 seats with audio/visual setup and air-conditioning units (Williams 2012, April 5). The former Lions Clubs International Foundation Chairman and Indian national, Lion Rohit C. Mehta, laid the foundation stone in 1993, and the final building was inaugurated in 1996 by Dr. Carl Kupfer who, at the time, was still the director of the National Eye Institute (USA) and past president of IAPB (2016; Williams 2012, April 5). The presence of an esteemed Indian business-man acting as representative of a Western organization, and a promi-nent Western ophthalmologist suggests that, in addition to Aravind's self-initiative and funds, Western funds and clout helped create LAICO as a semi-periphery of calculation.

Through translation, a country that is peripheral (Nepal, Kenya) or semi-peripheral (India, Mexico) in the world-system can serve as an important source of knowledge, skills, and technology. Tilganga and Aravind believe sharing their work practices is transferring knowledge, technology, and skills. This transfer involves the south–south extraction and circulation of medical and allied health professionals to transform them into community ophthalmology professionals. This transformation occurs by enrolling such professionals, and the institutions where they practice, into the autonomous global network to eradicate and control blindness (thereby accumulating niches).

Enrolling people into a network involves unilaterally imposing power. Unlike the network-builders, enrollees do not shape the network, but are indoctrinated into a preexisting network (Latour 1987). Therefore, an asymmetric division of power exists between the network-builders (trainers) and the enrollees (trainees). Trainers may learn just enough about the particular context of each trainee in order to better convince him or her how the interlocking innovations might be usefully adapted to fit their particular context. Otherwise, the trainers mainly perform training activities to convince the trainees of interlocking innovations' utility, and to enroll the trainees in the autonomous global network dedicated to eradicating and controlling blindness. In this chapter, I present several examples of training activities that are initiated by Aravind or Tilganga and utilized by Sala Uno, Loresho, and other eye clinics from around the world.

LAICO coordinates extensive training activities on-site across the Aravind system. These include: non-credit and accredited post-graduate courses for ophthalmologists, paramedics, and optometrists; instrument maintenance courses for biomedical engineers and instrument technicians; management courses for hospital managers and outreach camp managers; and an internal fellowship program for hospital managers. Through these training activities, the semi-periphery of calculation acts unilaterally, it collects funds and temporarily collects medical personnel before re-circulating the medical personnel outwards again back to their respective countries.

Because the world-system developed unevenly, a semi-periphery of calculation becomes authoritative through designation by a higher authority in addition to the traditional method of accumulating knowledge and mistakes. Centers of calculation in the global field of science attract respect, credit for their achievements, conference attendees, research trainees, and funds. Additionally, such centers of calculation attract recognition beyond what is expected considering their research productivity (Schøtt 1998). In Latour's theory of translation (1983, 1987), centers of calculation form through their credibility in the scientific field, through the accumulation of knowledge and mistakes in science. I argue that merit alone does not determine the high status enjoyed by centers of calculation. Considering that the historical location of such centers of calculation has most frequently been in the center of the world-system (earlier in Europe, and recently in North America; see Englander 2014), there is a case for an additional formation mechanism that is based in geo-political power between nation-states.

To illuminate what additional formations mechanisms might be present, I describe the formation of a World Health Organization Collaborating Center for the Prevention of Blindness that epitomizes calculation on the semi-periphery of modern science. When I use the terminology of periphery or semi-periphery, I am loosely using world-systems theory (Wallerstein 1974). Primarily, I am referring to the economic ranking of less economically developed countries (based upon gross domestic product purchasing power parity per capita) in comparison with the industrialized economic powerhouses such as the USA and the E.U. (see Table 7.1). The purchasing power parity (GDP PPP) per capita for India and Nepal ranks them among the lowest one-third of the list of approximately two hundred and thirty countries worldwide. GDP PPP per capita is the worth of the goods and services produced within a nation-state's borders divided by its population, normalized to reflect local cost of living.

Using these economic measures to rank countries makes it clearer why an official designation by a multilateral non-governmental organization with international authority, such as the WHO, helps promote training activities at LAICO.

Table 7.1 Ranking countries using GDP (PPP) per capita; in the world system, core countries have low number ranks while peripheral countries have high number ranks (Central Intelligence Agency 2012; United Nations Development Programme 2017)

Country	GDP per capita (PPP) rank	GDP per capita (PPP) in 2011 US dollars	Total GDP (PPP) in 2011 US dollars	Human development index (2012)
Nepal	207	1200	0.03808 trillion	0.545
Kenya	198	1700	0.07121 trillion	0.541
India	165	3700	4.42100 trillion	0.599
Mexico	86	14,700	1.66700 trillion	0.753
European Union	38	34,100	15.48000 trillion	Not calculated
Australia	21	40,800	0.91510 trillion	0.933
USA	11	48,300	15.08000 trillion	0.915

GDP is gross domestic product; PPP is purchasing power parity; Human development index combines measurements such as life expectancy, income and education where 1 is the ideal number

The World Health Organization has aided Aravind's translation efforts by recognizing them as a Collaborating Center for the Prevention of Blindness. This official title allows Aravind to use the WHO logo in their signage, advertising, and marketing materials (WHO 2014). The expectation is that Aravind will serve as a resource for other eye clinics in the region. Aravind is one among several eye hospitals identified as collaborating centers by the WHO, such as the high-volume eye hospital L. V. Prasad in southern India and other eye hospitals in Russia, Japan, Australia, Pakistan, Saudi Arabia, the USA, Iran, and Italy (WHO 2016). However, while this official designation comes with specific requirements for submitting data to the WHO, and serving regionally as a resource center for a particular disease, it does not come with any monetary funds to support such work. Essentially, this designation by the WHO puts a globally recognized brand name on research and teaching that is already well known regionally.

The global brand name provided by the WHO likely brings more international attention to Aravind. For instance, in my first several days at Aravind, I joined a visiting group of medical and technical professionals from He Eye Hospital (in north east China). They came expressly to learn about the "Aravind model," including the interlocking innovations. The first thing we did together was watch the *Infinite Vision* video (see Krishnan 2004). It is a comprehensive (and short, only thirty-five minutes) introduction to the history of the Aravind Eye Care System. One quote from the video is particularly memorable because Dr. Venkataswamy is commenting on the efficient production and scale processes of US franchises, such as McDonald's, and suggesting something similar is necessary to bring eye health care to the rural poor people around the world. Dr. Venkataswamy's words illuminate the role that the Aravind Eye Care System and, in particular, the Lions Aravind Institute of Community Ophthalmology have played in the translation of a new "systems thinking" in eye health care.

The formation of the Lions Aravind Institute of Community Ophthalmology provides a new understanding of how a semi-periphery of calculation forms in the world-system. In addition to accumulating knowledge and mistakes, LAICO's formation required recognition by a higher status authority, the WHO, and partial funding from the LCIF.

7.3   Training in a Semi-periphery of Calculation: South–South Circulation

Aravind believes that training is integral to providing high-volume high-quality eye health care. An ophthalmologist and administrator at Aravind explains (2012), "Places such as L.V. Prasad or Tilganga or Lions SightFirst Eye Hospital–Loresho also train; however, we do more training because we have more patients." The training activities at LAICO fall into on-site classes and off-site consulting activities. In their curriculum preparations, faculty at LAICO also must consider the local context(s) of whichever eye hospital unit they are attempting to train or consult with.

Tilganga and Loresho also regularly offer courses, however, the greatest number and variety are offered by LAICO. Tilganga, Loresho, and Aravind regularly train ophthalmologists in SICS, and Tilganga regularly trains outreach microsurgical eye camp managers. In addition to the SICS course, the majority of trainees come to LAICO for a regularly scheduled course in, e.g., phacoemulsification, instrument maintenance and repair, outreach camp management, or eye hospital management. LAICO is not the only community ophthalmology training facility in India or in the global south. Like Aravind, L. V. Prasad, another large Indian multi-campus eye hospital system, also provides certified training programs for ophthalmologists, optometrists, and ophthalmic assistants.

The classes on-site at LAICO involve a mixture of learning activities typical of what one might find in any training department of any large institution: lectures, tours of Aravind's Madurai campus, educational videos, observations (of surgical wards, eye camps, eye clinics), group discussions, group in-class exercises, group homework exercises, etc. Short-term visitors participate in a 1-day or half-day superficial introduction to the "Aravind model," which LAICO offers free of cost. Such introductions typically start with the overview session (including the *Infinite Vision* video), followed by a tour and individual meetings, or observations as appropriate. LAICO will also create a special tailored several day course for eye hospitals upon request by those willing to pay.

Translation involves physical circulating medical personnel: first extracting them from other countries in the global south and global north, followed by tabulating and transforming them through a semi-periphery of calculation, and finally rotating them back to their place of origin. During my fieldwork at Aravind in 2012, I was one among many US researchers, business students, and physicians whose visits were coordinated through LAICO. Some visitors from the Indian government or Lions Clubs might come for a half-day overview session. Reporters also come for an overview session and to conduct interviews. Very few stayed longer than a week without being involved in a course, or workshop.

While overview sessions are typically without cost, most trainees will pay fees for whatever course they are taking, and also to stay in an Aravind-owned hostel. Additionally, while perusing the LAICO's official visitors list, I realized that quite a few visitors in the Aurolab-owned hostel where I lodged were not on the list because they came to Aravind through a personal contact not through LAICO. Despite the numerous short-term visitors, this quantity pales in comparison beside the hundreds who attended courses, conferences, and workshops organized by LAICO over the same time period.

LAICO tracks and tabulates the international visitors and trainees. For example, there were thirty-five groups of visitors that came through LAICO (not including trainees or conference attendees) from March 1, 2012, through July 31, 2012. They ranged in size from twelve groups of 1 person, to one group of 58 people, for a minimum total of one hundred and sixty-three individual visitors during those five months. This averages 1.5 new people per business day (24 business days per month in India). Of those thirty-five groups, their purposes were as follows: Aravind Overview (19); Press (4); MBA internship (2); Research (2); Volunteer (3); and Other (5). The country origins of those thirty-five groups were as follows: India (18); USA (9); Nepal (1); Japan (1); China (1); Chile (1); Spain (1); Unknown (3). Clearly, translation involves the circulation of medical, management, and technical personnel from other countries in the global south and global north bidirectionally through a semi-periphery of calculation. This relates to a debate about the advantages and disadvantages of circulating expert scientists who are from the global south.

Development scholars have commented on the trend where the elite experts from LEDCs are lost to more economically developed countries in a process of extraction (Commander et al. 2004). Others have offered the counter-argument that the process is more complicated: There are gains and losses by both the northern centers of industry and education, and the underdeveloped peripheries of the global south (Commander et al. 2004). Science and technology studies scholars have studied the importance of circulating scientists for facilitating scientific collaborations and helping to develop regional economies (Schøtt 1998; Shenhav and Kamens 1991; Shrum and Shenhav 1995; Ynalvez and Shrum 2011). Much of this literature's weakness is its narrow focus on the unilateral and unidirectional south–north migration as opposed to the south–south development and circulation of experts (Hujo and Piper 2007).

This chapter, and the book overall, contributes to an emerging understanding that south to south expert transformation is key to development and innovation. One estimate suggests that south–south migration is responsible for 50% of outward migration from South Asia, and 69% of outward migration from sub-Saharan Africa (Ratha and Shaw 2007, 7). Additionally, between 10 and 29% of LEDC remittances (money sent home to LEDCs by foreign workers) come from other less economically developed countries (Ratha and Shaw 2007, 11–14). Consequently, the circulation of community ophthalmology experts from Ghana, Nigeria, Mexico, northern India, Bangladesh, and Nepal through a training center in southern India repeats larger existing patterns of south–south translation.

7.4   South–South Alignment and Transformation Through Training

Translation also occurs immaterially as knowledge, skills, and ideologies flow between South Asian trainers and their trainees from around the world. In this section, I argue that these community ophthalmology professionals who come for training in SICS, community outreach course design, and eye hospital management leave transformed: enthusiastic about "systems thinking" and how their new knowledge will improve their hospital or clinic.

Ophthalmologists come from both the global north and the global south come to Aravind and Tilganga to learn SICS. Therefore, SICS dissemination occurs through training, journal publications, and conference presentations. Also, Tilganga and Aravind both have published their own curriculum materials, e.g., DVDs, books, and pamphlets to extend their interlocking innovations outwards. Such distribution has several aims: (1) entering the system of merit-based reward in ophthalmology (Latour 1987); (2) advocating the excellent free (or subsidized) services that Aravind and Tilganga are providing to rural poor patients as part of their humanitarian mission; and (3) advertising the courses they are teaching to trainees from the global south and the global north.

Dr. James Clarke (2011) and his wife (who is also his business partner) started Crystal Eye Clinic in 2003. He was first exposed to SICS at an American Academy of Ophthalmology meeting. He then learned

SICS through DVDs and by shadowing Dr. Ruit who was demonstrating the procedure in Utah. He therefore expanded his surgical repertoire, which already included ECCE and Phaco.

Dr. Clarke started using SICS on his patients in 2007. He purchases IOLs from Sri Lanka and the UK—not Tilganga-FHIOL or Aurolab. His rural eye healthcare services depend upon cost recovery through the following diverse sources of income: a donation of 50% of costs (in supplies only) from the US NGO Unite for Sight; the sale of gently used eyeglass frames donated by Unite for Sight volunteers; and income from high-income urban patients in Accra, Ghana. However, his Crystal Eye Clinic in Ghana is not financially self-sufficient with the same degree of autonomy as Aravind and Loresho. His social entrepreneurship model works well enough, although Dr. Clarke and his wife occasionally have some reservations about having enough funds to continue doing all of their work with rural patients. This demonstrates that the standardized packages (i.e., Tilganga's SICs DVDs and Aravind's eye hospital management software) serve to align actors with the global autonomous network, but do not entirely enroll actors into the accumulated niches. This exemplifies how standardized packages enable alignment, and piecemeal learning about the South Asian interlocking innovations.

The work of Tilganga Institute of Ophthalmology and other high-volume eye hospitals to train community ophthalmology professionals helps explain the "systems" discourse that has permeated the autonomous global network. Tilganga is so committed to a discourse of "systems thinking" that they use it to evaluate who is eligible for their in-demand scarce training slots for the SICS course. For an interested ophthalmologist, attending a course at Tilganga is not as easy as exchanging payment for training and making travel arrangements. Potential trainees for the SICS course at Tilganga are screened to determine their future ability to continue using the newly learned technique for the benefit of future patients. An ophthalmologist at Tilganga (unpublished interview, 2009) explains,

> We will not train doctors unless they already have resources to work with (e.g., surgical tools and supplies, a well-equipped facility, etc.) for when they return home; we make this a condition of training. Doctors pay [Tilganga] for training; they find the funds from somewhere.

Over time at Tilganga, they found that they were not just training ophthalmologists in the surgical technique or even in the cost recovery
method, but in their entire surgical delivery system.

Tilganga does not appear daunted by the difficult conditions existing
in other countries that try to implement their surgical delivery system.
The same ophthalmologist at Tilganga said (unpublished interview, 2009),

> We are interested in giving assistance directly to the people and not to
> the government. For example, we have a program in North Korea; their
> doctors come once a year and we go to North Korea once a year and work
> with them. When they came, they had more exposure to high volume
> surgery and their hands were sharpened and their skill increased.

The community ophthalmology professionals at Tilganga continued practicing SICS locally and globally during the Nepalese civil
war, despite Nepal's poverty and government instability. Thus, they
are strong advocates for community-embedded science, technology,
and infrastructure development. This also meant Tilganga's community ophthalmology professionals were not shy about participating in
Himalayan Cataract Project's ophthalmologist training program for the
United Nations Millennium Villages Project. HCP circulated Nepalese
ophthalmologists and ophthalmic assistants to African villages to conduct training, and African ophthalmologists to Nepal to be trained
(Sachs 2007; Tabin and Newick 2008; Hayden 2010). The outcome
of Tilganga's careful trainee selection is that they are using training to
reproduce new high-volume eye hospitals and contributing to infrastructure creation for eye health care in the global south.

In addition to training outreach camp managers, LAICO teaches
experienced outreach camp managers how to design their own training programs to reproduce more outreach camp managers through. An
example is Loresho's ongoing development into a training center for
outreach camp managers.

Dr. Fayaz Khan came to Aravind in the late 1990s, a few years
after establishing Loresho, to upgrade his surgical skills from ECCE
to M-SICS. Although he learned M-SICS, what he came away most
excited about was Aravind's Taylorist and Fordist approach to an

efficient surgical systems approach. Trainees may return to Aravind for a new course or a refresher course. Some trainees may proselytize to their eye unit about sending more employees for training at LAICO. Frequently, trainees at Aravind end their course with the desire to consult with faculty at LAICO about how to better mirror the Aravind model in their own clinics. In 2008, Loresho (funded by LCIF and the Irish NGO Right to Sight) asked LAICO to help them become a training center.

Included among several years of LAICO documents about Loresho was a report that the marketing director, Peter Ndigwa (2008), prepared for Loresho board members about his training at Aravind Eye Care System and his participation in the Eye Excel program in October 2008,

> Though the Aravind set up is quite different from ours....Due to the high population in India, both trainers and trainees are easily available.
>
> The implication of the above is that we have to tailor our training centre [sic] to suit our African setup. We need to adapt some of the ways they conduct their training and at the same time adopt the training to suit the manpower and resources available.
>
> ....
>
> ...to make Lions SightFirst Eye Hospital an African Model of Aravind and our Training Centre a small LAICO.

In this report, it becomes clear that Peter Ndigwa is interested in appropriating the Aravind model for Kenya. His interest results in part from LAICO faculty's careful work to align what Aravind does with what is possible in other contexts.

With help from LAICO, Loresho now has the ability to train new outreach camp managers, but they are still strengthening this program. In 2008, Loresho's outreach camp manager, Joseph Macharia, received funding from the NGO Right to Sight (Ireland) to go through his second training at LAICO; he is now certified by Aravind to train other outreach camp managers. Subsequently, Macharia created the Loresho outreach camp management training manual. He then started training more outreach camp managers for Loresho, as well as one for a different eye unit in Kenya, and another for an eye unit in Cameroon.

By conducting courses for foreign trainees, the staff at LAICO and Tilganga unilaterally transfer "systems thinking" in community ophthalmology from South Asia outwards. Sociologist Bradford Gray (1992) writes in a population and public health journal that there is a core difference between public health medicine and clinical medicine: While public health medicine focuses on community-wide outcomes, clinical medicine focuses on individual patient outcomes. Therefore, this South Asian "systems thinking" is unique because it melds the global public health emphasis on community-wide outcomes, with the Western clinical medicine emphasis on the doctor's responsibility to provide the best outcome for each individual patient. The message from South Asia is that, if one cares to think systematically, one can come up with excellent individual outcomes that are community wide. Trainees take up this message with enthusiasm,

> I went for a hospital administrator's management training program. I really enjoyed the training and I think it is very useful. Sala Uno is inspired by Aravind; I almost feel like I am meeting Sala Uno's mother. (Juan Carlos Rodriguez, unpublished interview, 2012)

Enrolling trainees in courses is a process for transforming them into systems thinkers within community ophthalmology. In these courses, the trainees practice solving population health problems while thinking systematically about individual patient outcomes, hospital outcomes, and global disease eradication efforts. They can also purchase training materials (pamphlets and books created by Aravind), or pick up other standardized packages, such as blank forms from the Aravind Eye Hospital-Madurai records department, at no cost.

Juan Carlos Rodriguez (unpublished interview, 2012) illustrates this by describing his experience in the forty-five-day eye hospital management course at LAICO, saying, "It was a very interesting training program. It really helped me to have a wider point of view of an eye hospital.... They gave us a wide range of topics in order to have a more comprehensive point of view on how to manage these kinds of systems."

I participated in one full day of the course in which Juan Carlos was enrolled. That day, the class was taught by Sanil Joseph (MHA), who is a faculty member at LAICO. In an interactive exercise, he carefully led us to the conclusion that the hospital infrastructure problem that we management trainees had to solve was actually a hospital operations problem in disguise. At the exercise's beginning, Sanil showed us a picture of a hospital waiting area and provided some statistics. Long story short, the waiting room was too small and thus congested; patients were complaining. The question that we had to answer was about infrastructure, how could the hospital get more space to relieve the crowd?

We had time to brainstorm and talk to each other in small groups to arrive at an answer. However, the correct answer had little to do with expanding the space and everything to do with utilizing the existing space more effectively. By opening the hospital one half hour earlier, closing one half hour later, and giving patients that live locally and walk-in that morning an appointment the same afternoon, we could achieve two results: (1) higher patient satisfaction from a more spacious waiting room and (2) more even patient load distribution throughout the day instead of a high influx in the morning with few to no patients in the afternoon and evening. With this new schedule, there would be less chance of a patient arriving in the morning and waiting in a crowded room all day, without being seen by a doctor.

This is just one small example what LAICO teaches hospital management trainees. As illustrated above, this training is not always tailored to the specific problems of managing eye diseases. Yet, eye hospital managers in the global south find the operations management expertise LAICO instills both desirable and useful.

Juan Carlos's training at LAICO first demonstrated to him the necessary technologies and processes to incorporate at Sala Uno to create improvements. Eye hospital managers find such details important, and LAICO has trained many eye hospital managers, including, in the late 2000s, the accountant turned hospital manager from Loresho, Shamsherali Datoo, and the human resources manager at Sala Uno, Andrea Portilla.

Aravind is not the only institution that provides training for eye hospital managers. Additionally, L. V. Prasad, other high-volume eye hospitals in India, and the Kilimanjaro Center for Community Ophthalmology in Tanzania offer such training (Mehta and Shenoy 2011). However, when I asked some management trainees why they chose Aravind, they told me that either: (1) it was the cheapest program; (2) their INGO partner sponsored them and chose Aravind for training; or (3) they had not heard of the other programs. As discussed throughout this book, cost is not a trivial consideration for community ophthalmology professionals. Also, one can see Aravind's early and prominent role in the autonomous global network to eradicate blindness, and the invisible work of disseminated standardized packages which align professionals to be interested in further knowledge from Aravind. Finally, the third answer indicates the influence of the WHO's recognition of Aravind as a collaborating center.

From the above examples I can infer that, transforming trainees and enrolling them (as part of the accumulation of niches) requires teaching them a few of the autonomous global network's emerging rules: sarvodaya, community-embedded, high volume. This is why before I ever visited LAICO, I could go to the Unite for Sight Global Health & Innovation conference in the USA, and learn about "systems thinking" in eye health care from the eye hospital director of Kalinga Eye Hospital from Odisha (Orissa), India. The Kalinga Eye Hospital's director was presenting how, over the eleven years since starting, his institution had learned economic self-reliance and to eliminate redundancy in their systems (note: They too had trained at Aravind).

7.5   South–South Extension of the Eye Hospital

The south–south circulation of expert personnel through the semi-periphery of calculation and their subsequent transformation into systems thinker is not the only example of niche alignment. Frequently, in their efforts to extend their interlocking innovations, LAICO faculty travel outside India to consult with eye hospitals and clinics. In other words, the LAICO and Tilganga physically extend themselves outside South Asia.

LAICO's emphasis on reproducing eye hospitals also means they are focused on endogenous infrastructure for eye health care in the global south. Thulasiraj Ravilla explains (unpublished interview, 2012),

...[S]o that largely comes from that true commitment saying that we need more people involved in this. You know, if we really want to reduce blindness. So our dissemination has happened through that or [has been] driven by that energy, I would say ...

LAICO is unique because of its consultancy services where, as part of a site visit, a faculty member prepares an individualized, step-by-step guide for how to improve an eye hospital's productivity and efficiency. Whether LAICO faculty are designing a national eye care program in Rwanda (Mehta and Shenoy 2011, 189–98), or, helping increase the patient volume at a small Lions Eye Hospital an hour or two from Madurai within Tamil Nadu, they go through the same careful and methodical process. First, they perform research to evaluate the context that shapes the specific conditions for the institution with which they will consult (be it a corporate eye hospital, an NGO eye hospital, an eye unit in a government hospital, or even, perhaps, a government council or a national advisory board). They might have several phone conversations and e-mail communications with the potential clients. In some cases, the LAICO faculty members have already met key staff from the client institution in previous months, most likely when they came for a training seminar. Frequently, trainees find the LAICO faculty approachable and the training seminar useful, precipitating their request for further training services for their institution. Second, after collecting the necessary background information, the LAICO faculty member then performs a site visit where they: tour the facilities, note instruments (those present and those needed), and ask specific questions about inputs and outputs, i.e., "How many patients do you typically have? How many full-time staff? What are your working hours?" They use the answers received, together with the previously collected information, to develop a new plan or program. Essentially, this plan or program takes an idea previously developed at the Aravind Eye Care System and redefines it to fit the specific institution. It includes a method to monitor the results (often with the help of LAICO faculty at the early stages), etc.

The nonprofit arm of a foreign business consultancy group trained LAICO faculty members in consulting work. In 2006, the British finance consulting firm Westcott Williams, inspired by Dr. Venkataswamy, decided to spend 10% of their time (and their profits) performing consulting services for NGOs that perform social work that helps persons with disabilities. Every year since that time, they have come and performed a three-day workshop for LAICO faculty and other interested medical and non-medical staff across the Aravind Eye Care System (Herzlinger 2010). In 2012, the coordinator for Westcott Williams' work with Aravind was Sanil Joseph. He and other LAICO faculty were trained in the art of influencing clients to bring about sustainable changes in their work spaces and work practices. Sanil emphasized that the first key step is building rapport and credibility. Also, he insisted that you cannot just casually tell your client what to do; performing careful background research about their particular situation helps you to understand the complete picture as fully as possible so that you can get "buy-in" from your client. Both Sanil and another faculty member at LAICO dislike the word "argument" when discussing the consultant work that they perform with eye units. As this other faculty member explains,

> It is not necessary to argue with them. Our objective is to make them understand the need for changes or the need for improvement.... Perhaps they say, 'So that is possible for Aravind and that is not possible for us'... then we have to explain the level of possibilities for some changes. .... Suppose someone comes from Cambodia, from China, from [an] extreme part of India? I should not argue with them ... I can insist but I cannot make an argument. (LAICO Faculty Member 2012)

As shown in the above excerpted quote, faculty members are strategic. They demonstrate respect for the management trainees' authority and local knowledge, and attention to difficulties due to local politics. They also attempt to connect the trainees' knowledge to the faculty's evidence-based examples of successful innovations inside and outside of Aravind.

The trainers' care and attention to local knowledge is to better impose their own authoritative knowledge on the trainees.

The LAICO faculty's sensitivity to cultural context means that they are deliberate in trying to adapt interlocking innovations into strategies, plans, and training materials. One LAICO faculty member (unpublished interview, 2012) explains,

> Whatever the strategy we develop for any place, we need to fine tune for the local condition. We cannot fix any strategy to achieve. At the time of implementation we have to be a little flexible to operate ... Modification may be required
>
> ...
>
> I remember ... for Malawi we considered ... first what is the potential there? ....So we looked at data to get a sense of market potential; when we fixed the target we considered the available resources ... to convert the resources into utilization part we need to do some kind of strategies .... We oriented the stakeholders, particularly the technicians working in different areas....

A second LAICO faculty member (unpublished interview, 2012) described three examples of how to modify previous plans or programs to fit a specific context. First, the surgical theater opening and closing times are essential to the high-volume patient throughput. However, while this is standard at 7:30 a.m. across the eye hospitals within the Aravind Eye Care System in India, there may be less assurance of personal safety for community ophthalmology professionals who will not travel during when there is not daylight in other places around the world. Therefore, it is necessary to adjust the schedule to fit what is best for the local context.

Second, in Africa the eye camps cannot be conducted in the same manner as in India. The population density is very high in India with a short distance between two towns. In comparison, while individual towns in African countries may have a large population, there is frequently a large distance between two towns. Therefore, the frequency and location of outreach camps may need adjustment.

Third, Aravind assumes that the eye unit can both generate and control its funds when it teaches the Robin Hood model. However, clients may be working in eye units within larger government or private hospitals, where they cannot keep the funds their work has generated. This second LAICO faculty member points out that, in the absence of direct control over the revenue stream, the clients may usefully adapt the pricing structure that Aravind has developed. By making their eye unit a source of revenue to the larger institution, the clients might "command respect from the central hospital administration, they will be able to say, 'we need this or we need that'," says the second LAICO faculty member (unpublished interview, 2012).

After gathering data on-site at the client eye institution, and creating a plan to fit the local context, LAICO faculty present this plan to the client's upper-level administrators and staff. During their presentation, they leverage examples from their previous work in eye health management within India, and from their previous consulting experiences, in order to convince these clients of their proposed plan's viability.

In the examples above, LAICO's goal was to teach eye hospital managers how to improve the efficiency and productivity within their respective eye units. Thulasiraj Ravilla (TedIndia 2009) was delighted to report that,

> We created competition for ourselves, ...We proactively and systematically promoted these practices to many hospitals in India, many in our own backyards and then in other parts of the world as well. The impact of this has been that these hospitals, in the second year after our consultation, are double their output and then achieve financial recovery as well [sic].

Dr. S. Aravind estimates only 20% of the 300 hospitals currently using the "Aravind model" are actually using the full model (Mehta and Shenoy 2011; Rosenberg 2013). This indicates the work LAICO faculty must undertake to extract useful background data and cases, and use them to create strategies, plans, and curriculum about interlocking innovations that are adaptable for a specific biophysical and psychosocial context outside of southern India. While the interlocking innovations are known in piecemeal and partial ways, the overarching ethos of a systems approach is emerging and dominating in the accumulating niches, stretching from India and Nepal, to Ghana, Kenya, and Mexico.

7.6 Conclusion: Translation of Interlocking Innovations and Niche Accumulation

In this chapter, I have argued that translation is unilateral, operating through bidirectional movement of data, people, knowledge, and technology to accumulate niches and reproduce interlocking innovations.

A semi-periphery of calculation can translate its own interlocking innovations, thereby enrolling more allies into the autonomous global network dedicated to eradicating and controlling blindness, and furthermore accumulating more niches. This chapter primarily discussed two semi-peripheries of calculation which were recognized by a higher status authority in the world-system. LAICO's authority to share knowledge with other community ophthalmology clinics and hospitals around the world was highlighted and accentuated by their official designation by the WHO as a Collaborating Center for the Prevention of Blindness. Likewise, Tilganga's surgical systems approach was made more authoritative with official recognition from the UNDP.

In addition to LAICO's courses, other training activities are provided by Tilganga Institute of Ophthalmology and Lions SightFirst Eye Hospital, -Loresho. All three of these sites serve as knowledge-sharing platforms that cater primarily to community ophthalmology professionals from the global south. Community ophthalmology trainers are translating this idea of "systems thinking," but this is enacted through standardized packages, alignment, and transformation.

South Asian supralocal standards are disseminated among the larger autonomous global network through standardized packages. Knowledge about patients, surgical techniques, and ophthalmic consumables is produced and then packaged in one place (e.g., Aravind or Tilganga) as DVDs, hospital management software, pamphlets, or books. Subsequently, this knowledge is disseminated unilaterally to many other places, e.g., other eye hospitals in the global south. The American Academy of Ophthalmology and other ophthalmic member association meetings serve as important sites for disseminating standardized packages. The simplicity of a standardized package does not make for easy transfer of science and technology-practice from one location to another.

Most frequently, a standardized package inspires new allies to apply to Aravind or Tilganga for training; this begins their alignment to the rules of the global autonomous network to eradicate blindness.

Alignment involves careful selection and extraction of trainees. Extraction refers to the circulation of people, data, etc., from a subordinate position to the more dominant semi-periphery of calculation and back again. At the local level, this involves extracting patients from rural areas to urban centers. Globally, this involves extracting tabulated data about patients from semi-peripheries of calculation to the WHO, as well as circulating professionals from the global north and other countries in the global south to South Asian semi-peripheries of calculation for training. Tilganga is guided by the "systems thinking" ideology to preselect trainees that will have local support to implement what they will learn.

The imposition of power through alignment and transformation is typical of the translation mode of circulation. Tilganga and LAICO employees share a "systems thinking" ideology through their: targeted courses "teaching the trainers," other management courses, and site-based consulting activities. On the one hand, these trainers and consultants are interested in transforming the local context to fit their own models. They selectively extract data from interactions with trainees and clients to demonstrate how the local context might successfully be adapted to fit their models. On the other hand, the trainees and client institutions are well aware that the model must be adapted to their local context. The trainees and client institutions adopt interlocking innovations in piecemeal yet context-appropriate ways.

Inculcating enthusiasm for interlocking innovations is also part of transforming trainees and clients. Aravind's founder and other Aravind employees had an early enthusiasm for improving productivity and efficiency within their organization that they also used to train other community ophthalmology professionals outside their organization. Transformation involves changing the trainees' or clients' expectations and knowledge. Before leaving Aravind or Tilganga, they are interested in solving the problem of avoidable blindness through the interlocking innovations of: management strategies, surgical techniques, surgical theater logistical practices, cheap South Asian ophthalmic consumables, and an ideology of sarvodaya.

Aravind and Tilganga deliberately set out to reproduce smaller versions of themselves. This transformative work is essentially what Latour might call a laboratory "extension." In order to reproduce cheap eye health care for individual patients, a translation process occurs where the eye hospital itself is extended into a new context: from India or Nepal to another country less economically developed country. "But how can laboratory practice be extended? .... [T]he answer is simple: only by extending the laboratory itself" (Latour 1983, 150–51). Thus, it seems that for these interlocking innovations to successfully extend on "rails" (to borrow from Latour's vocabulary), the local context must be shaped to become more in alignment with the context from which the interlocking innovations have emerged (Fujimura 1987).

Finally, the increasing number of links between interlocking innovations, specialized groups, infrastructures, government departments, agencies, professional organizations, higher education institutions, factories, etc., "leads to irreversibility, mutual dependencies and path dependence" (Geels 2005a, 92), that is technological momentum. Dr. Venkataswamy's dream to perfect patient eyesight through the spread of an efficient, productive model for providing eye health care is coming to fruition.

In the next chapter, I will discuss how community ophthalmologists, in pursuit of the best science and technology at the lowest cost to serve their rural poor patients, have initiated a struggle between phacoemulsification versus the SICS; this has launched them into the spotlight in the global field of ophthalmology.

References

Bakker, Sjoerd, Pieter Leguijt, and Harro van Lente. 2015. "Niche Accumulation and Standardization—The Case of Electric Vehicle Recharging Plugs." *Journal of Cleaner Production* 94 (May): 155–64.
Basalla, George. 1967. "The Spread of Western Science." *Science* 156: 611–22.
Central Intelligence Agency. 2012. "The World Factbook — Central Intelligence Agency." Central Intelligence Agency Library, The World Factbook. https://www.cia.gov/library/publications/the-world-factbook/.

Commander, Simon, Mari Kangasniemi, and L. Alan Winters. 2004. "The Brain Drain: Curse or Boon? A Survey of the Literature." In *Challenges to Globalization: Analyzing the Economics*, edited by Robert E. Baldwin and L. Alan Winters, 235–78. Chicago: University of Chicago Press.

Englander, Karen. 2014. "The Rise of English as the Language of Science." In *Writing and Publishing Science Research Papers in English*, edited by Karen Englander, 3–4. Dordrecht: Springer Netherlands. http://link.springer.com/10.1007/978-94-007-7714-9_1.

Fujimura, Joan H. 1987. "Constructing 'Do-Able' Problems in Cancer Research: Articulating Alignment." *Social Studies of Science* 17 (2): 257–93.

———. 1988. "The Molecular Biological Bandwagon in Cancer Research: Where Social Worlds Meet." *Social Problems* 35 (3): 261–83.

Geels, Frank W. 2005a. "Conceptual Perspective on Systems Innovations and Technological Transitions." In *Technological Transitions and System Innovations: A Co-evolutionary and Socio-Technical Analysis*, 75–102. Cheltenham and Northampton, MA: Edward Elgar.

———. 2005b. "The Dynamics of Transitions in Socio-Technical Systems: A Multi-level Analysis of the Transition Pathway from Horse-Drawn Carriages to Automobiles (1860–1930)." *Technology Analysis & Strategic Management* 17 (4): 445–76.

———. 2005c. "Processes and Patterns in Transitions and System Innovations: Refining the Co-evolutionary Multi-level Perspective." *Technological Forecasting and Social Change*, Transitions Towards Sustainability Through System Innovation, 72 (6): 681–96.

Geels, Frank W., and Johan Schot. 2007. "Typology of Sociotechnical Transition Pathways." *Research Policy* 36 (3): 399–417.

Gray, Bradford H. 1992. "World Blindness and the Medical Profession: Conflicting Medical Cultures and the Ethical Dilemmas of Helping." *The Milbank Quarterly* 70 (3): 535.

Harding, Sandra. 2008. *Sciences from Below: Feminisms, Postcolonialities and Modernities*. Durham, NC: Duke University Press.

Hayden, Faith A. 2010. "Expanding Outreach: A Look at the Himalayan Cataract Project's Past, Present & Future." *Eyeworld*, December. https://www.eyeworld.org/article-expanding-outreach--a-look-at-the-himalayan-cataract-project.

Herzlinger, Regina. 2010. *The Global Sight Network Initiative*. Harvard Business School. Retrieved December 9, 2012. http://papers.ssrn.com/sol3/papers.cfm?abstract_id=1991930.

Hess, David J. 1995. *Science and Technology in a Multicultural World: The Cultural Politics of Facts and Artifacts*. New York: Columbia University Press.

Hughes, Thomas Parke. 1987. "The Evolution of Large Technological Systems." In *The Social Construction of Technological Systems: New Directions in the Sociology and History of Technology*, edited by Wiebe E. Bijker, Thomas Parke Hughes, and Trevor J. Pinch, 51–82. Cambridge: The MIT Press.

Hujo, Katja, and Nicola Piper. 2007. "South–South Migration: Challenges for Development and Social Policy." *Development* 50 (4): 19–25.

IAPB. 2016. "IAPB History." IAPB History | International Agency for the Prevention of Blindness. http://www.iapb.org/about-iapb/iapb-history.

Jöns, Heike. 2011. "Centre of Calculation." In *The SAGE Handbook of Geographical Knowledge*, 158–70. London: Sage.

Kleinman, Daniel Lee. 1998. "Untangling Context: Understanding a University Laboratory in the Commercial World." *Science, Technology, & Human Values* 23 (3): 285–314.

Krishnan, Pavithra. 2004. *Infinite Vision: Dr. Govindappa Venkataswamy*. Aravind Eye Care System.

Latour, Bruno. 1983. "Give Me a Laboratory and I Will Raise the World." In *Science Observed: Perspectives on the Social Study of Science*, edited by Karin D. Knorr-Cetina and Michael Mulkay, 141–70. London: Sage.

———. 1987. *Science in Action: How to Follow Scientists and Engineers Through Society*. Cambridge, MA: Harvard University Press.

Marseille, Elliot. 1994. "Intraocular Lenses, Blindness Control, and the Hiding Hand." In *Rethinking the Development Experience: Essays Provoked by the Work of Albert O. Hirschman*, edited by Lloyd Rodwin and Donald A. Schön, 147–75. Washington, DC and Cambridge, MA: Brookings Institution and Lincoln Institute of Land Policy.

Medina, Leandro Rodriguez. 2014. *Centers and Peripheries in Knowledge Production*. 1st ed. Vol. 115. Routledge Advances in Sociology. New York, NY: Routledge.

Mehta, Pavithra K., and Suchitra Shenoy. 2011. *Infinite Vision: How Aravind Became the World's Greatest Business Case for Compassion*. San Francisco, CA: Berrett-Koehler Publishers.

Ndigwa, Peter. 2008. "A Report by Peter Ndigwa on the Education Trip to LAICO." Report Prepared for the Board of Members, Lions SightFirst Eye Hospital–Loresho, Nairobi, Kenya.

Nye, David E. 2013. *America's Assembly Line*. Cambridge: MIT Press.

O'Connell, Joseph. 1993. "Metrology: The Creation of Universality by the Circulation of Particulars." *Social Studies of Science* 23 (1): 129–73.

Pigg, Stacy L. 1995. "Acronyms and Effacement: Traditional Medical Practitioners (TMP) in International Health Development." *Social Science & Medicine* 41: 47–68.

Raj, Kapil. 2006. *Relocating Modern Science: Circulation and the Construction of Knowledge in South Asia and Europe, 1650–1900.* New Delhi: Permanent Black.

Ratha, Dilip, and William Shaw. 2007. "South-South Migration and Remittances." World Bank Working Paper 102. World Bank, Washington, DC.

Raven, Rob. 2007. "Niche Accumulation and Hybridisation Strategies in Transition Processes Towards a Sustainable Energy System: An Assessment of Differences and Pitfalls." *Energy Policy* 35 (4): 2390–400.

Ritzer, George. 1996. "The McDonaldization Thesis: Is Expansion Inevitable?" *International Sociology* 11 (3): 291–308.

Rosenberg, Tina. 2013. "A Hospital Network with a Vision." *The New York Times.* Opinion Pages—Opinionator. Retrieved April 16, 2013. http://opinionator.blogs.nytimes.com/2013/01/16/in-india-leading-a-hospital-franchise-with-vision/.

Rubin, Harriet. 2001. "The Perfect Vision of Dr. V." *Fast Company*, January 31. Retrieved May 1, 2009. http://www.fastcompany.com/42111/perfect-vision-dr-v.

Sachs, Jeffrey D. 2007. "A Global Coalition of Good." *Time*, September 6. Retrieved May 3, 2010. http://www.time.com/time/magazine/article/0,9171,1659725,00.html.

Schøtt, Thomas. 1998. "Ties Between Center and Periphery in the Scientific World-System: Accumulation of Rewards, Dominance and Self-Reliance in the Center." *Journal of World-Systems Research* 4 (2): 112–44.

Shenhav, Yehouda A., and David H. Kamens. 1991. "The 'Costs' of Institutional Isomorphism: Science in Non-Western Countries." *Social Studies of Science* 21 (3): 527–45.

Shrum, Wesley, and Yehouda Shenhav. 1995. "Science and Technology in Less Developed Countries." In *Handbook of Science and Technology Studies*, edited by Sheila Jasanoff, Gerald E. Markle, James C. Petersen, and Trevor J. Pinch, 627–51. Thousand Oaks, CA: Sage.

Tabin, Geoffrey, and Emily R. Newick. 2008. "Eye Care for the Millennium Villages." *Cataract & Refractive Surgery Today*, April. Retrieved February 27, 2010. http://bmctoday.net/crstoday/2008/04/article.asp?f=CRST0408_05.php.

TedIndia. 2009. Thulasiraj Ravilla: How Low-Cost Eye Care Can Be World-Class | Video on TED.Com. India: TED Conferences LLC. Retrieved November 2, 2012 (http://www.ted.com/talks/thulasiraj_ravilla_how_low_cost_eye_care_can_be_wowor_class.html).

United Nations Development Programme. 2017. "Human Development Index (HDI) | Human Development Reports." United Nations Development Programme Human Development Reports. http://hdr.undp.org/en/content/human-development-index-hdi.

Wallerstein, Immanuel. 1974. "The Rise and Future Demise of the World Capitalist System: Concepts for Comparative Analysis." *Comparative Studies in Society and History* 16: 387–415.

Williams, Logan D. A. 2012, April 5. "Direct Observation Fieldnotes. SF 1588-Enhance Eye Care Services at Lions Eye Hospitals in India Vision Building, Strategic Planning Workshop." Lions Aravind Institute of Community Ophthalmology, Madurai, India.

———. 2012, July 17. "Direct Observation Fieldnotes. Eye Excel: Expanding Global Eye Care Workforce Excellence in Training." Lions Aravind Institute of Community Ophthalmology, Madurai, India.

WHO. 2014. "Terms and Conditions for WHO Collaborating Centres." World Health Organization. http://www.who.int/collaboratingcentres/Terms_and_conditions_for_WHOCCS.pdf.

———. 2016. "WHO | WHO Collaborating Centres Database." WHO Collaborating Centres Database, April 14. http://www.who.int/collaboratingcentres/database/en/.

Ynalvez, Marcus Antonius, and Wesley M. Shrum. 2011. "Professional Networks, Scientific Collaboration, and Publication Productivity in Resource-Constrained Research Institutions in a Developing Country." *Research Policy* 40 (2): 204–16.

8

Evidence-Based Medicine: Contesting the Phaco-Regime

Politics. Not just national politics, but also politics between you and me. If you are bringing a new thing, then the established ones are always wondering [about] it. Then we had to keep fighting; we had to be on our toes to negate whatever comes out. (Community Ophthalmologist at Tilganga Institute of Ophthalmology 2012)

When ophthalmologists in Mexico learned about Sala Uno, many became very upset. Co-CEO Javier Okhuysen (2012) explains, "The model has been very disruptive. [Our competitors] think we are dumping our costs. They don't understand how something can grow so fast." Sala Uno's director of community outreach, Jorge Léon de La Barra, further explains:

> So you get the love and hate. We try to make them understand we are not trying to take their patients; rather we are trying to make services available to those [low-income people] who do not have service. But yeah it is a collateral damage that some [high-income] patients do say 'hey it is cheaper here,' and they come.

Sala Uno's experience of "the love and the hate" in Mexico City, Mexico, exemplifies how contesting the Phaco-regime plays out locally.

© The Author(s) 2019
L. D. A. Williams, *Eradicating Blindness*,
https://doi.org/10.1007/978-981-13-1625-8_8

While in Mexico, like elsewhere, the user fee for service model prevails, individual private physicians will treat a few patients, charging each a high price. In contrast, Sala Uno follows the high-volume practices they learned from Aravind; their numerous counselors, optometrists, and ophthalmic nurses work together with their few ophthalmologists to treat many patients, charging each a low price. "By doing that we will be just as profitable and sustainable," says co-CEO Carlos Orellana.

Traditional ophthalmic competitors are very angry because Sala Uno has lowered prices for cataract surgery—so angry that rumors have been spreading that Mexican medical societies have banned Sala Uno's ophthalmologists from membership. Dr. Juan Pablo Olivares (2012), the chief medical officer of Sala Uno, explains,

> First of all, it hasn't been really that Sala Uno has been, or its doctors have been, banned from any medical society for doing SICS. It is more like a gossip thing that you know that some doctors are not very fond of the procedure. And word of mouth is preying inside the ophthalmologist community against Sala Uno. That's been mostly what's been happening.

However, in emails between the two co-CEOs, prestigious Western ophthalmologists, friends of Sala Uno, and friends of the Aravind Eye Care System, it appears that the contentious elements of this SICS versus Phaco debate in Mexico may have not started out as just rumor. In them, Okhuysen and Orellana solicit practical advice because the president of a major ophthalmic society that is important in Mexico is threatening their physicians. The co-CEOs receive some strategies on how to win allies for Sala Uno within the field of ophthalmology in Mexico. They are told to emphasize that they serve the "bottom of the pyramid" and that their model is different, but not wrong. However, when interviewed, Sala Uno employees have suppressed the debate's contentiousness. This is likely a strategic decision to continue the work of treating patients and collecting evidence in the face of the local outcry in the field of ophthalmology, which, while loud, does not appear to have teeth. Former adversaries in the field of science may later become advocates after the emotional furor of the debate shifts into the territory negotiation, ally enrolling, and evidence building of agonistic engagement (Delborne 2008). This was certainly true when South Asian ophthalmologists developed their own intraocular lens-manufacturing facilities (Chapter 5) and can likely be generalized to acrimonious epistemic debates in science or medicine overall.

The intent of this chapter is to demonstrate how community ophthalmology professionals engage in epistemic and material contestation that is concurrent with their shift from a subordinate to a more dominant position in the global field of science. The remainder of this chapter has the following structure: Sect. 8.1 starts by introducing the concepts of contestation and breakthrough of innovations. Section 8.2 analyzes the status position of community ophthalmologists in the world-system and how this connects to their practices. Next, Sect. 8.3 discusses the difference between evidence-based medicine and the cost-effectiveness movement as it relates to the global debate between the Phaco-regime and community ophthalmologists. Section 8.4 illuminates the unique scientific management and assembly line features of operating theater practice by community ophthalmologists; these unique practices invented in South Asia have been celebrated within the autonomous global network as the surgical systems approach. Subsequently, Sect. 8.5 discusses the debate initiated globally when Aravind and Tilganga take a stand against Western aseptic techniques by using evidence to confirm that their own surgical systems approach, with its different aseptic technique, provides more efficient outcomes with the same safety level. Section 8.6 indicates that this stance indicates breakthrough in the multi-level perspective; community ophthalmologists, after accumulating niches, have now birthed their own SICS-regime from the interstices of the Phaco-regime. Finally, Sect. 8.7 concludes with a discussion for how this informs the conceptualization of contestation and systemic technology choice.

8.1 Theory: Contestation and Breakthrough from Niche to Regime

In this chapter, I argue that repeated contestation creates a fracture point in the old regime, which subsequently becomes two regimes. Challengers contest the incumbent regime's rules and technological trajectories. Most of the challenges remain private between actors. The few public challenges help to broadcast (and thus validate) the global existence of dual regimes.

Contestation has long been an important part of science and technology studies. Scholarship on contestation has previously focused on public controversies in science (Epstein 1995; Nelkin 1992; Wynne 1992), public controversies in technology (Mazur 1975; Jasper 1988), controversies and scientific change (Collins and Restivo 1983; Delborne 2008; Griffith and Mullins 1972; Hess 2016), and controversies and technological change (Hess 2005; Hård 1993). These controversy studies have critiqued Kuhnian paradigms and Mertonian institutionalism as providing insufficient explanation for scientific and technological change over time.

Previous work by science and technology studies scholars determined that controversies are integral to produce novel science and technology (Delborne 2008, 511; Epstein 1995; Hård 1993; Nelkin 1992; Nieusma 2007). However, the degree that controversies are integrated with the circulation of science and technology remains unknown.

[T]he successful design of appropriate technology recognizes that design, implementation, and use of the technology are not separate and linear phases, but rather simultaneous and circular processes… technical change brings about social change and vice versa–… this is the only way in which a sustainable sociotechnical arrangement can be achieved. (de Laet 2002, 4)

Anthropologist Marianne de Laet (2002) argues above that separating scientific knowledge production from its circulation is not easy. Yet, with globalization shifting how scientists cooperate and compete to disseminate their knowledge products, it is important to contextualize scientific controversies within a global field of science. The shifts in political-economic ideology, technical communication, social organization, and status hierarchies between expert scientists (or technologists) must necessarily correspond to shifts in what knowledge and artifacts circulate across the globe, to whom, and why. In addition to contestation being integral to production processes of knowledge and artifacts, contestation is also integral to science and technology circulation.

Conflict studies can enhance the study of change in socio-technical systems. Instead of offering the technological determinist argument that technologies induce social change, some scholars have struggled to explain how social change induces technological change: First, social constructivists argued that the social interests of relevant groups select scientific problems and stabilize technology design (Pinch and Bijker 1987); second, Hård (1993) combined constructivism and conflict sociology to suggest that social groups with greater resources use technology selection to apply power, that is, subordinate, control, or exclude other groups; and third, Hess (2005, 2016) extended conflict sociology to demonstrate that the new product and technology design suggestions arising from industrial transition movements are selectively incorporated by corporations, and therefore, the end result is a limited industrial reform. Conflict studies describe change within the incumbent regime in one of three ways: "Stability (powerful actors suppress change), incremental change ('reform' to accommodate protests) and radical change ('overthrow' by challengers)" (Geels 2010, 504). However, this does not explain how challengers employ interlocking innovations to fracture an incumbent regime into dual socio-technical regimes.

Some scholars using the multi-level perspective draw upon political ecology to inform their definition of power in socio-technical regimes. They suggest that power is reflected in decision-making processes, both by who controls participant selection and involvement, as well as, which language and discourse are used to support arguments and influence allies (Lawhon and Murphy 2012, 367). They remind us of inequality's durability: Those dominant actors who already have a high-status position in the landscape and regime are more likely to have their interests supported (Lawhon and Murphy 2012, 364; Hess 2016; Hess et al. 2016). Indeed, transitions are less likely to happen when such incumbents have the power to oppress or ignore challengers to the incumbent regime (Geels 2010, 502; Hess 2016). Therefore, socio-technical transitions require shifts in the balance of power between incumbents and challengers. One way to shift the balance of power is if the challengers gather allies through niche-accumulation (Geels 2010, 502). Challengers begin this process through normative contestation, where social movements or expert activists who want to change performance criteria in the incumbent regime oppose incumbent actors using a variety of commonly used collective action strategies (Elzen et al. 2011, 263; Hess 2016).

I argue that contestation is the movement of knowledge and artifacts from challengers in a subordinate position in the world-system to incumbent actors in the dominant position that involves an acrimonious bidirectional and bilateral exchange between the two positions. Contestation and scientific change in the various sciences has occurred with the following dynamics: A group of highly creative challengers form around a new theory, practice, or radical technology in opposition to incumbents (Griffith and Mullins 1972); the challengers propagate their new theory in part because they have high levels of in-group communication and solidarity (Collins 2012; Griffith and Mullins 1972; Mullins 1975); charismatic leadership and proselytizing (Mullins 1975); and ability to leverage allies (Collins 2012; Griffith and Mullins 1972; Mullins 1975) and material resources (Collins 2012; Griffith and Mullins 1972).

The high degree of bitter and hostile behavior and rhetoric directed by the incumbents against the challengers during contestation contrasts with conventional scientific change where agonistic engagement involves debate that remains within polite scientific norms (Delborne 2008). Instead, contestation's acrimonious nature points toward sociologist Randall Collins' (2012) more general theory of conflict escalation and de-escalation where face-to-face interaction is common to evaluate the enemy, ramp up anger and fear, and display symbols of group solidarity. In science, the challenger and incumbent may engage in their bitter debates largely out of the public eye but in a way that is internally transparent to their field. This means that the rancorous debate is displayed through attacks on the credibility of the challengers: after conference presentations, in anonymous referee reports, in published letters responding to earlier publications, etc. In order to expose the unequal power relationships that are inhibiting their creation of new knowledge and artifacts the public might desire, the challengers may also search out allies outside their scientific specialty, or within the public (Delborne 2008, 511).

The example of the autonomous global network to eradicate blindness reveals that the challengers can create their own opportunity for socio-technical transition. In this chapter, I will use conflict sociology to showcase how challengers employ interlocking innovations as a wedge to divide an incumbent regime into both a new challenger regime and a new incumbent regime. These dual regimes have different technological trajectories, but each solves the same technical problem as the old regime.

8.2 Challenging Dominant Ideologies and Biases

The majority of the community ophthalmology professionals I have described in this book were born in the global south; all have spent many years living and working there on the issue of avoidable blindness. Community ophthalmology professionals are expert elites in their own countries but are frequently marginalized in the global field of ophthalmology. These ophthalmologists, managers, and engineers experience a dissonance or "status inconsistency" (Lenski 1954, 1956) in the global field of science. They are, on the one hand, elite experts that typically have garnered high esteem in their places of work in the global south (Adams 1998). At home, they have high status from their success in treating patients, through inventing new surgical techniques and orphan drugs, or by designing ophthalmic technologies (Williams 2017, 2018). Yet, on the other hand, they are still very cognizant of the economic and cultural differences between themselves and their peers from the global north (Hwang 2008). Dr. G. Venkataswamy's self-reflection provides insights into how such a status inconsistency positions such experts in the global field of science (Mehta and Shenoy 2011, 64),

> Lots of times I suffer from inferiority complex. I feel I am not an upper caste like the Brahmins. Then in the West that I am not the white class…. Being brought up in a colonial country, you are all the time looked down upon….When I was a student and when I was a doctor, the British were ruling us. It didn't occur to us to feel that we could do something as well or better than them. We had to work hard in our own way and build that feeling of, 'Oh! We are as good as people in London'.

Above, Dr. Venkataswamy points out that his liberation from colonization is tied to his praxis (Fanon 1961, 21). Professionals in the global south, such as Dr. Venkataswamy, have developed their own expertise and specialized knowledge based upon their position in the world-system which shapes their ability to perform their work.

I found that innovation from "below," a subordinate position of power in the scientific field, is a deliberate choice of elite experts in less economically developed countries. They also had access to other, potentially higher-paying and more prestigious, professional opportunities. For example, community ophthalmologists, while not poor like their patients, are marginalized by a different measure. They frequently make less money and have less prestige than clinical ophthalmologists within both: urban settings in the global south and wealthy industrialized countries in the global north. Many chose the less-prestigious career of community ophthalmology due to family ties, or because they found the (initially unquantified) public health problem of avoidable blindness to be strikingly important and its remediation a personally satisfying challenge. However, the ability to make such a choice is premised upon earlier privilege from high-quality secondary education and supportive family networks. The fact that these local elites choose to start with the opinions and perspectives of locally marginalized groups is a form of strong objectivity (Harding 1992, 2015; Chapter 4).

The logic of research, design, and development by community ophthalmology professionals emerges from the problems and the perspectives of the marginalized on different levels. Firstly, their research, design, and development focus on poor rural patients in less economically developed countries. These rural patients are marginalized because of inadequate health care especially in comparison with wealthy urban patients in the same country or in wealthy industrialized countries. Community ophthalmologists frequently used a logic of research (Harding 2009) that started from the perspective of the marginalized. This perspective was non-Western as opposed to Western, rural rather than urban, elderly instead of young, and poor not rich. This is a form of "decolonization, which sets out to change the order of the world...summed up in the well-known words: 'The last shall be first'" (Fanon 1961, 2).

Thus, decolonization acts to dismantle Mertonian cumulative advantage (Merton 1988 [1968]).

Secondly, the knowledge that these community ophthalmology professionals have is geo-politically and geo-physically situated in peripheral nations of the world-system. This highly scientific and technical knowledge is therefore endogenous, but it is not in any way "traditional." However, the endogenous knowledge these community ophthalmology professionals produce is frequently considered local in comparison with local knowledge from the West, which is frequently viewed as universal.

The very novelty of their ideas causes disruption among their local peers and additionally in the global field of science. As the founder of Grameen Bank and Nobel Peace Prize winner, Muhammad Yunus puts it, "So the process works like this: that our indigenous ideas have to be validated by the West before we can accept them. We don't know how to sell our own ideas" (Roy 2010, 125 citing Grameen Trust 2003). This is because developmentalism as a discourse not just is present among Westerners, but also is commonly present among local bourgeoisie, especially those educated in Western institutions of higher education (Fanon 1961; Grosfoguel and Cervantes-Rodríguez 2002; Pigg 1992). Therefore, sometimes a fight is necessary. Community ophthalmologists did indeed have rhetorical battles to fight at home and abroad; decolonization is violent (Fanon 1961).

In the early stages of trying out their new ideas, community ophthalmologists encountered significant resistance from their local community, which deferred back to the global standard of universal Western knowledge. Likewise, on the global stage, community ophthalmologists also found that they were disputed by their Western peers whom also defer back to the global standard of universal Western knowledge. Such local and global scientists are supposedly objective: dedicated only to the neutral, detached, and disinterested evidence-based practices created by uncovering truth from nature (Harding 1992; Merton 1973). However, Fanon (1961, 37) wryly observes that such sincere objectivity typically works against the marginalized. This neutral objectivity contains an unrecognized bias that privileges Western scientific knowledge over local scientific knowledge. Therefore, this second aspect of margin-alization is more insidious because it goes unrecognized. These unrecog-nized ideologies and biases must be challenged in order for science and technology to flow from a subordinate to a dominant position in the global field of science.

> We break the rule... Dr. Ruit was there in the beginning; I agree with his concept ....He couldn't follow the rules; he always want to break the rules for better society and better community. (Community ophthalmology professional at Tilganga Institute of Ophthalmology 2012)

Challenging dominant ideologies and biases is a critical, if often implicit, element of contestation as a mode of science and technology flow.

8.3   Challenging the Sole Emphasis on Evidence-Based Medicine

Phacoemulsification functions in the incumbent regime as a form of evidence-based medicine. Evidence-based medicine involves using the most current, reliable, science to increase an individual patient's life span and quality of life, even if this intercession might increase the patient's costs (Sackett et al. 1996, 71). Evidence-based medicine uses scien-tific research to create medical guidelines and is thus distinct from the cost-effectiveness movement (Timmermans and Berg 2003). While evi-dence-based medicine may frequently include a consideration of costs, this is not central to how it defines the best medical care for individual patients. Instead, the primary emphasis of evidence-based medicine is on scientifically verified best practices for high-quality patient outcomes (Sackett et al. 1996; Timmermans and Berg 2003). In evidence-based medicine, clinically established evidence is more influential than a phy-sician's individual opinion about a medical practice or a group of physi-cians' consensus about a medical practice (Solomon 2015).

Community ophthalmologists work to change the global field of ophthalmology with a newer emphasis on both cost-effective and evi-dence-based medicine. This is apparent by a systematic review published by the Cochrane Group comparing Phaco and SICS (Riaz et al. 2013). The Cochrane Group is a well-known British nonprofit that provides systematic reviews to inform evidence-based health care (Timmermans and Berg 2003). Among the ten journal articles describing clinical trials that compared the two techniques (Riaz et al. 2013), this systematic review included: a journal article for SICS by Dr. Ruit (Ruit et al. 2007) and a journal article for M-SICS by Dr. Ravindran (Venkatesh et al. 2010). The Cochrane systematic review synthesizes all ten peer-reviewed articles to determine that phacoemulsification has better three-month outcomes and equivalent six-month outcomes when compared to SICS (Riaz et al. 2013). Additionally, the Cochrane systematic review article suggests that SICS is much lower in cost than phacoemulsification; this is based on costs presented in Dr. Ruit's journal article.

The newer focus on both cost-effective and evidence-based medicine is also apparent in South Asian community ophthalmology professionals' decision to manufacture low-cost IOLs in the 1990s (Chapter 5). At Aravind's Aurolab, and Tilganga's Fred Hollows Intraocular Lens laboratory, they decided to produce low-cost, high-quality intraocular lenses. This early emphasis on cost-effective evidence-based medicine has continued to steer these two manufacturing units. An Aurolab employee (unpublished interview, 2012; **Williams emphasis**) clarifies,

> [T]hese innovations, these medical devices all these ideas and new products – it's all developed in the West and priced for [the] Western economy…These technologies they don't even percolate to southern hemisphere, where [the] majority of the population lives … **they don't even travel, they don't even benefit the others, [on the] other side of the globe**….So how technology can be used for a larger population … I see an opportunity even for Aurolab.

Bala Krishnan (unpublished interview, 2012) explains: "Aurolab wanted to play that role of being the catalyst of bringing down the price; we priced it intentionally low in order to make that change; that is the continuing role we see for Aurolab." By 1996, Aurolab had been producing IOLs for four years, and Tilganga-FHIOL had just started producing commercially available lenses. By choosing to define low cost as a necessity, these organizations demonstrate "mission stickiness" (Rangan 2004). In each country, they continued to proceed with creating their own laboratories, despite the furor in the global field of ophthalmology about the impossibility of their task. While they allowed the furor to die down, they quietly continued their process of contesting developmentalism.

Their decision to make high-quality eye care low in cost was an ethical and moral choice intended to make a difference in the field of ophthalmology, particularly for poor rural patients. While my interlocutors describe their decision as a "catalyst" in the global field of ophthalmology, I argue that their decision caused a dual socio-technical regime in the global field of ophthalmology because it made the most scientifically effective medical intervention (an implanted biomedical prosthetic) available to poor rural blind patients at the same time as it was made available to wealthy urban patients.

It took me some time to reach this conclusion. The conundrum I encountered as I wrapped up my fieldwork was that my interlocutors had not described any problems in making the cost of intraocular lenses and ambulatory surgery low. Instead, the difficulties they encountered were in: challenging developmentalism; and finding Western manufacturing partners for the turnkey process of technology transfer. I incorrectly concluded that making the implantable biomedical prosthetic low in cost was a simple thing for them to do considering their access to cheap labor.

However, when I presented this analysis to the senior leadership at Aravind, the Chairman, Dr. R. D. Ravindran, refuted it, insisting that the low cost of the ophthalmic consumables was the innovation. He stated that any gains from cheap labor were actually eclipsed by the high costs of customs duties on imported raw materials in India, purchasing electric power and transporting raw materials and finished goods (Williams 2012, June 27). Therefore, making the ophthalmic consumables low cost is a significant innovation produced by the staff at Aurolab and Tilganga's TFHIOL. It was significant because it challenged evidence-based medicine due to its newer emphasis on medical practice being both cost-effective and informed by the most current, reliable science. It also challenged Schumacher's (1973) definition of appropriate technology as small-scale.

8.4   Inventing New Aseptic Technique and Operating Theater Practices

The "assembly line" innovation is a feature of the interlocking innovations in community ophthalmology that is central to the Robin Hood model. The principles of the Fordist assembly line and Taylorist scientific management (Nye 2013) appear repeatedly in the operating theater, the outpatient visits, and the eye screening camps. Aravind is well known for using Sisters in various roles such as: janitorial staff, vision counselors, eyeglass grinders, operating theater assistants, and ophthalmic technicians (similar to optometrists), instrument maintenance technicians, canteen cooks, etc. Whether patients come to Aravind's rural eye camps, their village-based vision centers, their city-based surgical centers, or their city-based tertiary eye hospitals, these Sisters provide the majority of their care. The result is that they carefully feed the patients with white cataract into an assembly line within the operating theater.

This assembly line illustrates Fordism and flexible specialization: Each ophthalmic assistant is responsible for a limited range of tasks and are interchangeable. Taylorist scientific management yields routinized checklists specifying: what is done, when, and how. Community ophthalmology units combine increased efficiencies from Fordism and Taylorism with intensive labor for low costs. This avoids the common critique that Schumacher (1973) had for high technology, which produced high wages through the efficient use of limited labor.

The operating theater is the most visible example of the Fordist assembly line and Taylorist scientific management in community ophthalmology. It is in the operating theater that every morning, for several hours, a large number of proficient ophthalmic assistants (working for low to medium wages) feed cataractous patients to the central team-member, the surgeon, who works very quickly and efficiently (for medium wages) to provide those blind patients with sight.

A case in point is the operating theater in the Aravind Eye Hospital-Madurai's "Free Hospital" (for non-paying and walk-in paying patients), which usually opens at 7:30 a.m. and finishes before noon

Monday through Saturday every week (Mehta and Shenoy 2011). Before entering the operating theater, the doctors and ophthalmic assistants scrub very thoroughly, especially underneath their fingernails. The trainees learn how to do this according to Aravind's standard, regardless of their previous training in aseptic technique, to minimize the risk of patient infection (Williams 2012, June 21). Then, they put on gloves.

In the operating theater, an ophthalmologist sits before two operating tables. Her microscope is on a lever positioning system, which allows her to maneuver it between the two surgical tables. She does so in between surgeries, sliding between surgical tables on her wheeled stool with a pit stop (two out of three times when I observed) to rinse her gloves in antiseptic solution. Everything comes to her. Her ophthalmic assistants deliver a steady stream of patients to one operating table while she works on a patient at the other table and vice versa. Specially trained ophthalmic assistants place and remove various items directly into her hand, including: instruments, intraocular lenses, sutures, and so on. I watched for almost an hour one morning and was able to record the following notes directly after exiting the operating theater (Williams 2012, July 16):

> … I saw either 10 or 12 surgeries performed by one person. I estimate that I entered the OT around 8:55 a.m. and I left the OT around 9:45 a.m.
>
> When I came in the senior medical officer was finishing (my count) number 1 and when I left she was starting (my count) either number 11 or number 13. Let's go with the lesser number, say she did 10 while I was there. That is 10 in 50 minutes, or on average 5 minutes per surgery. I think that some took a lot less than that, like 2 minutes. Whereas others took more time like 6 minutes. I did not have a stop watch or anything, so I cannot be sure. Anyway, it was really fast.
>
> The 3 longer surgeries involved:
>
> • A small very dark (and I assume dense) cataract for a bent-over slow shuffling delicate looking old woman in a purple sari.
> • When the ophthalmic assistant dropped the lens, and another ophthalmic assistant was sent for a replacement lens (this happened twice)
>
> …

I remember being surprised that the senior medical officer spoke gently to the ophthalmic assistant after she dropped the lens the second time, and then demonstrated how to hold the tweezers (forceps?) in order to properly hold and secure the lens.

However, I noticed that after the second time, she no longer let the nurse ophthalmic assistant give her the lens, but instead took it herself from the packaging before placing it into the [patient's] eye.

Actually the only time that I saw the senior medical officer raise her voice was when the ophthalmic assistant she was talking to was across the room (having just escorted a patient out of the operating theater) and the senior medical officer needed the ophthalmic assistant to read her the case sheet before she started the surgery. To make sure she was operating on the correct eye I guess.

The sketch I noted of my observation has been recreated as Fig. 8.1. It demonstrates that there are key differences between the aseptic techniques followed by cataract surgeons in community ophthalmology and the standard practice of most Western surgeons. There are multiple patients and physicians per operating theater.

At Aravind and Tilganga, the operating theater practices are not the Western standard; however, they maintain low postoperative infection rates. For example, at Aravind, the surgeons reuse the same gloves for ten surgeries, just rinsing their gloved hands with antiseptic solution between patients. They also remain in the same gown. Once per day, ophthalmic assistants clean wrapped instruments using a conventional long-cycle (75 minutes) steam and high-pressure autoclave sterilizing process. Between surgeries, ophthalmic assistants clean unwrapped instruments using a rapid short-cycle (17 minutes) steam and high-pressure autoclave sterilizing process (Ravindran et al. 2009). There are multiple surgeons, patients, and nurses per theater. Several other surgical consumables that are expensive to constantly replace but present a low-chance for cross-contamination are reused in the operating theater, including irrigation/aspiration tubing and bottles of irrigation fluid and Ringer's lactate intravenous solution (Ravindran et al. 2009). The patients in the Camp Hospital, Free Hospital, or the Executive Tier Hospital all wear their street clothes covered by a hospital gown.

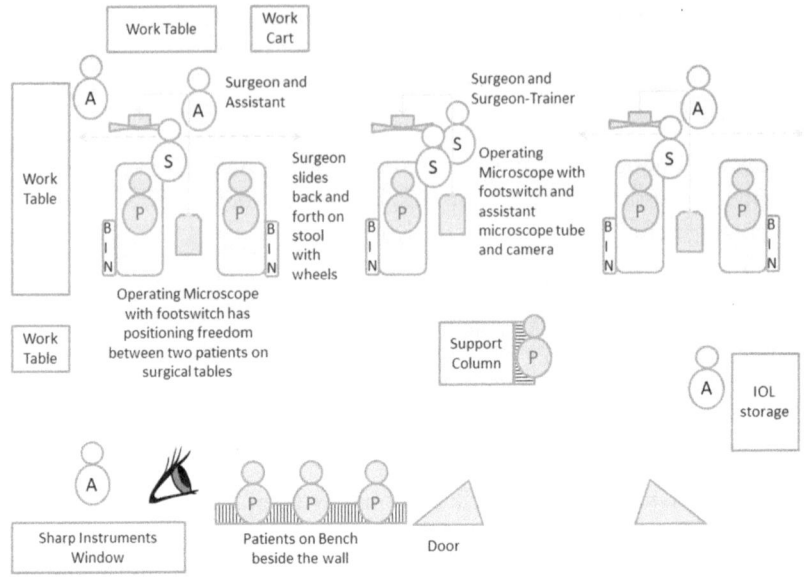

Fig. 8.1 Drawing of my observation in the Aravind "Free Hospital" (Walk-in Hospital) Operating Theater. I stood by the instruments window and ophthalmic assistants came past me every few minutes to the window near my left shoulder to drop off a tray, with its set of used instruments, so they could be quickly sterilized and used again (Williams 2012, July 16)

Many people might assume that, with such deviance from universal (read: Western) aseptic technique, the postoperative infection rates at Aravind and Tilganga should be higher than the infection rates in clinical ophthalmology eye units.

One reason why postoperative infection rates could be higher is that malnourished and stressed patients are more prone to infections. Aravind predominantly serves low-income patients who are receiving cataract surgery for free or a deeply subsidized rate. Community ophthalmologists acknowledge that the unique bio-physical context of poverty, e.g., "poor personal hygiene, malnutrition, poor sanitation, and lack of access to clean water," are risk factors that increase chances for postoperative infection (Ravindran et al. 2009, 633–34). Arguably, infection rates for poor patients should be high because of their likely malnutrition. The chief of ophthalmology at Albany Medical Center

(USA), Dr. John Simon, visited an eye surgical camp in India in 1991. Dr. Simon (2010) recalled that, because of the impoverished state of their primarily rural patients, ophthalmologists at that eye hospital had to admit them, "a few days ahead of time so that you can [feed] [them] up enough so that [they] have the ability to heal wounds because these people are malnourished. They have signs all over the place 'be sure to eat some fat every day.'"

At Aravind, the postoperative infection rate is indeed higher among poor patients (who typically have ECCE or M-SICS procedures); infection rates are lower among middle income and wealthy patients (who typically have phacoemulsification; Ravindran et al. 2009). One reason for this might be the increased risk of infection that comes from poverty, where the patient is the most likely source of infectious organisms. Aravind tries to mitigate this risk factor by cleaning each patient's face with iodine three times before surgery and applying iodine drops in the eye just before surgery (Ravindran et al. 2009). This is in contrast with the clinical ophthalmology standard of deploying expensive antibiotics in the irrigation fluid during surgery (Ravindran et al. 2009). Another reason for the increased infection risk might be that the SICS micro-incision is slightly larger than the Phaco micro-incision, which might allow more microorganisms into the eye organ. However, Aravind believes it more likely that the differences in infection rate between rich patients who undergo Phaco as compared to poor patients who undergo SICS is related to the fact that only experienced full-time surgeons perform the Phaco cases on rich patients, whereas both trainees and full-time surgeons perform SICS on poor patients.

Thus, the operating theater technology-practice for Aravind and Tilganga, to include a variety of standards and protocols, is different than in clinical ophthalmology organizations. Dr. R. D. Ravindran et al. (2009) discussed these operating theater practices. He also discussed the fact that Aravind maintains the same order of magnitude of postoperative infection rates: His study demonstrated infection rates of 0.09% compared to 0.21% for US Medicare patients from 1994 to 2001 (Ravindran et al. 2009 citing West et al. 2005). Aravind's low infection rates were present in a study that included 42,426 cataract surgeries.

8.5   Challenging Eurocentric Operating Theater Practices

The sharp contrast between aseptic technique in South Asian community ophthalmology units and Western clinical ophthalmology has initiated a debate that has remained largely within the scientific field of ophthalmology and included diatribes against Aravind and Tilganga.

Professionals at Aravind and Tilganga put their "heads on the block" by releasing details of their efficient processes that challenge the dominant regime's operating theater aseptic technique (Larkin 2010, 4). In the October 2010 magazine of the European Society of Cataract and Refractive Surgery (ESCRS), *Eurotimes*, they were featured in a provocatively titled article, "What can be learned from the developing world?" In this article, doctors from India and Nepal advocated the South Asian surgical system approach, and European doctors shared their own particular appropriation of this approach. Dr. Parikshit Gogate (former medical director of the Desai Eye Hospital, Pune, Maharashtra, India) argued that industrialized nations might learn how to safely reuse instruments to improve efficiency (Larkin 2010). Consultants from the Nordic Healthcare Group discussed how, after their time-motion study of an Aravind Eye Hospital, six Finnish hospitals adopted some of Aravind's scientific management for decreased surgical times. By fast-tracking surgical cases based on known surgical complexity, using structured checklists and using standardized instrument sets, the Finnish hospitals could cut down on their waiting lists for eye surgery, while also continuing to use Western aseptic techniques in the operating theater (Larkin 2010). These basic medical protocols and guidelines are typical of evidence-based medicine (Timmermans and Berg 2003; Prentice 2018).

The Spanish president of ESCRS, Dr. José Güell (MD, Ph.D.) challenged the Nordic Healthcare Group, Aravind Eye Care System, and Tilganga Institute of Ophthalmology, about the safety of their practices (Larkin 2010). His challenge was surprising because, in a February 2010 interview with *Eurotimes*, right after he assumed the presidency, Dr. Güell revealed that he was cognizant of the large scale of the problem of avoidable blindness around the world. Looking through the 2010 issues of *Eurotimes*, you can see that Dr. Güell exhorted his fellow Western ophthalmologists to give, not just money, but also time, to low-income areas of the world where patients do not have access to eye health care. Therefore, his dismissal of the practices of South Asian and Finnish ophthalmologists to address the backlog of blindness does not jibe well with his sympathy and advocacy efforts, unless one understands that South Asian ophthalmologists are challenging the dominant regime in the field of ophthalmology.

Aravind's aseptic technique challenges the dominance of Western surgical aseptic techniques in the global field of ophthalmology. While ostensibly focused on the utility of seventeen-minute short-cycle autoclave sterilization as a mechanism for saving time (and thus saving money), in fact Dr. Ravindran's et al. (2009) article describes all of the internally standardized operating theater practices performed at Aravind. The paper concludes that unwrapped short-cycle sterilization technique used to clean instruments between surgeries at Aravind neither increases nor decreases the incidence of postoperative endophthalmitis infection (Ravindran et al. 2009). However, the certainty of this careful conclusion downplays the more controversial implication: Aravind's internally standardized operating theater practices, achieved through the application of scientific management to decrease costs, neither increases nor decreases the incidence of endophthalmitis infection compared to the Western standard for surgical practices in ophthalmology. This implication is likely to resonate powerfully with ophthalmologists already oriented toward evidence-based medicine because the data set that Aravind uses in the article is so very large, more than 42,000 patients. Coincidentally, the same year that Dr. Ravindran's paper was published, the US Department of Health and Human Services reminded its inspectors in a memo that short-cycle rapid autoclave sterilization for wrapped instruments was an acceptable practice for ambulatory surgical units in the USA (Hamilton 2009).

Aravind's operating theater practices have, in turn, been challenged by Indian ophthalmologists in a contentious debate. One of the more skeptical responses came from ophthalmologists at a competing high-volume cataract surgical system, the L. V. Prasad Eye Institute (Hyderabad, Telangana, India) who asked reasonable questions about the study design and challenged its rigor (Khanna and Garudadri 2010). This exchange of logical scientific arguments published in peer-reviewed scholarly journals fits the scientific norm of organized skepticism (Merton 1973).

In contrast, Dr. Ravi Thomas (2009, 2010), a self-proclaimed proponent of M-SICS (formerly from L. V. Prasad Eye Institute but writing from Queensland Eye Institute in Australia; Houck 2009), used dismissive rhetoric when discussing Aravind's aseptic techniques. In his reply letter in the *Indian Journal of Ophthalmology*, Dr. Ravindran et al. (2011) quotes some of Dr. Thomas' letter saying,

> Finally, although we acknowledge that our efforts to reduce unnecessary costs may raise controversy, we take exception to the disdainful tone of this letter, such as in the use of terms such as 'short cuts' and the insinuation that we are suggesting … '…less rigor …' In fact, there are major differences among these procedures and imposing universal rigid standards for every procedure across all of medicine probably does result in unnecessary and wasteful practices.…

In the above excerpt, Dr. Ravindran et al. (2011) points out that the aseptic technique should not be universal, but context-specific to the surgical procedure being performed. More or less, he is arguing that the cost-effective aseptic techniques used at Aravind are certainly different than Western aseptic technique, but difference is not negligence. In fact, results from Aravind's large volume of cataract surgery patients provide new evidence that suggests their aseptic techniques still provide excellent outcomes. Additionally, because Aravind reuses consumables they significantly reduce environmental pollution from medical waste: Cataract surgeries at Aravind have a carbon footprint equivalent to 5% of the carbon footprint for cataract surgeries performed in the UK (Thiel et al. 2017).

One sympathetic foray into this contentious debate denounces reuse of consumables as unethical, but kindly suggests that as India trains more ophthalmologists and becomes increasingly more industrialized,

Indian ophthalmology will move away from high volume to focus on high quality (Gogate and Kulkarni 2011). Dr. Gogate's new response is a reversal of his position one year earlier in *Eurotimes* and highlights ophthalmologists' awareness that operating theater practices are part of a socio-technical regime that can change over time.

Finally, an Australian ophthalmologist, Dr. Janice Ku et al. (2012), demonstrated she is well-aware of the controversial implication that is implicit in Dr. Ravindran's et al. (2009) paper. She wrote in a letter published in the *Journal of Cataract Refractive Surgery* (Ku et al. 2012, 1301),

> The Aravind Eye Hospital … convincingly indicates that disposable single-use surgical equipment is not the key to the prevention of acute postoperative bacterial endophthalmitis.

From the perspective of Dr. Ku et al. (2012), Dr. Ravindran's et al. (2009) paper serves primarily as evidence to further advance her own potentially field-changing idea for cataract surgery: the end of sutureless surgery, and the return to suturing all microsurgical wounds to prevent endophthalmitis.

This illustrates a larger point noted by historian of science Everett Mendelsohn (1987): In some scientific controversies, there is no closure of the debate where all scientists come to a consensus about the phenomenon in dispute. Instead, "it appears that scientific work is able to continue and that the knowledge and explanatory modes used by both parties of a conflict … can be, and often are, used even while disagreement persists" (Mendelsohn 1987, 101). Yet, this disagreement is entirely fruitful to the scientific enterprise (Solomon 2015). Therefore, dissent, like consensus, is a very important part of advancing scientific knowledge.

However, many Western ophthalmologists might become more convinced once they have participated in SICS training themselves (including the grand rounds where they learn about the complication rates for themselves and their fellow trainees). Such training best demonstrates the efficacy of the South Asian surgical systems approach.

In response to my question about Aravind's operating theater practices, Dr. Bruce Spivey (2013) commented, "Multiple patients in one theater ... In one operating room? .... I don't know if we'd be allowed to do that....There are lots of rules that exist in the U.S." In addition to his past presidency of the International Council of Ophthalmology, Dr. Spivey was the executive officer of the American Academy of Ophthalmology. He is an ally of community ophthalmologists, but has not necessarily been inside Aravind's operating theater himself.

In contrast, an American ophthalmology resident (2012) that came to the Tilganga Institute of Ophthalmology for a two-week observership explained that, in the USA,

> We have very strict protocol for sterile technique and you are trained and re-trained in it all through medical school and our internship in ophthalmology. And if you see somebody doing something outside of that protocol, it's your obligation to tell them to do otherwise. And a lot of it's evidence-based medicine. So what we are using to wash our hands every time has been shown to be very efficacious. We change gloves be-tween every procedure. You know, where you hold your hands is important. All these things. How we sterilize instruments with autoclave is standard.

> Then obviously here it's different. There isn't washing with some kind of special product or using soap and water between each case, or the gel that we use, or changing gloves between procedures. But, the outcomes, from the literature I've been exposed too, don't seem to be significantly different.

> So I feel like this is an incredible program that is highly efficient here with great outcomes. People can see and everything works well; it's just vastly different. And when you are just indoctrinated into a standard system—if you go anywhere in the United States it's exactly the same. If you go into any hospital you know what to do, this is how it's done. This is just the accepted way. And to come to [a] hospital that's very different, it has an impact.

In the above example, the US ophthalmology resident recognized that American aseptic technique is not universal. Indeed, epistemological plurality is possible (Healy 2003). She has experienced a third-order change in thinking, where she now recognizes that the epistemic sovereignty of particular organizational practices can be altered (Dotson 2014). However, her change in thinking was likely abetted by whatever interest brought her to Nepal for an observership in the first place. Many Western ophthalmologists who come for training in SICS at Aravind or Tilganga are already fairly open-minded, as I found that all of them intend to practice the technique in less economically developed countries (not at home).

Universal standards do not necessarily have to be Western, although they often have been in recent history. Quark (2012) argued that scientific regulation in the global cotton industry formalizes unequal power relationships between countries. She followed the cotton global commodity chain and found that fiber science in the capital-intensive US cotton industry differed from the fiber science suitable for the labor-intensive Chinese cotton industry (Quark 2012). By integrating world-systems theory with the new political sociology of science (see Wallerstein 1974; Frickel and Moore 2006), she showed the process by which the "universal" fiber science, as represented by the US classificatory system, came to dominate the global cotton industry and was eventually adopted by Brazil, Germany, African countries, and China (Quark 2012).

Similar to Quark's study (2012), this book showcases the contextual and historically contingent power of certain countries to frame standards, regulations, and research-agendas in the global field of science. Where our studies differ is that this chapter additionally demonstrates that there are times when the universal (read: Western) standards of science and technology are successfully disputed "from below"—from countries positioned as subordinate within the global field of science. However, this is not a case of a particular nation asserting sovereignty by rejecting regulation by Western agencies. Instead, this occurred regionally in South Asia through an emergent process where an autonomous global network of physicians, health educators, policy-makers, and engineers worked within the global field of ophthalmology to create and circulate new values, norms, ideologies, standards, practices, sciences and technologies.

The struggle for dominance between Western and South Asian aseptic technique in the global field of ophthalmology demonstrates that global epistemological plurality is always local: It is tied to regionally similar cultures and supported by national epistemic sovereignty. This national epistemic sovereignty is partially shaped and enforced by state regulation and the scientific norms of domestic civil society organizations.

8.6   Breakthrough of a SICS-Regime in the Global South

When community ophthalmologists are challenging the dominant use of phacoemulsification and Western aseptic technique, they are challenging a socio-technical regime. SICS is not just a new surgical technique, it serves as proxy for a new model of eye health care, and it incorporates many other things besides itself into a SICS-regime. As it grows in popularity in the global south, the SICS-regime grows into the interstitial spaces left wide open by an expensive Phaco-regime that cannot, by itself, serve the needs of the world's poor rural blind people.

The SICS-regime replaces expensive phacoemulsification equipment with ophthalmologists' increased surgical skill and keeps many of the same surgical instruments. Additionally, the SICS-regime replaces personalized doctor–patient interaction in small clinics with a high volume of patients who see their ophthalmologist for five minutes and likely have a different surgeon in large tertiary eye hospitals. The growth of the SICS-regime into the Phaco-regime's interstitial spaces has meant they are economically connected if geo-politically and geo-physically separate. The two regimes are economically connected because the SICS-regime subsumes the Phaco-regime in the global south. This is demonstrated in two ways: first, because incremental innovations in the Phaco-regime are implemented for wealthy patients in the SICS-regime for the Robin Hood model; and second, because the social responsibility departments of multinational biotechnology companies in the Phaco-Regime (i.e., Alcon) will donate pharmaceutical drugs (Samsky 2012), instruments, ophthalmic consumables, or funds to eye clinics in the global south. For example, Alcon donated a $225,000 surgical simulator to the WetLab at Aravind Eye Hospital, Madurai, where trainees practice both phacoemulsification and SICS on either: the simulator or eye organs freshly harvested from deceased humans or animal models. Also, one popular Alcon phacoemulsification machine is the Centurion® Vision System. Aravind Eye Care System has installed this machine in four eye hospitals across the system: Madurai, Tirunelveli, Coimbatore, and Puducherry (Aravind E-News 2013). Individual chief medical officers in those four eye hospitals approved sourcing the Centurion® over the more affordable Pegasus phacoemulsification machine produced by Aurolab for sale in India only. This choice seems to contradict Aravind Eye Care System's goal of providing inexpensive or free cataract surgery for poor patients, but ultimately can be justified by the conspicuous consumption of its wealthier patients that subsidizes the poor patients.

Community ophthalmologists in the global north and the global south believe the SICS-regime is better for patients. The emerging SICS-regime increases its relevance and stature as it increases the high numbers of patients treated with good visual outcomes. The Irish ophthalmologist of the NGO Right to Sight, Dr. Kate Coleman (2011), demonstrated this in her presentation at the Unite for Sight Global Health and Innovation Conference when she suggested that the "Indian model" is the best model for addressing the cataract backlog in Africa.

The SICS-regime is therefore challenging the power of northern multinational companies with the power of southern nonprofit companies. The dominant surgical technology-practice of Phaco+IOL has been challenged, but not eliminated. Instead, phacoemulsification becomes absorbed into the radical finance model created by these South Asian institutions. The growth of the SICS-regime to subsume the Phaco-regime in India, Nepal, Kenya, and Mexico involved changes in: the science of surgery; the biomedical prosthetics for surgery; national tax policy regulating imported biotechnologies; laws, and other policies governing surgical eye camps and government health insurance schemes (including remittances for eye hospitals).

Meanwhile in South Asia, where the SICS-regime started growing approximately ten years after the Phaco-regime started gaining traction around the world, proponents of the SICS technique believe that expertise in both SICS and Phaco is central to systematically addressing the backlog of blindness. Community ophthalmologists in the SICS-regime argue it is the responsibility of community ophthalmologists to think beyond what brings personal prestige to what will reduce the backlog of blindness. At Tilganga, a community ophthalmologist (unpublished interview, 2012) reflects,

> New things come and we keep changing. I think that is typical human nature; But [what] you have to keep in mind is... Let's say now in China and India; we always talk about these two nations worldwide these days. [In] India ... cataract surgical rate is very high while in China it is very low. Whatever approach you take, whether a mass approach or an individual approach, whether I want to upgrade myself; my upgrade is contributing towards...a kind of system... The surgeons who are learning the Phaco should do [SICS/ECCE] also. That is why India went ahead [and] the surgeons are learning the Phaco while also doing the mass [ECCE]. While in China, 'I learn Phaco for myself ... I learn Phaco to be superior.' While in China [they have all] those cataracts that need to be done with SICS. In India they did both. I think that's the difference...

Community ophthalmologists in the SICS-regime believe that a good surgeon (a high-volume surgeon) knows both the gold standard technique of Phaco and the equivalent outcome technique of small-incision cataract surgery. This is for reasons of fiscal sustainability, patient safety, and prestige. Aravind-trained ophthalmologists are SICS enthusiasts, while stating that Phaco is scientifically (or technically) superior. "I would say that I am a small-incision enthusiast as well as Phaco. Both are great techniques and both give good results and there are advantages and disadvantages to both," declares Dr. Juan Pablo Olivares (unpublished interview, 2012). Dr. Olivares believes that if ophthalmologists become enthusiasts for SICS they will look for the training and start doing it. He would like to start doing some publishing in medical journals to encourage Mexican ophthalmologists to adopt the technique. He believes that he can help Sala Uno can become influential in Mexico by talking about their results, including their low complication rates, at meetings, conferences, and courses. Thus, Dr. Olivares is active in agonistic engagement to build up evidence, within Mexico, of SICS' efficacy.

Meanwhile, another Aravind-trained Indian ophthalmologist, Dr. Tulika Kar, performs high-volume cataract surgery (mostly SICS, but some Phaco to keep her skills honed) for an Indian NGO in Africa. Dr. Kar (unpublished interview, 2012) says that Phaco is better if you have a good Phaco machine and you are a good surgeon. A third Aravind-trained ophthalmologist, Dr. Jyotee Trivedy (unpublished interview, 2011), works at Loresho and refuses to say that one technique is better than the other; instead, she points to her publication in the *Nepal Journal of Ophthalmology* as evidence that a good ophthalmologist should be able to do both (Trivedy 2011). She claims that SICS is her favorite but, like Dr. Kar, emphasizes that the quality of the surgery depends upon the surgeon's experience (Trivedy, unpublished interview, 2011). A US Health and Human Services Agency for Healthcare Research and Quality fellow at Stanford University, ophthalmologist Dr. Suzanne Pershing, suggests that manual small-incision cataract surgery should be a part of every surgeon's "overall skill set" (Pershing and Kumar 2011).

Community ophthalmologists are advocating a new socio-technical regime for the field of ophthalmology that also follows evidence-based medicine. Dr. Spivey explains (unpublished interview, 2013), "When you see you can make an improvement and there's some impediment in a rule or because of a rule. Then argue against it....you don't want to destroy the whole system because it's based on some good reasons. [However], [s]ometimes those reasons are no longer applicable or they're out of date. Hence, then you argue." The key insight to understand here is that community ophthalmologists argued against the efficacy of phacoemulsification for low-income rural patients, and thus, the SICS-regime subsumed the Phaco-regime in the global south, but did not eliminate it in the global north.

8.7 Conclusion: Contestation and Systemic Technology Choice

In this chapter, I have argued that the process of contestation is a mode of science and technology flow and that this bidirectional mode of flow involves bilateral power relationships between subordinate and dominant positions in a field. This is evident by the growth of dual socio-technical regimes in the global south. Community ophthalmologists created the SICS-regime which, unlike the Phaco-regime, primarily exists in less economically developed countries.

Their heterogeneous technology choices maintain the Schumpeterian-Gandhian approach to eye health care, but they also demonstrate systemic technology choice. They are leading a shift in the appropriate technology movement from considering just the politics of singular artifacts in context to additionally consider the importance of a heterogeneous collection of innovations in scientific knowledge, technology-practice, and organizational processes that are linked ideologically. Systemic technology choice is a form of democratic technology choice used by social movement activists that understands technology transfer to involve a system of artifacts and rules (i.e., values, norms, and ideology). By shifting to such systems thinking, they provide an interesting insight into studies of science and technology transfer about the importance of considering the politics of transferring a system of artifacts.

This example demonstrated how once the interlocking innovations formed, then the new SICS-regime began to quickly emerge through translation and niche-accumulation. Finally, repeated iterative contestation—first challenging developmentalism and cost-insensitive evidence-based medicine, and second challenging a supposedly universal Western aseptic technique for cataract surgery—was the wedge for the SICS-regime to breakthrough as a stable and acknowledged alternative to the Phaco-regime. The SICS-regime solves the same technical problem as the Phaco-regime, but emphasizes: non-users as the market, a radical rule-set, and particular geo-political and geo-physical areas of the world.

Conflicts in science and technology-practice are concomitant with the creation and circulation of new knowledge and technology from subordinate to dominant positions in a field. The process of contestation provides analytical insight at three levels:

1. At the micro scale, this process describes how some actors in subordinate positions of power use new forms of science and technology to challenge existing knowledge hierarchies and social relations. This is a normal and productive mode of scientific knowledge technology creation and dissemination.

2. At the mesoscale, this process may contribute to the development or destruction of an incumbent socio-technical regime in an interstitial process. After interlocking innovations have accumulated a few niche-markets, then the challengers have a stronger base from which to challenge the incumbent regime. Through repeated contestation, the incumbent regime is fractured into dual regimes: one very similar to the original incumbent regime, and a second based upon interlocking innovations that monopolized the interstitial spaces of the original incumbent regime.
3. At the macroscale, this process facilitates the movement of some actors from positions of subordinate power to positions of dominant power in the world-system or global socio-technical landscape.

In this chapter, I have argued that the contestation mode of science and technology flow allows individuals (or groups) that were previously dominant and subordinate to each other to change their social relationships, especially in the case of scientists engaged in contestation who are producing and circulating the field-changing innovations from below. In this case, community ophthalmologists, who are predominantly located in the global south, have been able to approach equity in their relations with their wealthier colleagues in clinical ophthalmology (who are predominantly located in the global north or in the urban centers of the global south).

By exploring the SICS-regime through the network preventing blindness that includes Aravind, Tilganga, Loresho, and Sala Uno, I have found clear concurrence of various modes of science and technology circulation (diffusion, appropriation, translation, and contestation). Each mode helps practitioners and scholars to understand interrelating power dynamics. Thus, a new understanding emerges that, in any global field of science, knowledge and artifacts are affected by ideologies, geo-physical context, and geo-political context during the process of technology transfer, that is, "[u]niversals … fall apart, and regroup differently, when they travel" (de Laet 2002, 1).

In the final chapter of this book, I summarize how insights gained from this case of community ophthalmology professionals inform the dual regime thesis as a general theoretical model, and the three new concepts: interlocking innovations, contestation, and systemic technology choice.

References

Adams, Vincanne. 1998. *Doctors for Democracy: Health Professionals in the Nepal Revolution.* Cambridge: Cambridge University Press.

Aravind E-News. 2013. "Aravind News." *Aravind E-News,* December. http://www.aravind.org/default/aravindnewscontent/NI00000133.

Coleman, Kate. 2011. "Proof of Sustainable Eye Care Systems in Africa, the Only Way to V2020." Unite for Sight 2011 Global Health & Innovation Conference, Yale University, New Haven, CT. Retrieved January 17, 2013. http://www.uniteforsight.org/conference/speaker-schedule-2011.

Collins, Randall. 2012. "C-Escalation and D-Escalation: A Theory of the Time-Dynamics of Conflict." *American Sociological Review* 77 (1): 1–20.

Collins, Randall, and Sal Restivo. 1983. "Robber Barons and Politicians in Mathematics: A Conflict Model of Science." *Canadian Journal of Sociology/ Cahiers Canadiens de Sociologie* 8: 199–227.

de Laet, Marianne. 2002. "Introduction: Knowledge and Technology Transfer or the Travel of Thoughts and Things." In *Research in Science and Technology Studies: Knowledge and Technology Transfer, Vol. 13, Knowledge and Society,* edited by Marianne de Laet, 1–9. New York: JAI Press.

Delborne, Jason A. 2008. "Transgenes and Transgressions: Scientific Dissent as Heterogeneous Practice." *Social Studies of Science* 38 (4): 509–41.

Dotson, Kristie. 2014. "Conceptualizing Epistemic Oppression." *Social Epistemology* 28 (2): 115–38. https://doi.org/10.1080/02691728.2013.782585.

Elzen, Boelie, Frank W. Geels, Cees Leeuwis, and Barbara van Mierlo. 2011. "Normative Contestation in Transitions 'in the Making': Animal Welfare Concerns and System Innovation in Pig Husbandry." *Research Policy* 40 (2): 263–75.

Epstein, Steven. 1995. "The Construction of Lay Expertise: AIDS Activism and the Forging of Credibility in the Reform of Clinical Trials." *Science, Technology & Human Values* 20 (4): 408–37.

Fanon, Frantz. 2004 [1961]. *The Wretched of the Earth.* Translated by Richard Philcox. New York: Grove Press.

Frickel, Scott, and Kelly Moore, eds. 2006. *The New Political Sociology of Science: Institutions, Networks, and Power.* Madison: University of Wisconsin Press.

Geels, Frank W. 2010. "Ontologies, Socio-Technical Transitions (to Sustainability), and the Multi-level Perspective." *Research Policy,* Special Section on Innovation and Sustainability Transitions, 39 (4): 495–510.

Gogate, Parikshit, and Anil Kulkarni. 2011. "Pearls and Pitfalls of High Quality High Volume Cataract Surgery." *Indian Journal of Ophthalmology* 59 (5): 414.

Grameen Trust. 2003. *Notes from Grameen Dialogues*. Dhaka: Grameen Bank.

Griffith, Belver C., and Nicholas C. Mullins. 1972. "Coherent Social Groups in Scientific Change." *Science* 177 (4053): 959–64.

Grosfoguel, Ramón, and Ana Margarita Cervantes-Rodríguez, eds. 2002. *The Modern/Colonial/Capitalist World-System in the Twentieth Century: Global Processes, Antisystemic Movements, and the Geopolitics of Knowledge*. Westport, CT: Greenwood Press.

Hård, Mikael. 1993. "Beyond Harmony and Consensus: A Social Conflict Approach to Technology." *Science, Technology & Human Values* 18 (4): 408–32.

Harding, Sandra. 1992. "After the Neutrality Ideal: Science, Politics, and 'Strong Objectivity.'" *Social Research* 59 (3): 567–87.

———. 2009. "Postcolonial and Feminist Philosophies of Science and Technology: Convergences and Dissonances." *Postcolonial Studies* 12 (4): 401–21.

———. 2015. *Objectivity and Diversity: Another Logic of Scientific Research*. Chicago and London: University of Chicago Press.

Healy, S. 2003. "Epistemological Pluralism and the 'Politics of Choice.'" *Futures* 35 (7): 689–701.

Hess, David J. 2005. "Technology- and Product-Oriented Movements: Approximating Social Movement Studies and Science and Technology Studies." *Science, Technology & Human Values* 30 (4): 515.

———. 2016. *Undone Science: Social Movements, Mobilized Publics, and Industrial Transitions*. Cambridge: The MIT Press.

Hess, David J., Sulfikar Amir, Scott Frickel, Daniel Lee Kleinman, Kelly Moore, and Logan D. A. Williams. 2016. "11. Structural Inequality and the Politics of Science and Technology." In *The Handbook of Science and Technology Studies*, edited by Ulrike Felt, Rayvon Fouché, Clark A. Miller, and Laurel Smith-Doerr, 4th ed., 319–47. Cambridge: The MIT Press.

Houck, Kristine. 2009. "Physician Works to Improve Several Educational Programs in Ophthalmology." *Ocular Surgery News India Edition*, March 2009. https://www.healio.com/ophthalmology/news/print/ocular-surgery-news-india-edition/%7B0d87d543-3673-40b6-a330-12636ec08a74%7D/physician-works-to-improve-several-educational-programs-in-ophthalmology.

Hwang, K. 2008. "International Collaboration in Multilayered Center-Periphery in the Globalization of Science and Technology." *Science Technology & Human Values* 33 (1): 101–33.

Jasper, James M. 1988. "The Political Life Cycle of Technological Controversies." *Social Forces* 67 (2): 357–77.

Khanna, Rohit C., and Chandrasekhar Garudadri. 2010. "Incidence of Postcataract Endophthalmitis at Aravind Eye Hospital." *Indian Journal of Ophthalmology* 58 (6): 562.

Ku, Janice J. Y., Michael C. Wei, Shahriar Amjadi, Jessica M. Montfort, Ravjit Singh, and Ian C. Francis. 2012. "Role of Adequate Wound Closure in Preventing Acute Postoperative Bacterial Endophthalmitis." *Journal of Cataract and Refractive Surgery* 38 (7): 1301–1302.

Larkin, Howard. 2010. "What Can Be Learned from the Developing World?" *European Society for Cataract and Refractive Surgery EUROTIMES* 15 (10): 4–6.

Lawhon, Mary, and James T. Murphy. 2012. "Socio-Technical Regimes and Sustainability Transitions: Insights from Political Ecology." *Progress in Human Geography* 36 (3): 354–78.

Lenski, Gerhard E. 1954. "Status Crystallization: A Non-vertical Dimension of Social Status." *American Sociological Review* 19 (4): 405–13.

———. 1956. "Social Participation and Status Crystallization." *American Sociological Review* 21 (4): 458.

Mazur, Allan. 1975. "Opposition to Technological Innovation." *Minerva* 13 (1): 58–81.

Mehta, Pavithra K., and Suchitra Shenoy. 2011. *Infinite Vision: How Aravind Became the World's Greatest Business Case for Compassion.* San Francisco, CA: Berrett-Koehler Publishers.

Mendelsohn, Everett. 1987. "The Political Anatomy of Controversy in the Sciences." In *Scientific Controversies: Case Studies in the Resolution and Closure of Disputes in Science and Technology*, edited by Hugo Tristram Engelhardt and Arthur L. Caplan, 93–124. New York: Cambridge University Press.

Merton, Robert K. 1973. "The Normative Structure of Science." In *The Sociology of Science: Theoretical and Empirical Investigations.* Chicago: University of Chicago Press.

———. 1988. "The Matthew Effect in Science, II: Cumulative Advantage and the Symbolism of Intellectual Property." *Isis* 79 (4): 606–23.

Mullins, Nicholas C. 1975. "New Causal Theory: An Elite Specialty in Social Science." *History of Political Economy* 7 (4): 499–529.

Nelkin, Dorothy, ed. 1992. *Controversy: Politics of Technical Decisions.* Newbury Park, CA: Sage.

Nieusma, Dean. 2007. "Challenging Knowledge Hierarchies: Working Toward Sustainable Development in Sri Lanka's Energy Sector." *Sustainability: Science Practice and Policy* 3: 32–44.

Nye, David E. 2013. *America's Assembly Line.* Cambridge: The MIT Press.

Pershing, S., and A. Kumar. 2011. "Phacoemulsification Versus Extracapsular Cataract Extraction: Where Do We Stand?" *Current Opinion in Ophthalmology* 22 (1): 37–42.

Pigg, Stacy L. 1992. "Inventing Social Categories Through Place: Social Representations and Development in Nepal." *Comparative Studies in Society and History* 34: 491–513.

Pinch, Trevor, and Wiebe E. Bijker. 1987. "The Social Construction of Facts and Artifacts: Or How the Sociology of Science and the Sociology of Technology Might Benefit Each Other." In *The Social Construction of Technological Systems: New Directions in the Sociology and History of Technology*, edited by Wiebe E. Bijker, Thomas Parke Hughes, and Trevor Pinch, 159–87. Cambridge: The MIT Press.

Prentice, Rachel. 2018. "How Surgery Became a Global Public Health Issue." *Technology in Society*, Technology and the Good Society 52 (February): 17–23.

Quark, Amy A. 2012. "Scientized Politics and Global Governance in the Cotton Trade: Evaluating Divergent Theories of Scientization." *Review of International Political Economy* 19 (5): 895–917.

Rangan, V. Kasturi 2004. "Lofty Missions, Down-to-Earth Plans." *Harvard Business Review* 82 (3): 112–19.

Ravindran, Ravilla D., Rengaraj Venkatesh, David Chang, and Sabyasachi Sengupta. 2011. "Reply to 'Reducing Endophthalmitis in India: An Example of the Importance of Critical Appraisal'." *Indian Journal of Ophthalmology* 59 (5): 412–14.

Ravindran, Ravilla D., Rengaraj Venkatesh, David F. Chang, Sabyasachi Sengupta, Jamyang Gyatsho, and Badrinath Talwar. 2009. "Incidence of Post-cataract Endophthalmitis at Aravind Eye Hospital: Outcomes of More Than 42,000 Consecutive Cases Using Standardized Sterilization and Prophylaxis Protocols." *Journal of Cataract & Refractive Surgery* 35 (4): 629–36.

Riaz, Yasmin, Samantha R. de Silva, and Jennifer R. Evans. 2013. "Manual Small Incision Cataract Surgery (MSICS) with Posterior Chamber

Intraocular Lens Versus Phacoemulsification with Posterior Chamber Intraocular Lens for Age-Related Cataract." Edited by The Cochrane Collaboration. *Cochrane Database of Systematic Reviews*, no. 10 (October).

Roy, Ananya. 2010. *Poverty Capital: Microfinance and the Making of Development*. New York: Routledge.

Ruit, Sanduk, Geoffrey Tabin, David Chang, Leena Bajracharya, Daniel C. Kline, William Richheimer, Mohan Shrestha, and Govinda Paudyal. 2007. "A Prospective Randomized Clinical Trial of Phacoemulsification vs Manual Sutureless Small-Incision Extracapsular Cataract Surgery in Nepal." *American Journal of Ophthalmology* 143 (1): 32–38. e2.

Sackett, David L., William M. C. Rosenberg, J. A. Muir Gray, R. Brian Haynes, and W. Scott Richardson. 1996. "Evidence Based Medicine: What It Is and What It Isn't." *BMJ* 312 (7023): 71–72.

Samsky, Ari. 2012. "Scientific Sovereignty: How International Drug Donation Programs Reshape Health, Disease, and the State." *Cultural Anthropology* 27 (2): 310–32.

Schumacher, Ernst F. 1973. *Small Is Beautiful: Economics as If People Mattered*. London: Blond & Briggs.

Solomon, Miriam. 2015. *Making Medical Knowledge*. Oxford: Oxford University Press.

Thiel, Cassandra L., Emily Schehlein, Thulasiraj Ravilla, R. D. Ravindran, Alan L. Robin, Osamah J. Saeedi, Joel S. Schuman, and Rengaraj Venkatesh. 2017. "Cataract Surgery and Environmental Sustainability: Waste and Lifecycle Assessment of Phacoemulsification at a Private Healthcare Facility." *Journal of Cataract & Refractive Surgery* 43 (11): 1391–98.

Thomas, Ravi. 2009. "Role of Small Incision Cataract Surgery in the Indian Scenario." *Indian Journal of Ophthalmology* 57 (1): 1.

———. 2010. "Reducing Endophthalmitis in India: An Example of the Importance of Critical Appraisal." *Indian Journal of Ophthalmology* 58 (6): 560–62.

Timmermans, Stefan, and Marc Berg. 2003. *The Gold Standard: The Challenge of Evidence-Based Medicine and Standardization in Health Care*. Philadelphia: Temple University Press.

Trivedy, Jyotee. 2011. "Outcomes of High Volume Cataract Surgeries at a Lions SightFirst Eye Hospital in Kenya." *Nepalese Journal of Ophthalmology: A Biannual Peer-Reviewed Academic Journal of the Nepal Ophthalmic Society: NEPJOPH* 3 (5): 31–38.

Venkatesh, Rengaraj, Colin S. H. Tan, Sabyasachi Sengupta, Ravilla D. Ravindran, Krishnan T. Krishnan, and David F. Chang. 2010. "Phacoemulsification Versus Manual Small-Incision Cataract Surgery for White Cataract." *Journal of Cataract & Refractive Surgery* 36 (11): 1849–54.

Wallerstein, Immanuel. 1974. "The Rise and Future Demise of the World Capitalist System: Concepts for Comparative Analysis." *Comparative Studies in Society and History* 16: 387–415.

West, Emily S., Ashley Behrens, Peter J. McDonnell, James M. Tielsch, and Oliver D. Schein. 2005. "The Incidence of Endophthalmitis After Cataract Surgery Among the U.S. Medicare Population Increased Between 1994 and 2001." *Ophthalmology* 112 (8): 1388–94.

Williams, Logan D. A. 2012, June 21. Participant Observation Fieldnotes. Lunch. Inspiration Hostel. Aravind Eye Care System, Madurai, India.

———. 2012, June 27. Participant Observation Fieldnotes. Community Ophthalmology NGOs and Transnational Circulation of Innovation Produced in LEDCs. Lions Aravind Institute of Community Ophthalmology, Madurai.

———. 2012, July 16. Direct Observation Fieldnotes. Cataract Operating theater. Aravind Eye Hospital—"Free Hospital", Madurai.

———. 2017. "Getting Undone Technology Done: Global Techno-Assemblage and the Value Chain of Invention." *Science, Technology and Society* 22 (1): 38–58.

———. 2018. "Mapping Superpositionality in Global Ethnography." *Science, Technology, & Human Values* 43 (2): 198–223.

Wynne, Brian. 1992. "Misunderstood Misunderstanding: Social Identities and Public Uptake of Science." *Public Understanding of Science* 1 (3): 281–304.

9

Conclusion: Innovation from Below

This book offers a feminist postcolonial multi-level perspective analysis: It pairs an explicit attention to the imposition of power through modes of science and technology circulation with new insights into the multi-level perspective on socio-technical system change. This makes it particularly useful for understanding technology transfer or innovation in the global south. Throughout this book, I have provided examples of the production of novel surgical sciences, technologies, finance models, and management sciences in the economic periphery, along with the circulation of these context-appropriate innovations from Nepal and India outward to Kenya and Mexico (and elsewhere in South America, Europe, and Africa).

In Chapter 1 of this book, I argued that phacoemulsification and Western aseptic technique together with their respective governmental policies, regulatory institutions, and incremental innovations constitute an entire socio-technical regime built around addressing immature cataracts in wealthy white-collar patients. In 1967, the radical innovation of phacoemulsification began incubating in a technology niche, and by 1984 the Phaco-regime dominated the global field of ophthalmology. This Phaco-regime has built up momentum over time (Hughes 1987, 1994).

© The Author(s) 2019
L. D. A. Williams, *Eradicating Blindness*,
https://doi.org/10.1007/978-981-13-1625-8_9

It has become the gold standard procedure for cataract surgery in many wealthy urban areas around the world, but for a variety of reasons, was not appropriate to meet the needs of poor rural patients in the global south.

My findings, based on this global ethnography of an autonomous global network formed to eradicate and control blindness, suggest that there has been a transition in the global field of ophthalmology. This transition started in 1975 with an autonomous global network and continued with the creation of a variety of eye hospitals utilizing a new Robin Hood finance model (Chapters 2 and 3). These eye hospitals developed rules emphasizing high-quality, high-volume, health services for all (Chapters 3 and 4). They deliberately focused on a marginalized group, rural poor prospective patients. To achieve their aims, they connected with local and global partners to develop new health education and data collection practices to make these patients into health consumers and to better define the problem of avoidable blindness (Chapter 4). Inside two South Asian eye hospitals, Aravind Eye Care System and Tilganga Institute of Ophthalmology, new innovations incubated in appropriate technology niches: intraocular lenses as a technology innovation (Chapter 5); SICS, a surgical science innovation that provided most of the same benefits as Phaco at lower cost (Chapter 6); and the knowledge of how to use interlocking innovations altogether to create efficient eye health infrastructure that produces good patient health outcomes (Chapter 7). Incubation in Aurolab and Tilganga-FHIOL occurred from 1996 onward, which points to the emergence of the new SICS-regime. However, this transition is unique in that it has primarily occurred geo-politically in the less economically developed countries of the global south, starting with India and Nepal. Therefore, the incumbent Phaco-regime and the new SICS-regime coexist in the global landscape.

The intent of this chapter is to synthesize insights from previous chapters and illuminate the features of a general theoretical model: the dual regime thesis. The remainder of this book's conclusion has the following structure: Sect. 9.1, summarizes two new concepts. The first concept, systemic technology choice, contributes to studies of appropriate technology movements; the second concept, interlocking innovations, contributes to the multi-level perspective and specifically understanding the dual regime thesis. Section 9.2 highlights the book's conceptual contribution to understanding contestation in a global field of science while reiterating the transition to dual regimes in the global field of ophthalmology through circular causality and multiple modes of circulation. Next Sect. 9.3 examines the theoretical implications of the dual regime thesis for socio-technical transition pathways in the multi-level perspective. This examination continues in Sect. 9.4, which reviews the ramifications of the dual regime thesis for understanding multi-regime interactions. Subsequently, Sect. 9.5 suggests new questions and future work for new industrial sectors and international relations theory. Finally, Sect. 9.6 focuses on the potential for further transition in the global field of ophthalmology.

9.1   Systemic Technology Choice, Kaplinsky's Dilemma and Interlocking Innovations

The concept of systemic technology choice helps to explain changes in the appropriate technology movement that are linked to Kaplinsky's reflection on the policy dilemma inherent in scaling-up appropriate technology. This concept and reflection are essential to better understand how interlocking innovations form in appropriate technology niches.

This book has described a new shift in the appropriate technology movement in less economically developed countries where self-sufficient NGOs in the global scientific field of ophthalmology are addressing the diseases of avoidable blindness. Systemic technology choice represents a shift from analyzing the failure of high technology transfer and proposing intermediate technology as the solution, to strategically considering how any knowledge or technology transfer is in fact the transfer of a socio-technical system. Persons engaged in the practice of systemic technology choice are very much aware that high or low technology transfer can be equally problematic and for the same reason—the narrow focus on the movement of a singular artifact. Therefore, systemic technology choice emphasizes the transfer of a system of artifacts (e.g., instruments, knowledge, practices, and products) along with values, policies, etc.

This book offers new insights into appropriate technology at a large scale demonstrating power relationships and economic logics. While Kaplinsky's dilemma juxtaposes mass production or mass participation, I have described community ophthalmology units taking a third approach that combines the benefits of both for community members. Community ophthalmology professionals working in South Asia reinterpreted ideological influences from both neoliberal market capitalism and local Gandhian philosophy through:

- COMMUNITY OWNERSHIP or LOCAL TRUSTEESHIP (Gandhi): Reinvesting profits from sales to elite community members for the benefit of marginalized community members;
- HIGH TECHNOLOGY and LARGE SCALE (Schumpeter): Using low-labor, large-scale, high technology to create high-quality, inexpensive, products;
- LOW-COST and LOW PROFIT MARGINS (Schumacher and Gandhi): Selling high-quality, inexpensive, products below market rates primarily to benefit marginalized community members;
- LABOR INTENSIVE and LARGE SCALE (Schumacher, Schumpeter, and Gandhi): Employing numerous secondary school-educated assistants and technicians for many specialized, routinized tasks that were previously performed by postgraduate-educated professionals;
- LIVING WAGES (Schumacher and Gandhi): Paying living wages to secondary school-educated marginalized community members trained as assistants and technicians, while, paying postgraduate-educated elite professionals below market rate wages.

In order to do this, they had to work simultaneously across the biotechnology industry sector, the civil society sector, and the healthcare industry sector to produce interlocking innovations.

Interlocking innovations are multiple, complimentary, and sub-system composed knowledge and artifacts. Typically, interlocking innovations include new radical innovations in knowledge, technology, or process that are closely linked with existing incremental innovations and black boxed. For the SICS-regime, the interlocking innovations include the Robin Hood finance model, SICS surgical technique, and IOLs and additionally, organizational innovation of standards and benchmarks for routinization of high-volume patient throughput (Chapters 4 and 8); science innovation of South Asian aseptic technique (Chapter 8); a clean laboratory for manufacturing IOLS as a technology sub-system (Chapter 5); an ideology of sarvodaya or working for the good of all, but especially those who are marginalized; and the Buddhist economic philosophy of enoughness (Chapter 3). In short, South Asian interlocking innovations combined an emphasis on serving the marginalized with: an IOL laboratory; a surgical systems approach; and hospital management practices.

Interlocking innovations were first produced inside of a variety of niches as separate and singular knowledge and artifacts. These multiple innovations and sub-systems were complimentary and came together to form interlocking innovations with their own politics, ideology, and values that transfer along with them. Once linked and black boxed, they then circulated outside of the niche through translation and contestation.

9.2   Socio-Technical Transitions, Circular Causality, and Contestation

The multi-level perspective on socio-technical transitions is sometimes misread as advocating for linear phases of transition because it typically divides technological phases into periods. However, socio-technical change is known to occur simultaneously across niches, the socio-technical regime, and landscape (Geels 2005c, 2007; Raven 2007; Raven and Verbong 2007; Sutherland et al. 2015). The multi-level perspective is unique because it argues for the explanatory power of circular causality, when processes link up across multiple dimensions and levels, with multiple, complimentary effects, to drive socio-technical regime change (Geels 2005c, 686).

In this book, I have explained how four modes of science and technology circulation occurred simultaneously in the autonomous global network dedicated to eradicating and controlling blindness from the mid-1990s onward. This is another way of thinking about circular causality in socio-technical transitions. Like Shepherd (2006, 421), I too argue that translation and appropriation occur simultaneously. Furthermore, I have demonstrated the concurrence of diffusion, appropriation, translation, and contestation which, together, allow for both a bilateral power dynamic and a bidirectional circulation of science and technology.

In Chapter 5, I exposed how South Asian community ophthalmology professionals acted as challengers and used diffusion to bring incremental innovations into their appropriate technology niches. Diffusion is a unilateral and unidirectional process that increases the power of the knowledge or technology purveyor. To bring IOL manufacturing laboratories to India and Nepal, community ophthalmology professionals paid firms in the USA and Australia to perform turnkey technology transfer. However, this temporary technological dependency furthered the more radical agenda of endogenous development and technological sovereignty. Community ophthalmology professionals had to contest developmentalist ideas about appropriate technology for the rural poor from peers at home and abroad before they started the turnkey technology transfer.

In Chapter 6, I revealed how challengers created radical surgical science innovations through a bilateral and unidirectional process of appropriation by which a consumer becomes a producer and increases in power. Inside their appropriate technology niche, Nepalese community ophthalmologists perfected SICS for the hard case of white cataracts. They adapted it from an Israeli ophthalmologist and made SICS on par scientifically with the state-of-the-art phacoemulsification procedure created in the USA.

In Chapter 7, I illuminated how the autonomous global network to eradicate and control blindness accumulated niches through translation. Translation is bidirectional and unilateral; the dominant knowledge or technology purveyor imposes power over time and space through extraction, selection, and transformation in a two-way exchange. Aravind and Tilganga's dissemination of their interlocking innovations is a unilateral imposition of power: They increase their economic and social power by circulating their innovations from their protected niches in India and Nepal outward. As they train others to use their techniques, they also extract information from trainees and from patients. Their training efforts are validated by recognition from the more powerful World Health Organization and United Nations Development Programme.

Finally in Chapter 8, I reveal how repeated contestation creates a fracture point in the incumbent regime, which is subsequently revealed as dual: the incumbent regime and the challenger regime. Contestation is the movement of knowledge and artifacts from challengers in a subordinate position in the world-system to incumbent actors in the dominant position, and this involves an acrimonious but bidirectional and bilateral exchange between the two positions. Ophthalmologists, engineers, managers, and other community ophthalmology professionals do not participate in traditional forms of collective action (i.e., protests and marches) against governments or corporations. Instead, those involved in community ophthalmology organizations are very much interested in utilizing scientific evidence or technological design to press forward with their social agendas (Hess 2016; Williams 2017). The community ophthalmology professionals could fracture the incumbent regime because they contested practices and rules that influenced its technological trajectory.

Community ophthalmology professionals completed this fracturing with new cognitive and normative rules that challenged the incumbent regime. They followed a new technical trajectory of endogenous development through a radical emergent radical rule-set:

- cognitive rules of eradicating blindness, self-sufficiency, self-reliance, sarvodaya, and economic enoughness to guide the organization
- formal rules of community-embeddedness (both local and global) and high volume negotiated with the state and philanthropists
- unwritten normative rules of anti-developmentalism and local sovereignty to shape values and behavior.

For this case of systemic technology choice by community ophthalmologists, they used contestation to circulate their interlocking innovations which acted as a wedge to divide the incumbent socio-technical regime of Phaco into dual regimes: one Phaco-regime in the global north and another SICS-regime in the global south. They did so by challenging knowledge hierarchies (Nieusma 2007): They disputed the knowledge paired with authority of other experts. This did not result in closure of the debate between which surgical technique, or aseptic technique, provides the patient with the best outcomes. However, it allowed community ophthalmologists to establish the existence and dominance of the SICS-regime to solve the problem of avoidable blindness for low-income rural patients all over the world.

Circular causality occurs through concurrent diffusion, appropriation, translation, and contestation. The outcome is that within the global field of ophthalmology, there are dual socio-technical regimes acting in parallel.

9.3 Socio-Technical Transition Pathways and the Dual Regime Thesis

This book also offers a new general theoretical model for the multi-level perspective on socio-technical system change: the dual regime thesis. "By accepting that transition need not entail the displacement of one universal system by another, one can consider a broader range of configurations" (Furlong 2014, 145). The dual regime thesis is particularly useful to understand socio-technical change initiated by appropriate technology movements to innovate on behalf of marginalized people. This new theoretical model adds to the multi-level perspective of socio-technical transitions: an extended understanding of four ways that landscape is differentiated and the new coexistence transition pathway.

The work of community ophthalmologists has informed a new theory of socio-technical change in regimes using the multi-level perspective. In a transition pathway, we may not start and end with a single dominant regime; instead, structural inequality and other differences in the landscape may lead to a situation where we have dual and complimentary regimes, each able to solve the same socio-technical problem. In the case of community ophthalmology, that problem was blindness due to cataract disease. The two regimes interact with each other, but the incumbent regime controls the technological trajectories of ophthalmology innovations in the global north, while the challenger regime controls the technological trajectories of ophthalmology innovations in the global south (see Fig. 9.1).

In prior work on socio-technical transitions, the landscape was seen as monolithic. Therefore, it typically had two states: stable and disturbed. Stable landscapes provide moderate pressure on the socio-technical regime. In stable landscapes, transitions started through internal changes in the regime, such as the reconfiguration and transformation pathways. In contrast, disturbed landscapes meant transitions relied on significant change in the landscape to trigger change in the regime, such as the technological substitution pathway and the dealignment and realignment pathway (Geels 2005b).

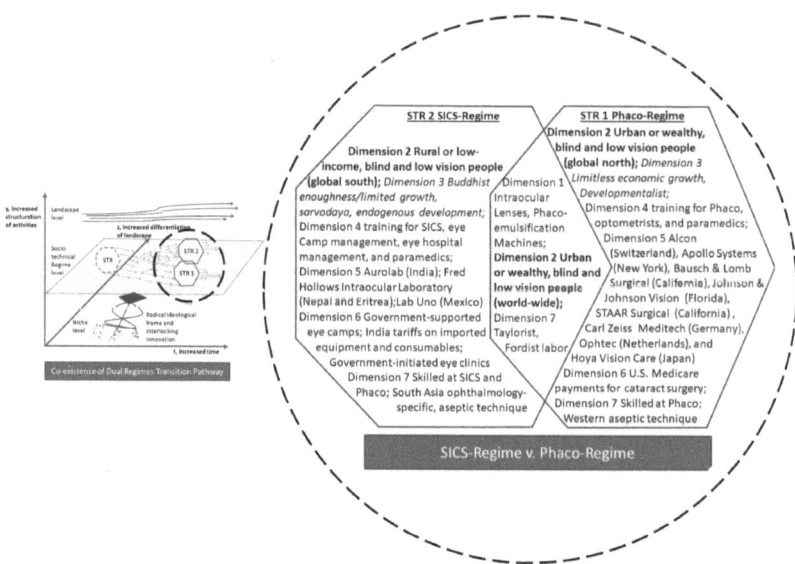

Fig. 9.1 Coexistence of dual regimes, SICS v. Phaco, in the differentiated landscape. Each of the two regimes has the typical dimensions: Dimension 1 Technology; Dimension 2 Markets, user practices; Dimension 3 Culture, symbolic meaning; Dimension 4 Infrastructure; Dimension 5 Industry; Dimension 6 Policy; and Dimension 7 Scientific knowledge

Additionally, previous work has emphasized that landscapes can be heterogeneous and include aspects that are material, environmental, political, and technological including "broad political coalitions, …values, environmental problems…wars… the material and spatial arrangements of cities…and electricity infrastructures" (Geels 2005a, 78–79). Thus, a landscape can be an earlier socio-technical regime that is so entrenched and ossified as to serve as the gradually changing background for investigating a active new socio-technical regime (Geels 2005a; Geels and Schot 2007). Most transition studies tacitly rely on these entrenched elements without explicitly referencing them.

The dual regime thesis extends a new understanding of differentiation in the landscape, where "[S]tatic landscape structures create different affordances and action possibilities" (Geels et al. 2016, 901). In this book, the 1980 event of global smallpox eradication impacts various parts of the landscape differently. In the global north, it serves as a form of moderate landscape pressure on US and UK ophthalmologists who ignore it; they are already occupied with the technical problem of smaller incisions for cataract surgery using the new phacoemulsification. In contrast, in the global south, smallpox eradication serves as an exogenous shock that ignites a sense of optimism among a small social network of epidemiologists and clinical ophthalmologists which subsequently grows into an autonomous global network interested in eradicating blindness (Chapter 2).

While actors in the socio-technical regimes cannot implement short-term change in the landscape, they are affected by long-term and short-term changes in the landscape (Geels 2005a, 79). The global network to eradicate blindness, which eventually grew to become appropriate technology niches and then the SICS-regime, has always been geopolitically dispersed globally (although not worldwide). This autonomous global network has primarily created infrastructure, technology, and new knowledge in the global south.

This ethnographic study demonstrated that the landscape was differentiated in four ways. The most prominent form of landscape differentiation was geo-political. This was exemplified by the member-state governments sending representatives to WHO and IAPB committees and setting policies on: establishing charitable organizations (Chapters 2, 3, and 11);

training personnel (Chapter 7); repairing roads, bridges, telephone poles, and electricity transmission wires (Chapter 4); and practicing surgical aseptic technique (Chapter 8).

Another form of landscape differentiation was geo-physical where differences in altitude, temperature, etc., placed different demands on instruments and human personnel. The differences in eye camps point to this form of differentiation although this was not elaborated upon in detail (Chapter 4).

A third way that the landscape was differentiated was epistemic. There were differences in how types of knowledge were perceived by local ophthalmic societies, versus national ophthalmic societies, and versus regional ophthalmic societies and international ophthalmic societies. For example, the Asian-Pacific Academy of Ophthalmology highlighted the challenge that SICS brought to the Phaco-regime (Chapter 1). Meanwhile, the European Cataract and Refractive Surgery instead emphasized the challenge that South Asian ophthalmologists' aseptic technique brought to clinical ophthalmology, and an ophthalmic society in Mexico wanted to ban Sala Uno ophthalmologists (Chapter 8).

The final form of landscape differentiation is population density. While previously the multi-level perspective has considered population demographics an important part of the landscape (Geels 2005a), this book has illuminated how population density shapes regimes and niches. This was true for community ophthalmologists who found that their radical finance model for cost recovery, the Robin Hood model, works better in nation-states with high population density in rural areas (see Chapter 7).

The coexistence transition pathway reacts differently to landscape pressure than the previous four transition pathways. In the technological substitution pathway, the landscape provides an exogenous shock that stimulates new firms to develop novel technology and gradually accumulate more niches; this is also true for the coexistence pathway. However, technology break through in the coexistence pathway does not involve replacing the old regime.

Analogous to the reconfiguration pathway, coexistence involves internal cumulative changes guided by financial and design considerations as the initial social network emerges from the niche and grows into a regime

(Geels and Schot 2007). This is demonstrated by Aravind, Tilganga, Loresho, and Sala Uno; each eye hospital serves a different percentage of poor patients depending upon the income they are able to make from wealthy patients (Chapter 3 and 11). It is furthermore confirmed by the gradual technology-practice change in India from eye surgical camps to eye screening camps as a government-regulated standard that occured from 1976 to 2002 at Aravind (Chapter 4). Unlike the reconfiguration pathway, the coexistence pathway did not subsume the incumbent regime globally. Instead, the coexistence pathway created a new challenger regime that subsumed the incumbent regime in the global south, but otherwise continues in parallel to the incumbent regime.

Coexistence, like the dealignment and realignment pathway, involves multiple innovations that compete until one wins. I have only described two (Aravind's MSICS with irrigating vectis versus Tilganga's SICS with anterior chamber maintainer) of the many alternative versions of SICS that competed against each other in India, Nepal, and elsewhere in the global south. The dominant version, Dr. Ruit's SICS, was published early and is frequently cited. However, Dr. Ruit's SICS technique could not win on its own. In the coexistence pathway, the surgical science innovation was one among a set of interlocking innovations that distinguished it from the other surgical techniques.

Finally, the coexistence pathway is similar to the transformation pathway in that moderate landscape pressure ignites an institutional power struggle that changes cognitive and normative rules and technological trajectories (Geels and Schot 2007). In the transformation pathway, these power struggles would be internal to the incumbent regime. However, for the coexistence pathway, they result in breakthrough of interlocking innovations and the fracturing of the incumbent regime in two. The challengers, community ophthalmologists in South Asia, are outside the knowledge centers of the global north (Chapters 6 and 7). Nevertheless, they frequently challenge the Western knowledge touted by European (or local) clinical ophthalmologists (Chapters 6 and 8) in order to define appropriate technology and make appropriate decisions for their specific South Asian contexts. For example, South Asian community ophthalmologists scientifically validate their own aseptic technique practices as both evidence-based and cost-effective (Chapter 8). Instead of internally altering the incumbent regime, their struggles bolster their own novel practices and solidify their emergent radical rule-set. With the coalescing of the emergent radical rule-set, the new challenger regime is born.

In addition to the niche-regime interactions and landscape differentiation described above, the coexistence pathway comes out of the dual regime thesis and therefore must contend with multi-regime interactions.

9.4   Multi-regime Interactions and the Dual Regime Thesis

Coexistence is unlike other transition pathways because it involves multi-regime interactions that are simultaneously symbiotic and competitive. The dual regime thesis also highlights a new multi-regime interaction: interstitial birth.

Originally, there were five multi-regime interactions: disintegration, competition, symbiosis, fiat birth, and integration (Geels 2007; Raven 2007; Raven and Verbong 2007; Sutherland et al. 2015). Regimes typically operate on the scale of decades (Raven et al. 2012, 72). Therefore, when multi-regime interactions are typically of short duration (9 or fewer years), then they might be called an event. Meanwhile, if they are typically of long duration (10 or more years), then might be called a relationship. These multi-regime events and relationships can be defined along a spectrum from low to high levels of inter-regime reciprocity:

- Disintegration event (lowest inter-regime reciprocity)—one regime splits into two; an example would be when the telecommunications sector split into landline versus mobile (Raven and Verbong 2007, 503);
- Competition relationship—two or more regimes address the same societal problem, and therefore fight each other for resources resulting in a variety of solutions (Geels 2007; Raven and Verbong 2007, 502) and can lead to integration by one regime subsuming another (Raven and Verbong 2007, 502);

- Symbiosis relationship—two or more regimes work cooperatively to share resources, sometimes with mutual dependency; either one regime's products serve as the second regime's raw material or the cooperative relationship helps each regime provide a solution to the same societal problem (Geels 2007; Raven and Verbong 2007, 503);
- Fiat Birth event—landscape pressures force the birth of a third regime from two existing symbiotic regimes, such as EU policy directives creating a renewable electricity regime in Great Britain, Germany, and the Czech Republic that combined features of an agriculture regime and traditional electricity regime (Sutherland et al. 2015); and
- Integration event (highest inter-regime reciprocity)—two or more regimes combine into one regime, such as the merger of gas and electric companies in the Netherlands (Raven and Verbong 2007, 503).

An important feature of multi-regime interactions with high levels of inter-regime reciprocity is called spillover. Spillover refers to when two or more regimes share many of the same cognitive rules and technology (Raven and Verbong 2007, 501; Sutherland et al. 2015, 1551).

The dual regime thesis and coexistence transition pathway suggest a new multi-regime interaction event called interstitial birth. Interstitial birth involves the disintegration of the incumbent regime and emergence of a new regime and incumbent regime. The interstitial birth of the new regime depends initially on spillover from the incumbent regime. This spillover does not include the cognitive rules of the incumbent regime (i.e., unlimited economic growth), many of which are fiercely contested by the challengers in the autonomous global network and appropriate technology niches. However, it does include some technology transfer from the incumbent regime to the new regime. As the new regime emerges through interstitial birth, science and technology diffuses to the appropriate technology niches, or is appropriated by the challengers into their niches.

The early work of the autonomous global network from 1975 onward was an important foundation for the interstitial birth event. However, I argue that the interstitial birth event occurred over just four years. It began in 1996 with the presence of two intraocular lens laboratories producing low-cost ophthalmic consumables and the inauguration of the Lions Aravind Institute for Community Ophthalmology (Chapters 5 and 7) and ended with Dr. Ruit publishing his SICS microsurgical technique in 2000 (Chapter 6). The shared learning platform (LAICO) helped to enhance allies' enthusiasm and enabled more rapid niche accumulation. During those four years, the autonomous global network accumulated multiple niches from the interstices in the incumbent regime (Chapters 4, 7, and 8). These interstices were both the empty spaces and the "absences of action" (Debaise 2013, 102). The SICS-regime originated with local elites who focused narrowly on providing cost-effective eye health services to marginalized non-users. Their narrow focus encouraged the SICS-regime to grow in the interstices of the Phaco-regime.

Challengers to the incumbent regime generated a new regime that was simultaneously separate from the incumbent regime (differentiated in the landscape) and part of the incumbent regime (the empty spaces where the incumbent regime failed to act). By focusing on providing goods and services to non-users, the challengers could set their own technological trajectory because they had no competitors from the incumbent regime. This is in contrast to the incumbent regime which was bound by the momentum of the already existing infrastructures, policies, cognitive rules, and user parameters. Likewise, the challengers encountered little competition from incumbent actors in the geophysically and geo-politically differentiated landscape.

An interstitial birth event, as a multi-regime interaction, is one part of a multi-regime pattern of relationship change. While previous cases have discussed two patterns of change in multi-regime interactions, this book discusses a third pattern. Pattern 1 was demonstrated from 1930 to 1970 in the USA where two regimes (radio and music record) co-evolved from competition to symbiosis while introducing new music genres out of music niches: Rhythm & Blues, Country & Western, and Rock (Geels 2007). This first example demonstrates that two regimes can compete to solve the same problem with different innovations, but over time, can evolve to cooperatively address the problem.

Pattern 2 occurred from 1969 to 2003 in the Netherlands, where the waste regime and electricity regime co-evolved from separate to symbiotic and, finally, integrated (Raven 2007; Raven and Verbong 2007). This second example is premised on regimes being equivalent with industrial sectors (Raven 2007, 2198; Raven and Verbong 2007). Therefore, the shift from symbiotic to integrated is premised on multi-industrial sector interactions.

In contrast to the two cases described above, the coexistence transition follows a third pattern; it involves multi-regime interactions evolving over time from interstitial birth event to a final state this is simultaneously both symbiotic and competitive. The SICS-regime is not dependent upon the Phaco-regime although it uses Phaco technology. Thus, there is spillover from the Phaco-regime to the SICS-regime (Chapters 5 and 6), illustrating a symbiotic relationship between the SICS-regime and Phaco-regime. While the biotechnology industrial sector component of the SICS-regime and Phaco-regime is in symbiotic relationship, the medical science sector component of the two regimes has long been in a competitive relationship (Chapter 8).

9.5   New Questions and Future Work

This book has implications for how we think about socio-technical regimes. Prior work has suggested that the boundaries of a socio-technical regime are fuzzy. Here, we can see that a socio-technical regime can exist with a global market but not have control over all geo-political locations worldwide. That is, a socio-technical regime can simultaneously be global but not worldwide (Worthington 1993). A socio-technical regime can also be multi-sectoral. In this book, each regime involved the global fields of ophthalmology, international development, and biotechnology industry.

Also, the timescale of this multi-level perspective analysis of socio-technical change is from 1975 to 2017, of forty-two years; it is of long enough duration for a very detailed analysis. However, it is just short of the fifty years recommended for studying technological transitions in socio-technical systems (Geels and Schot 2007). Therefore, it is possible that other indicators beyond time length are more important to correctly identify technological transitions and their boundaries. For example, a significant indicator may be to identify that a socio-technical system has momentum in the way that Hughes (1987) has described, where it has economies of scope and scale. From that starting point, scholars can collect historical and sociological evidence to explain the socio-technical system's development.

The timing of creating interlocking innovations in an appropriate technology niche was nonlinear with two asynchronous sets of synchronous innovations. The first set of synchronous innovations was the development of the Robin Hood model concurrent with the development of the benchmarks and standards for eye camps (Chapter 3). A second set of synchronous innovations occurred after the first set. Through diffusion, these community ophthalmology organizations were creating endogenously produced IOLs. Simultaneously, through appropriation, the autonomous global network was creating the SICS technique. The nonlinear timing of the creation of multiple, linked, complimentary and sub-system innovations into an interlocking innovation may be worth future study.

Systemic technology choice and the dual regime thesis might be further applied to better understand the global mobile telephone industry as a socio-technical system undergoing technological transition. Odumosu (2009) has suggested that the Nigerian GSM mobile telephone system is structured in a manner that is significantly different than the European GSM mobile telephone system in terms of: policy, regulations, infrastructure, and technologies. It is therefore possible that Nigerian engineers engaged in systemic technology choice to produce a mobile telephone socio-technical regime that was more appropriate for Nigerian users.

Another industry that might be analyzed as the coexistence of dual regimes is the banking industry. Individuals without bank accounts in the global south can transfer money using M-Pesa in Kenya (Williams and Woodson 2012). Scholars are already pointing out that this is a socio-technical transition focused on inclusive innovation where Vodafone UK deliberately focused on creating a money transfer service for marginalized Kenyans without bank accounts. The result, after 15 years, was an increased number of Kenyans enrolled in both traditional banking as well as mobile banking (Onsongo and Schot 2017). Might this be another example of dual regimes?

A third industry that might be analyzed using the dual regime thesis is food systems. Member associations and other NGOs have sprung up for the purpose of certifying organic and Genetically Modified Organism (GMO)—free food in response to various levels of regulation and labeling of GMOs by nation-states around the world. What lay experts or professionals may have been involved in such certification efforts? What are the implications for understanding circuits of science, technology, capital, and ideology?

The coexistence of dual regimes might furthermore be used to analyze the importance of the state in science and technology transitions where challengers do not engage in traditional collective action. As sociology of technology is incorporated into international relations theory, recent questions have emphasized the importance of considering socio-technical regimes as part of a state's unique slate of powers (Herrera 2006). That is, in addition to the state's monopoly on violence, the state has a monopoly on cross-border communication and goods shipments (Herrera 2006). This requires that international relations scholars be attentive to different types of socio-technical regimes, to include electricity generation and supply (coal, nuclear, gas, etc.), telecommunications, or the transportation system (air, sea, and land). The international movement of knowledge and technologies occurs constantly and at different scales; this offers further opportunity for theorizing the explicit and tacit roles of multiple states in global socio-technical system change that relies upon science and technology circulation.

In international relations theory, the concept of contestation opens up new research avenues to explore the relationship between technology transfer and national sovereignty in its variety of forms, including biological (Stephenson 2011), cybered (Demchak and Dombrowski 2014), genomic (Benjamin 2009), or scientific (Mahony 2014; Samsky 2012). For such new research avenues, we might ask if specific modes of circulation, i.e., diffusion, translation, appropriation, or contestation, are more closely linked to one form of sovereignty over another? Considering that epidemics ignore national boundaries, what is the relationship between contestation of science and technology, sovereignty, and national security? How are the networks of bilateral and multilateral organizations that circulate development aid in the form of pharmaceutical drugs or technology transfer assistance contributing to endogenous development and scientific sovereignty?

The production and circulation of telecommunication knowledge, devices, and instruments are global in nature. This includes small electronics being fabricated in less economically developed countries and assembled in wealthy industrialized countries. It also includes countries that are politically not allied that participate in the long value-chain of inventions in telecommunications because of multinational corporations search for the most inexpensive labor. Does the global nature of telecommunications inflect discussions about cyber sovereignty?

The sub-concept of contestation also leads to new questions for future work, which include: Is challenging knowledge hierarchies always linked to a marginalized standpoint? Do elites (in comparison with the marginalized) also contest scientific knowledge and engage in technological conflict, or is such activity by elites always called oppression or subordination?

9.6 The Next Transition in the Global Field of Ophthalmology?

Community ophthalmologists' efforts to control costs have implications that reverberate throughout the global field of ophthalmology. Cataract surgeries are a major expenditure in ophthalmology clinics and departments around the world because of the high incidence of cataract disease among aging populations. For example, Medicare, a US government health insurance program for senior citizens, serves an aging population that is more likely than the average population to have cataract disease. The US Congress and the Health Finances Administration targeted the clinical ophthalmology community for an inquiry in the 1980s because cataract surgery accounted for 12% of the Medicare budget (Stark et al. 1989). The share of the Medicare budget attributed to cataract surgery has since decreased to 2.8% between 1996 and 2000: Of the US Medicare budget, 4% or approximately $6.67 billion went to four eye diseases including cataract disease while $4.75 billion dollars went to cataract disease alone, therefore cataract disease utilized (($4.75E9/$6.67E9) * 4%) = 2.8% of the Medicare budget from 1996 to 2000 (Salm et al. 2006). This percentage could increase again with the large population of baby boomers in the USA. Considering the prominence of cataract disease among the population of US senior citizens, and the necessity of surgery to treat the disease, it is likely that the US government would be interested in providing patients with the best visual outcomes for the cheapest cost.

An interesting question which requires further investigation is the timing and scale of a multi-regime integration event where dual socio-technical regimes combine into one socio-technical regime. This question may arise sooner rather than later as a singular innovation of the SICS socio-technical regime, the Robin Hood finance model, is circulating to a wealthy industrialized country, the USA.

The low-cost IOLs produced by Tilganga-FHIOL have the CE (Conformité Européene) mark and have already circulated from Nepal to Australia and Europe. However, once separated from the context of the global south and detached from the cognitive rule of reaching the unreached, might low-cost IOLs become just another cheap good that can be purchased in global markets? The circulation of the Robin Hood model, with its radical ideology of economic enoughness, from South Asia to the global north is more likely to reintegrate the Phaco and SICS regimes.

The Robin Hood model is being brought to the USA through the efforts of a nonprofit organization, Pacific Vision Foundation, in California. Ophthalmologists in San Francisco are thinking about how to use parts of the Robin Hood model to provide eye healthcare services to low-income people in the San Francisco Bay Area (Mehta and Shenoy 2011). In June 2007, the Pacific Vision Foundation was awarded approximately $10.6 million US Dollars in program and infrastructure development funds from the Robert Wood Johnson Foundation (and additional funds from other philanthropies) to develop a business plan and perform renovations on a building that they purchased downtown to turn it into a premiere medical training facility (Crum 2015). This new facility will serve both those who cannot afford to pay for eye health care, as well as those who have health insurance or can otherwise afford to pay (Crum 2015). The Eye Institute was inaugurated October 4, 2017 (The Pacific Vision Foundation 2017). The Pacific Vision Foundation ophthalmologists who created The Eye Institute are affiliated with the California Pacific Medical Center Department of Ophthalmology (est. 1870), the oldest US ophthalmology residency west of the Mississippi River. The Eye Institute will continue the work with low-income persons with eye disease that the California Pacific Medical Center Department of Ophthalmology Lions Eye Clinic had previously performed.

The founder of the Pacific Vision Foundation, Dr. Bruce Spvey (2013), explains that while the clinic cannot source lenses from Aurolab or Tilganga-FHIOL because they are not FDA-approved, they can use some of the other financial and scientific innovations from the SICS-regime as part of their own technology choices,

> We have a vision…that we'll provide proportionally more care to those people who can't pay for it ….There'll be people who can pay partially and there'll be people who can't pay anything. And we're going to take all comers …. But we're looking at how we can provide …equal care, but payment stratification…. There's stratified payment in various places around the United States, but never to the degree that we're looking for as purely free care …. So that's what's different. That is an Aravind model…. we're going to copy them in every way that fits. Obviously, this can't be the same as Aravind. Our health system is different … Expectations of the patients are different.

I predict that as The Eye Institute grows in influence in San Francisco it will, in a similar manner to the Mexican clinic Sala Uno, disrupt the existing medical establishment. The Eye Institute will have to navigate that mode of contestation as controversial production and circulation of science and technology.

Several technology transition outcomes are possible. In the first option, stable reproduction, the Robin Hood model as an incremental innovation (without being linked to the other complimentary innovations), will support another US-based node of the SICS-regime.

In this outcome, the SICS-regime and the Phaco-regime would be less geo-physically and geo-politically differentiated; therefore, they would likely have a higher degree of a symbiosis relationship.

In the second option, transformation, the Robin Hood model will precipitate spillover of cognitive and normative rules from the SICS-regime to the Phaco-regime that emphasize building science, technology, and practice around the most marginalized patients. This transfer of rules will stimulate radical socio-technical change in the Phaco-regime starting in the USA and later spreading to Australia, Japan, and Europe. This will result in SICS-regime reproduction, Phaco-regime transformation, and the multi-regime event of integration between the SICS-regime and the Phaco-regime.

A third option is that, without the other complimentary components of the interlocking innovations, the Robin Hood model will fail to stimulate radical socio-technical change in the Phaco-regime. Instead, the stable Phaco socio-technical regime will follow a reconfiguration pathway and modify its internal organizational processes slightly to add on this new incremental innovation while otherwise continuing with business as usual. This would involve technological spillover from the challenger SICS-regime to the incumbent Phaco-regime, and a higher degree of competitive relationship between the two coexisting regimes.

There are several possibilities for this next transition in the global field of ophthalmology as the Pacific Vision Foundation expands the reach and influence of The Eye Institute which may likely shed more insight onto socio-technical system change in global health.

References

Benjamin, Ruha. 2009. "A Lab of Their Own: Genomic Sovereignty as Postcolonial Science Policy." *Policy and Society* 28 (4): 341–55.

Crum, Robert. 2015. "An Innovative Ophthalmological and Financial Model for People at All Economic Levels." Program Results Report. Robert Wood Johnson Foundation. http://www.rwjf.org/content/dam/farm/reports/program_results_reports/2015/rwjf419225.

Debaise, Didier. 2013. "A Philosophy of Interstices: Thinking Subjects and Societies from Whitehead's Philosophy." *Subjectivity* 6 (1): 101–11.

Demchak, Chris C., and Peter J. Dombrowski. 2014. "Rise of a Cybered Westphalian Age: The Coming Decades." In *The Global Politics of Science and Technology—Vol. 1—Concepts from International Relations and Other Disciplines*, edited by Maximilian Mayer, Mariana Carpes, and Ruth Knoblich, 91–113. Global Power Shift: Comparative Analysis and Perspectives. Berlin and Heidelberg: Springer.

Furlong, Kathryn. 2014. "STS Beyond the 'Modern Infrastructure Ideal': Extending Theory by Engaging with Infrastructure Challenges in the South." *Technology in Society* 38 (August): 139–47.

Geels, Frank W. 2005a. "Conceptual Perspective on Sytems Innovations and Technological Transitions." In *Technological Transitions and System Innovations: A Co-evolutionary and Socio-Technical Analysis*, 75–102. Cheltenham, UK; Northampton, MA: Edward Elgar.

———. 2005b. "The Dynamics of Transitions in Socio-Technical Systems: A Multi-level Analysis of the Transition Pathway from Horse-Drawn Carriages to Automobiles (1860–1930)." *Technology Analysis & Strategic Management* 17 (4): 445–76.

———. 2005c. "Processes and Patterns in Transitions and System Innovations: Refining the Co-evolutionary Multi-Level Perspective." *Technological Forecasting and Social Change*, Transitions towards Sustainability through System Innovation 72 (6): 681–96.

———. 2007. "Analysing the Breakthrough of Rock 'n' Roll (1930–1970) Multi-regime Interaction and Reconfiguration in the Multi-level Perspective." *Technological Forecasting and Social Change* 74 (8): 1411–31.

Geels, Frank W., and Johan Schot. 2007. "Typology of Sociotechnical Transition Pathways." *Research Policy* 36 (3): 399–417.

Geels, Frank W., Florian Kern, Gerhard Fuchs, Nele Hinderer, Gregor Kungl, Josephine Mylan, Mario Neukirch, and Sandra Wassermann. 2016. "The Enactment of Socio-Technical Transition Pathways: A Reformulated Typology and a Comparative Multi-level Analysis of the German and UK Low-Carbon Electricity Transitions (1990–2014)." *Research Policy* 45 (4): 896–913.

Herrera, Geoffrey Lucas. 2006. "International Systems Theory, Technology and Transformation." In *Technology and International Transformation: The Railroad, the Atom Bomb, and the Politics of Technological Change*, 13–44. Albany: State University of New York Press.

Hess, David J. 2016. *Undone Science: Social Movements, Mobilized Publics, and Industrial Transitions*. Cambridge: The MIT Press.

Hughes, Thomas Parke. 1987. "The Evolution of Large Technological Systems." In *The Social Construction of Technological Systems: New Directions in the Sociology and History of Technology*, edited by Wiebe E. Bijker, Thomas Parke Hughes, and Trevor J. Pinch, 51–82. Cambridge: The MIT Press.

———. 1994. "Technological Momentum." In *Does Technology Drive History? The Dilemma of Technological Determinism*, edited by Merritt Roe Smith and Leo Marx, 101–114. Cambridge: The MIT Press.

Mahony, Martin. 2014. "The Predictive State: Science, Territory and the Future of the Indian Climate." *Social Studies of Science* 44 (1): 109–33.

Mehta, Pavithra K., and Suchitra Shenoy. 2011. *Infinite Vision: How Aravind Became the World's Greatest Business Case for Compassion.* San Francisco, CA: Berrett-Koehler Publishers.

Nieusma, Dean. 2007. "Challenging Knowledge Hierarchies: Working Toward Sustainable Development in Sri Lanka's Energy Sector." *Sustainability: Science Practice and Policy* 3: 32–44.

Odumosu, Toluwalogo B. 2009. *Interrogating Mobiles: A Story of Nigerian Appropriation of the Mobile Phone.* Troy, NY: Rensselaer Polytechnic Institute, Department of Science and Technology Studies.

Onsongo, Elsie Khakasa, and Johan Schot. 2017. "Inclusive Innovation and Rapid Sociotechnical Transitions: The Case of Mobile Money in Kenya." SWPS 2017-07. SPRU Working Paper Series. Brighton: Science Policy Research Unit (SPRU), University of Sussex.

Pacific Vision Foundation. 2017. "Thanks to Our Sponsors: The Eye Institute Grand Opening October 4, 2017." *Horizons: The Pacific Vision Foundation Newsletter*, December 2017.

Raven, Rob. 2007. "Co-evolution of Waste and Electricity Regimes: Multi-regime Dynamics in the Netherlands (1969–2003)." *Energy Policy* 35 (4): 2197–2208.

Raven, Rob, and Geert Verbong. 2007. "Multi-regime Interactions in the Dutch Energy Sector: The Case of Combined Heat and Power Technologies in the Netherlands 1970–2000." *Technology Analysis & Strategic Management* 19 (4): 491–507.

Raven, Rob, Johan Schot, and Frans Berkhout. 2012. "Space and Scale in Socio-Technical Transitions." *Environmental Innovation and Societal Transitions* 4 (September): 63–78.

Salm, Martin, Daniel Belsky, and Frank A. Sloan. 2006. "Trends in Cost of Major Eye Diseases to Medicare, 1991 to 2000." *American Journal of Ophthalmology* 142 (6): 976–82.

Samsky, Ari. 2012. "Scientific Sovereignty: How International Drug Donation Programs Reshape Health, Disease, and the State." *Cultural Anthropology* 27 (2): 310–32.

Shepherd, Chris J. 2006. "From in Vitro to in Situ on the Precarious Extension of Agricultural Science in the Indigenous 'Third World'." *Social Studies of Science* 36 (3): 399–426.

Stark, Walter J., Alfred Sommer, and Ronald E. Smith. 1989. "Changing Trends in Intraocular Lens Implantation." *Archives of Ophthalmology* 107 (10): 1441–44.

Stephenson, Niamh. 2011. "Emerging Infectious Disease/Emerging Forms of Biological Sovereignty." *Science, Technology & Human Values* 36 (5): 616–37.

Sutherland, Lee-Ann, Sarah Peter, and Lukas Zagata. 2015. "Conceptualising Multi-regime Interactions: The Role of the Agriculture Sector in Renewable Energy Transitions." *Research Policy* 44 (8): 1543–54.

Williams, Logan D. A. 2017. "Getting Undone Technology Done: Global Techno-Assemblage and the Value Chain of Invention." *Science, Technology and Society* 22 (1): 38–58.

Williams, Logan D. A., and Thomas S. Woodson. 2012. "The Future of Innovation Studies in Less Economically Developed Countries." *Minerva* 50 (2): 221–37.

Worthington, Richard. 1993. "Introduction: Science and Technology as a Global System." *Science, Technology, & Human Values* 18 (2): 176–85.

10

Appendix A:
The Extended Case Method
and Global Ethnography

Science and technology studies scholars are increasingly using ethnography in multiple research sites across geographical and economic scales. Ethnography typically involves, at minimum, "writing about the world from the standpoint of participant observation" (Burawoy 1998, 6). While science and technology studies scholars commonly used ethnography (Fuller 2006; Hess 2001; Marcus 2009), they most frequently used grounded theory methods (Fuller 2006), e.g., Marcus multi-sited ethnography or Clarke's situational analysis. In contrast, I used the extended case method (ECM)/global ethnography (GE; see Burawoy 1991, 1998, 2000; Gille and Ó Riain 2002) to examine how global forces shape micro-social processes.

Burawoy's extended case method differs from the Chicago School's grounded theory (Glaeser 2005); instead, the extended case method follows the Manchester School and expands Gluckman's work (Burawoy 1998). It posits that an ethnographer can comment on global processes by examining how global forces shape micro-social processes.

© The Author(s) 2019
L. D. A. Williams, *Eradicating Blindness*,
https://doi.org/10.1007/978-981-13-1625-8_10

Burawoy's ECM/GE differs from grounded theory by its emphasis on "bringing theory to the field" (Eliasoph and Lichterman 1999). Generally, ethnographies based upon grounded theory eschew such hypothesis testing. The grounded theory methodologies are entirely iterative-inductive (O'Reilly 2012); analysis is often concurrent with research in the field through theming or coding. An exception might be interpretive grounded theory where the sensitizing concept guides the initial research project design (Blumer 1954; Bryant and Charmaz 2007).

In contrast to typical ethnographies based upon grounded theory, the extended case method adds an early deductive step of structuring research questions to refute an existing theory of "great transformations" (Burawoy 1998). Thus, in the structure-agency debate, Burawoy's ECM examines both the agency of actors (e.g., individuals, communities, or organizations) and the structuring power of global forces (broadly defined as, e.g., "neoliberal globalization" to "modern development" to "science" to "American culture"). Global forces have their own internal logics by which they operate and reproduce social relations.

When Burawoy articulates the ECM/GE, he demonstrates extensions in space, time, and theory. Extensions in space involve selecting field sites to examine social processes. Ethnographers using the extended case method select similar field sites so that their small differences can illuminate the influence of macro-forces (Burawoy 1991; Glaeser 2005). Extensions in space and time occur through four mechanisms: observer and interlocutor co-presence within the field site; the interviewing process as an intervention into the field site; archival research; and field site revisits. The global ethnographer extends theory through three methods of reasoning: deduction, induction, and abduction.

In this appendix, I summarize the methods that I used to conduct a feminist postcolonial ethnography of community ophthalmology organizations. The remainder of the appendix is organized as follows:

First, Sect. 10.1 introduces the research paradigm for the project including the key features of the extended case method/global ethnography, which I am using. Next Sect. 10.2, illuminates how the field sites were chosen and how this relates to extending the case in space. Subsequently, Sect. 10.3 focuses on how I selected interlocutors for interviews, and my sample demographics. Section 10.4 explains how observation is equivalent to intervention through co-presence while also delineating the field notes that I created over many months. It also summarizes my archival research. Finally, Sect. 10.6 illustrates how I moved from data to theory generation through memos and theming.

10.1 Research Paradigm

My multi-sited ethnography is best described by Burawoy's ECM (1998), and Glaeser's ethnography of processes (2005). There are several features that are common to both ECM and ethnographic case methods more generally. Participant observation is central to any ethnography. Likewise, the development of emergent theory by iterating between qualitative data and causal hypotheses is a technique that is relevant to a variety of ethnographic case methods (Small 2009). Many ethnographic methods emphasize the deviant case because unique insights can be inferred (Small 2009). However, there are several key features of Burawoy's ECM/GE:

- Applying an a priori theory of society that is investigated; frequently, but not always, this is a theory of globalization (Burawoy 1991; Eliasoph and Lichterman 1999; Small 2009)
- Developing a historical understanding of the case (Burawoy et al. 2000)
- Revisiting the field site (Burawoy 2000; Gille and Ó Riain 2002)
- Refuting old theory, thereby generating new or improved theory (Burawoy 1998, 2000).

The a priori theory of society I investigated was developmentalism, including Western conceptualizations of technology transfer always moving from Western origins to the rest of the world (Basalla 1967; see Chapter 1). To start my pilot work, I chose a deviant case: Tilganga Institute of Ophthalmology, in the economically impoverished country of Nepal, was creating and disseminating both surgical science and technology products. Their technology products were sold in other less economically developed countries and also wealthy countries like Australia. Tilganga was likewise the site of my revisit.

I conducted all interviews for this project from 2009 to 2013. This included: my pilot study June–July 2009, and my dissertation fieldwork July 2011–May 2013. At the time, I was a doctoral student in an interdisciplinary social science graduate program called Science and Technology Studies. In my program, I was trained in ethnographic methods by anthropologist Kim Fortun and archival methods by historians Nancy Campbell and Atsushi Akera.

Before visiting each field site, I contacted an upper-level manager by email, forwarding my curriculum vitae and research proposal. In each site, I requested permission in advance to: conduct observation, share an office space, and (if I intended a long duration in that field site) work voluntarily with a supervisor on one of their projects. Upon entry and exit to the field site, I typically presented my research project to one or more upper-level managers.

I am a feminist postcolonial ethnographer; as such, I believe in sharing the results of my work with my interlocutors before publication for two reasons: (1) so that they can fact-check it and (2) so they can request that I redact specific facts that might be harmful to them. Due to this research paradigm, I signed a non-disclosure agreement with Aurolab to make this oversight more official according to Aurolab's standards as nonprofit biomedical manufacturing company. I later wrote about my early naiveté about my positionality, power, and access to field sites. My article offered a mapping tool for other ethnographers to use before and during fieldwork to help orient them to such issues (Williams 2018).

10.2   Extension in Space: Choosing Field Sites in Global Ethnography

Burawoy's extended case method extends the case in space through multiple field sites (1998, 2000); this makes it a novel approach to ethnography in science and technology studies which previously focused on one field site or laboratory. Burawoy's global ethnography extends ontologically to examine a process as it occurs within a network of relations (Glaeser 2005). It is a method of performing international ethnographic research in multiple field sites that offers clear guidance on site selection by looking at similarities and differences between formal organizations that are "highly similar at first glance" (Glaeser 2005; Lapegna 2009).

In contrast, the definition of a site in Marcus' multi-sited ethnography (1995) is not necessarily a function of place or nationality. Instead, ethnographers select sites for their potential discursive meanings, which are emergent (Marcus 1995). Some social scientists studying development are critical of the nominal guidance multi-sited ethnography offers for site choice (Lapegna 2009; Stirrat and Rajak 2011). Lapegna (2009) argues that, whereas Marcus' multi-sited ethnography (1995) and Burawoy's global ethnography (1991, 1998, 2000) are both middle-range theories, global ethnography offers more explicit direction in selecting sites, especially when examining the political economy of the world system.

In this research project, I extended the case spatially by selecting multiple field sites: my first site, Unite for Sight Global Health & Innovation Conference at Yale University; my second site, Lions SightFirst Eye Hospital in Loresho, Nairobi, Kenya; my third site, the Tilganga Institute of Ophthalmology in Kathmandu, Nepal; my fourth site, the Aravind Eye Care Systems in Madurai, India; and my fifth site, Sala Uno in Mexico City D.F., Mexico. All five are places where professionals can receive training in community ophthalmology; thus, they are excellent locations to study knowledge circulation. The Unite for Sight Global Health & Innovation Conference was important because it highlights transnational linkages between these community ophthalmology NGOs and other development organizations such as the UN.

At the other four field sites, I was immersed in the day-to-day social processes where these transnational linkages were perhaps less visible (Glaeser 2005, 35). The last four sites (all eye hospitals) are important because, while having the superficial appearance of similarity, they in fact offer slightly different but parallel insight into the production and circulation of science and technology.

I had learned about another high-volume eye hospital in southern India called L. V. Prasad before starting my primary fieldwork and data collection. Ultimately, I pursued funding specifically to study Tilganga and Aravind because of their uniqueness; in addition to reinventing surgical practice locally, they each had created their own biomedical prosthetic manufacturing laboratories. As Glaeser argues, "different locations may have different positions in networks of relations, and these need to be considered because they offer different perspectives on effect flows and interactions with other processes" (2005, 35). As a result, my main field sites for this study are the South Asian field sites. Also, I found to my surprise through the course of my research that Aravind emerged as my primary field site (Burawoy 2000).

I added the Mexican site to my study only after I had finished my fieldwork at Aravind where I met one of the managers from Sala Uno. Sala Uno contrasted sharply with the other community ophthalmology NGOs and government clinics I had learned were utilizing the Robin Hood model from Aravind. Its legal status as a for-profit clinic, and its semi-peripheral position in a middle-income country made it deviant compared to many other community ophthalmology clinics.

Burawoy's extended case method/global ethnography (1998, 2000) utilizes interviews, participant observation, and archival work across the similar field sites to extend the case in space and time through. In the next sections, I discuss these qualitative field methods as ethnographic interventions.

10.3 Extension in Space and Time: Intervening as an Interviewer

For this research project, I aimed for 60 interlocutors and collected interviews from 84 interlocutors. Two people withdrew informed consent, therefore, I discarded their transcripts for a total number of 82 interlocutors. The actual quantity of interview transcripts was slightly higher than the number of interlocutors because I interviewed a few people twice: once in 2009 for the pilot study at Tilganga and then again during 2011–2013 for my dissertation fieldwork (including a Tilganga revisit). I piloted my dissertation interview questions in 2010 by conducting interviews with prominent US ophthalmologists.

Prospective interlocutors were approached face-to-face and by email. I developed the interview schedule with semi-structured interview questions (Luker 2008, 169–72). Subsequently, I conducted my interviews in the style of a conversation (Heyl 2001). During the interview, I did not stick rigidly to the interview schedule; instead, I directed the most appropriate questions to each person based upon their role in the institution. If the interlocutor requested the interview schedule in advance, then I would give them a copy (usually by email). Unless the interlocutor preferred otherwise, I conducted my interviews, except for two in the USA, privately (with just myself and the interlocutor). I recorded interviews using a digital audio recorder; sometimes I additionally used my laptop as a backup recorder. Typically, each interview lasted about an hour (although some were as short as 20 minutes, and one was as long as 2 hours and twenty minutes). I conducted only four interviews by phone or by voice-over-Internet-protocol software (i.e., Skype); this was with US interlocutors.

I selected the interlocutors using a combined purposive and snow-ball sampling technique. This was a non-probabilistic sampling technique where initially I, as the expert, made a judgment about which people have the information that I need to answer my research questions. Therefore, I identified three target groups: group A, four local religious leaders and others working in eye health not affiliated with my field site; group B, sixty-five NGO medical and management professionals; and group C, fifteen medical technology manufacturers and repair technicians. I deliberate aimed for the highest percentage of interlocutors to be in group B. I also tried to interview people in comparable roles (where they existed) across the four eye hospital sites, including: the intraocular lens manufacturing unit manager, the eye donation unit manager, the eye hospital manager, the eye hospital founder(s), and the consultancy/training unit manager. Once I identified a handful of people within each field site as potential interlocutors, I relied in part upon their recommendations for other people to interview.

My interlocutors were physically present in the following cities during the interview: twenty-one in Kathmandu, Nepal; thirty-two in Madurai, India; ten in Nairobi, Kenya; seven in Mexico City, Mexico; and fourteen in various US cities. Other demographics of my sample include visually classified sex: twenty (24%) women and sixty-three (76%) men. I also tracked their geographic region of origin: forty-five (53%) South Asians (from Bangladesh, India, Nepal, and Sri Lanka); twelve Africans; one East Asian; one Latin-American; twenty-three North Americans; and two from the Oceanic region. I indexed the geographic region of origin based on birthplace (and nationality). Therefore, I counted Indian-Kenyans who were born in Kenya as African, persons born in India who worked in African countries as South Asian, and Mexicans as North American.

I correctly anticipated that I would conduct 90–100% of my interviews in English. English is an official language in both Kenya and India that is also taught to schoolchildren in Nepal. All the global health professionals (groups B & C) spoke English. I did require a translator for one interview with an astrologer (group A).

The interviews alone did not answer my research questions; the direct observation and the participant observation were also key to understanding the production and circulation of science and technology in this project.

10.4 Extension in Space and Time: Intervening as an Observer

Burawoy (1998) argues that participant observation provides insight into social processes through the co-presence of the ethnographer and interlocutor. Ethnographers using ECM describe and interpret the everyday practices and situations in which they are engaged through co-presence with their interlocutors at the field sites. These everyday practices and situations reproduce larger social relations. Therefore, such ethnographers "can compile situational knowledge into an account of social process because regimes of power structure situations into processes" (Burawoy 1998, 18).

For example, as a volunteer intern at the Aravind Eye Care Systems, I learned more about the internal power dynamics of this large NGO, as well as the power dynamics of its relationships with foreign non-profit organizations from wealthier countries, including the Lions Clubs International Foundation (USA/International), the SEVA Foundation (USA/Canada), and Right to Sight (Ireland). I also gained greater insight into community ophthalmology as an emerging network with particular tacit ideologies, explicit regulations, and unspoken behavioral norms that were reproduced and disseminated through training programs (see Chapter 7).

I directly observed or participated in field sites to make unstructured naturalistic observations (Given 2008, 551–52, 908–9). For the direct observations, I wrote copious notes in my research notebook or convertible tablet laptop and did not interact with the interlocutors as they conducted important tasks, i.e., surgery, or talking to an eye camp full of people. In contrast, my participant observations were premised upon the degree to which I was embedded in the formal organization as a volunteer intern. Therefore, I was only able to access such participant observation opportunities because I was intervening in the organization as a volunteer.

I conducted 10.25 months of participant observation at three field sites: Aravind, Tilganga, and Loresho. For my pilot study, I conducted participant observation at the Tilganga Institute of Ophthalmology in Nepal, where I worked in the Research Department in summer 2009 (1.5 months); at that time, I designed and implemented a survey on the satisfaction of guardians with pediatric patient care. Later as part of the primary data collection and global ethnography, I conducted participant observation at Lions SightFirst Eye Hospital—Loresho in Kenya in summer 2011 where I assisted the Information Technology and Marketing department with a small marketing project over 20 days (10 consecutive Fridays and Saturdays). Next, I returned to Tilganga's Research Department where from 2011 to 2012 (3.5 months), I edited reports Tilganga sent to funding partners such as The Fred Hollows Foundation and Project Orbis.

At the Aravind Eye Care Systems in India in 2012, I spent 4.5 months performing participant observation in multiple places, conferences, symposia, and so on through the Lions Aravind Institute of Community Ophthalmology (LAICO). I also participated in more mundane everyday activities, for example: attending approximately sixteen LAICO Operations Department's weekly meetings (12 h; March–July 2012); researching, writing, and disseminating an internal report on innovation at the Aravind Eye Care Systems (March–April 2012); acting as secretary of the monthly Innovation Club meeting (3 h; May–July 2012); eating three meals daily at the Aravind Inspiration Hostel Canteen with ophthalmologists, optometrists, biomedical engineers, and other visitors from India and around the world (March–July 2012); and leading a song at one of the monthly talent shows for the staff at the Madurai campus.

I was not embedded as a volunteer at Sala Uno; my visit there in 2012 only lasted four days. However, I enjoyed a few unique ethnographic moments of direct observation in-between conducting interviews where I could clearly see the forward momentum of this new community ophthalmology organization picking up steam.

My approximately 20.5 h of direct observation at the other three field sites included: cataract surgeries at the Tilganga Institute of Ophthalmology in Nepal (2 h; June 2009); conference sessions at the Unite for Sight Global Health and Innovation Conference (8 h; April,

2011); an eye camp, in a small town called Rironi an hour or so from Lions SightFirst Eye Hospital—Loresho (8 h; October 2011); and finally, at the Aravind Eye Care Systems in India in 2012, I observed cataract surgeries in the Free Hospital, Aravind Eye Hospital—Madurai, Madurai (2.5 h; July 2012). This observation complements the interviews with data gathered from directly watching the production and circulation of science and technology.

The extended case method extends through intervention; participant observation provides insight through distortion where formal organizations resist observation when the ethnographer enters and departs (Burawoy 1998, 16–17). My participant observation included formal meetings with colleagues, many informal discussions, and participation in the work-life of the two eye hospitals in South Asia. Typically, I found, throughout my participant observation, that the upper-level managers and my co-workers (in my volunteer internships) were happy to have me present as an observer. However, the many other professionals (especially doctors) I interviewed seemed less interested in my presence and our interview—I took up some of their precious time.

The historical contingencies of Nepal's formation as a country shaped Tilganga's institutional resistance to my observation. At Tilganga, the meetings, presentations, informal discussions, and so forth typically occur in Nepali. Thus, while I had access on paper (through my letter of affiliation), in practice, I only had access to the individuals willing to speak with me in the only language in which I am fluent, English. India's independence as a former British colony meant that there was a historical imposition of English on Indians in British India. An independent India continued the imposition of English, as well as Hindi, as official national languages. Therefore, my participant observation at Aravind was linguistically effortless as all the local staff and most of the foreign visitors spoke English. This was ironic because, of the two South Asian sites, Nepal was arguably more interesting because its global domestic product was substantially less than that of a "newly industrialized country" like India.

10.5 Extension in Space and Time: Contextualizing as Archivist

Most of my historical data came from physical archives and online repositories. I visited archives in three cities (Madurai, San Francisco, and Washington, DC) to learn more about clinical ophthalmology and community ophthalmologists.

In Spring 2011, I utilized a travel award from the Smithsonian Institutes and spent two days at the Patricia Bath collection at the Lemelson Center for Invention and Innovation, National Museum of American History in Washington, DC. While conducting fieldwork in Madurai, India during Spring 2012, I spent three days at the Resources Collection at the Govindappa Venkataswamy Eye Research Institute (GVERI) to collect archival material about the Aravind Eye Care System and its international and national partners. GVERI has source materials in English, Tamil, and Hindi to include: IAPB conference pamphlets, brochures from some of the 600 plus Lions clubs in India, and other organizational materials from other NGOs and eye hospitals. Lastly, in Spring 2013, I spent two days at the Foundation of the American Academy of Ophthalmology s Museum of Vision in San Francisco, California.

When writing and revising my results from 2013 to 2018, I also accessed the World Health Organization (WHO) Institutional Repository for Information Sharing (IRIS) available online. WHO IRIS materials included World Health Assembly notes, program budgets, etc., in English, French, Spanish, Russian, Chinese, and Arabic.

Other historical data came from local press coverage in English and also through organizational documents that I requested during my volunteer internships. These documents included: organization publications (including magazines and peer-reviewed journals) and organizational media (e.g., emails, pamphlets, newsletters, annual reports, websites, and videos).

I analyzed all of the data from interviews, observation, and archival work to find connective comparisons.

10.6 Extending Theory: Connective Comparisons

The extended case method ... deploys a ... comparative strategy, tracing the source of small difference to external forces. This might be called the integrative or vertical approach. Here the purpose of the comparison is to causally connect the cases. Instead of reducing cases to instances of a general law, we make each case work in its connection to other cases [sic]. (Burawoy 1998, 19)

Generally, ethnographies based on grounded theory have an inductive method of reasoning. In contrast, the ECM/GE as I describe it here involves the following methods of reasoning: (1) deduction—bringing theory to the field in order to confirm or refute it with certain facts (Given 2008, 208–09; O'Reilly 2012); (2) induction—data collection in the field to develop new probable theory (Given 2008, 430–31; O'Reilly 2012); and (3) abduction—the surprise of new facts being uncovered in the field generating plausible new hypotheses (Given 2008, 2–3).

During my fieldwork, I produced a variety of primary source ethnographic documents. Along with archival materials, organizational materials, and news media, my primary source documents included novel data that I collected: interview transcripts (created by myself or Accentance, LLC in Chantilly, Virginia) and observation field notes (Emerson et al. 2011). Primarily, I wrote field notes in twenty bound college rule composition notebooks. For the Aravind site only, I typed some of my field notes (500–1000 words each), especially during meetings. I also typed rough notes during interviews which I could use to start immediate analysis.

The reliability and validity of my primary source data came through saturation (when new data collection no longer yields new information or insights) and triangulation (the repetition of particular facts across different sources). For example, historical data for these multiple sites (derived through other primary source documents) helped to validate many of the facts repeated by my interlocutors during interviews.

Through induction, deduction, and abduction, I was developing non-obvious connections between my field notes, interview transcripts, and social theory. I generated inductive insights through 22 typed free-writing memos (500–1200 words each). The free-writing memos involved writing on any topic that was at the forefront of my mind (Lempert 2007). Usually, I wrote about something surprising or confirmatory I had observed that week.

Additionally, I created 9 typed analytic research memos which I prepared for meetings with dissertation committee chairs (500–2000 words each). These research memos combined iterative-induction with abduction (O'Reilly 2012). Iterative-induction is a practical process for moving between data collection and theory generation while in the field that acknowledges these stages are repetitive, uncertain, and inscription-dependent (O'Reilly 2012, 30). The research memos were semi-structured so that I could regularly reflect upon the theory I was re-constructing (a deductive approach) and any surprising empirical data that did not fit the known social science literature (an abductive approach). To generate insights from abduction, I asked myself about any surprises I encountered. My findings through abduction related to my theory, but also to my positionality and methods (Williams 2018).

Meanwhile, I generated further insights through four site narratives, one each for Aravind, Tilganga, Loresho, and Sala Uno (5000–26,500 words each). The site narratives were semi-structured; they were structured around my research questions (a deductive approach), but they also allowed space for new empirical data and for making new generalizations to emerge from that data (an iterative-inductive approach). Every time that I completed an interview, I added highlights from my notes that confirmed what was already written in the site narrative, or offered a startling contrasting perspective. Also, when I received a new interview transcript, I would add more to the site narrative.

For my site narratives, the dissertation, and this book, I chose representative quotes from my interview transcripts to exemplify particularly striking findings. Many of my interlocutors, especially women and men subordinate employees, preferred anonymity. In such cases, I used a very generic description of their professional role in their organization. I did use a pseudonym at the request of one man.

I started writing the site narratives in September 2011, after I had spent several months in Kenya. These site narratives were iterative-inductive (O'Reilly 2012), and they changed slightly over time as I gathered new data. For example, the Loresho site narrative took from September 2011 to November 2012 to complete; I was still working on it after I had left Kenya. Writing the different site narratives primarily overlapped with my time in that field site, but also extended to after I exited the field.

A major emergent theme, the importance of high volume as a formal organizational rule among community outreach managers and the eye units at large, only became obvious after I had finished writing the site narrative for my last site. While I had been aware that high volume was a minor theme, it was only upon reflection that I realized the need for high volume had been present in the discourse of all the sites, as demonstrated in my research memos and other site narratives. Something about how the staff of Sala Uno, the youngest organization, expressed their struggles with the Robin Hood model of cost recovery crystallized the importance of high volume for all the organizations.

A minor emergent theme, the idea of mitigating risk while developing "labs of their own," emerged from writing the site narratives for Aravind and Tilganga (see Chapter 5). Like other emergent themes, it was not part of my original research questions. While the idea of for-profit companies mitigating risk is not novel to entrepreneurship and business literature, it becomes a novel inductive generalization in this case of nonprofit technology companies. These two emergent themes are some of the many connective comparisons throughout this book.

References

Basalla, George. 1967. The Spread of Western Science. *Science* 156 (3775): 611–22.

Blumer, Herbert. 1954. "What Is Wrong with Social Theory." *American Sociological Review*, 18: 3–10.

Bryant, Antony, and Kathy Charmaz. 2007. "Grounded Theory in Historical Perspective: An Epistemological Account." In *The Sage Handbook of Grounded Theory*, edited by Antony Bryant and Kathy Charmaz, 31–57. London: Sage.

Burawoy, Michael. 1991. "Conclusion: The Extended Case Method." In *Ethnography Unbound: Power and Resistance in the Modern Metropolis*, edited by Michael Burawoy, 271–87. Berkeley: University of California Press.

———. 1998. "The Extended Case Method." *Sociological Theory* 16: 4–33.

———. 2000. "Introduction: Reaching for the Global." In *Global Ethnography: Forces, Connections, and Imaginations in a Postmodern World*, edited by Michael Burawoy, Joseph A. Blum, Sheba George, Zsuzsa Gille, Millie Thayer, Teresa Gowan, Lynne Haney, Maren Klawiter, Steve H. Lopez, and Sean Riain, 1st ed., 1–40. Berkeley and Los Angeles: University of California Press.

Eliasoph, Nina, and Paul Lichterman. 1999. "'We Begin with Our Favorite Theory…': Reconstructing the Extended Case Method." *Sociological Theory* 17 (2): 228–34.

Emerson, Robert M., Rachel I. Fretz, and Linda L. Shaw. 2011. *Writing Ethnographic Fieldnotes*. 2nd ed. Chicago Guides to Writing, Editing, and Publishing. Chicago: The University of Chicago Press.

Fuller, Steve. 2006. "Seeking Science in the Field: Life Beyond the Laboratory." In *The Sage Handbook of Fieldwork*, edited by Dick Hobbs and Richard Wright, 333–44. 1 Oliver's Yard, 55 City Road, London EC1Y 1SP United Kingdom: Sage.

Gille, Zsuzsa, and Seán Ó Riain. 2002. "Global Ethnography." *Annual Review of Sociology* 28: 271–95.

Given, Lisa. 2008. *The Sage Encyclopedia of Qualitative Research Methods*. Thousand Oaks, CA: Sage.

Glaeser, Andreas. 2005. "An Ontology for the Ethnographic Analysis of Social Processes: Extending the Extended-Case Method." *Social Analysis* 49: 16–45.

Hess, David J. 2001. "Ethnography and the Development of Science and Technology Studies." In *Handbook of Ethnography*, edited by Paul Atkinson, Amanda Coffey, Sara Delamont, John Lofland, and Lyn Lofland. London and Thousand Oaks, CA: Sage.

Heyl, Barbara Sherman. 2001. "Ethnographic Interviewing." In *Handbook of Ethnography*, edited by Paul Atkinson, Amanda Coffey, Sara Delamont, John Lofland, and Lyn Lofland, 369–83. London: Sage.

Lapegna, Pablo. 2009. "Ethnographers of the World United? Current Debates on the Ethnographic Study of Globalization." *Journal of World-Systems Research* 15 (1): 3–24. https://doi.org/10.5195/jwsr.2009.336.

Lempert, Lora Bex. 2007. "Asking Questions of the Data: Memo Writing in the Grounded Theory Tradition." In *The Sage Handbook of Grounded Theory*, edited by Antony Bryant and Kathy Charmaz, 245–65. London: Sage.

Luker, Kristin. 2008. *Salsa Dancing into the Social Sciences: Research in an Age of Info-Glut*. Cambridge, MA: Harvard University Press.

Marcus, George E. 1995. "Ethnography in/of the World System: The Emergence of Multi-sited Ethnography." *Annual Review of Anthropology* 24 (1): 95.

———. 2009. "Multi-sited Ethnography: Notes and Queries." In *Multi-sited Ethnography: Theory, Praxis and Locality in Contemporary Research*, edited by Mark-Anthony Falzon, 181–96. Surrey: Ashgate.

O'Reilly, Karen. 2012. *Ethnographic Methods*. London and New York: Routledge.

Small, Mario Luis. 2009. "'How Many Cases Do I Need?': On Science and the Logic of Case Selection in Field-Based Research." *Ethnography* 10 (1): 5–38.

Stirrat, R. L., and Dinah Rajak. 2011. "The Romance of the Field?" In *The Anthropologist and the Native: Essays for Gananath Obeyesekere*, edited by H. L. Seneviratne, 1000–25. London: Anthem Press.

Williams, Logan D. A. 2018. "Mapping Superpositionality in Global Ethnography." *Science, Technology, & Human Values* 43 (2): 198–223.

11

Appendix B: The Robin Hood Model

Chapter 3 demonstrated that Aravind Eye Care System started out, because of necessity, as completely self-sufficient (swadeshi) and self-ruled (swaraj); later, the eye hospital began accepting donations and government subsidies. Many community ophthalmology organizations have adoped or appropriated the Robin Hood model of soical entrepreneurship from Aravind. Below, the other organizations are described in more detail, to include: Tilganga Institute of Ophthalmology in Nepal (Sect. 11.1), Lions SightFirst Eye Hospital—Loresho in Kenya (Sect. 11.2), Sala Uno in Mexico (Sect. 11.3) and Unite for Sight in the USA (Sect. 11.4). These organizations are very similar to Aravind in India because they use cost recovery to be (more or less) self-sufficient in operating expenses through multiple revenue streams.

11.1 Tilganga Institute of Ophthalmology (Kathmandu, Nepal)

Tilganga Institute of Ophthalmology started out as self-ruled (swaraj), but not self-sufficient: It relied upon donations from many local and global partners to pay operating expenses. Over time, it has become more self-sufficient, but still worries about financial viability.

© The Author(s) 2019
L. D. A. Williams, *Eradicating Blindness*,
https://doi.org/10.1007/978-981-13-1625-8_11

The Nepal Eye Program was legally established by Nepalese ophthalmologist Dr. Sanduk Ruit in 1992 in Nepal. The Tilganga Institute of Ophthalmology (initially called Tilganga Eye Center) became the operating body of the Nepal Eye Program in 1994. With the help of the Queen of Nepal, they acquired a former golf course just across the street from the Pashupati temple, the most famous Hindu temple in Nepal, and built the eye hospital on this site. They later acquired an adjacent lot, at high cost, on which they built the second building of their two-building campus (see Fig. 11.1).

Similar to Aravind, Tilganga is a tertiary eye hospital and thus offers many ophthalmic specialties. Additionally, Tilganga operates several community vision centers outside of Kathmandu providing primary eye health care in more rural areas of Nepal.

The Fred Hollows Foundation paid the salaries of the Nepal Eye Program for the first three years until 1997. Afterward, Tilganga paid its

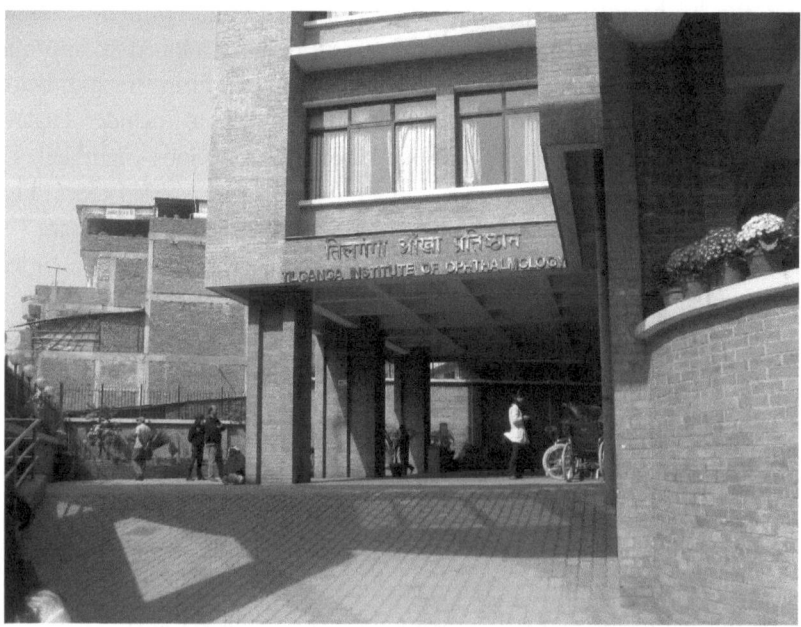

Fig. 11.1 New building on campus of Tilganga Institute of Ophthalmology (Photo by Logan D. A. Williams)

own salaries, while still benefiting from occasionally donated equipment or software.

In Tilganga's implementation of the Robin Hood model of social entrepreneurship, they have never had financial support from the government of Nepal in the form of remittances for patients. Aside from the institute's nonprofit status, which excuses it from paying taxes, Tilganga has relied entirely on its own profits and private largesse from local businessmen, local religious leaders, and foreign NGOs (see Table 11.1). For example, the Australian Agency for International Development (AUSAID) and the United States Agency for International Development (USAID) have each provided funds toward infrastructure creation at different historical moments. After a long civil war 1996–2008, the government of Nepal changed from a Hindu monarchy to a federal democratic republic. Neither during the transition, before, or after, has the state subsidized patients' eye health care. Without the security of consistent, reliable financial support via government remittances for patients, Tilganga has more anxiety about balancing their books in comparison with Aravind's sangfroid.

Tilganga started because of disagreements between Dr. Ruit and Dr. Pokhrel in Nepal about the importance of starting an intraocular lens-manufacturing facility (see Chapter 5).

Tilganga like Aravind relies upon close partnerships with international NGOs from the West to do some of its work inside and outside of Nepal. Two international NGOs have been the major partners of Tilganga: The Fred Hollows Foundation (Australia) and the Himalayan Cataract Project (USA). The Himalayan Cataract Project was co-founded by Dr. Ruit with US ophthalmologist and outdoor enthusiast Dr. Geoffrey Tabin. The Himalayan Cataract Project partners with both Tilganga and the United Nations Millennium Villages Project to bring the "Tilganga model" to Africa.

In addition to being leaders in the autonomous global network to eradicate and control blindness, both Tilganga and Aravind are embedded in the clinical ophthalmology network in the global field of ophthalmology. Judging by the composition of the editorial board of the *Nepalese Journal of Ophthalmology*, Tilganga is the premiere scientific institution for ophthalmology in Nepal.

Table 11.1 Diverse revenue sources pay for expenses at Tilganga Institute of Ophthalmology (Nepal)

Revenues from sales (+)	Revenues from donations (+)	Fixed expenses (−)	Recurring expenses (−)
Ophthalmic consumable Profits			Manufacturing and donating Ophthalmic consumables
Wealthy Patient Fees; Deeply Subsidized Low-income Patient Fees	Donations from INGOs (e.g.. LCIF, SEVA, HCP, etc.) and individuals	Hospital Equipment; Hospital Vehicles	Hospital staff training; no cost surgery for eye camp patients; district eye clinics
		Second Building Land Acquisition (2009)	Low-income patients deeply subsidized or No Cost Surgery; Staff Salaries
	Local: businessmen, community leaders, religious organizations, etc.	First Building Construction (1992)	Outreach Microsurgical Eye Camp
	Pashupati Temple Trust	First Building Land Acquisition (1992)	
	The Fred Hollows Foundation	First Building Construction (1992); the IOL Mfg. Laboratory	Staff Salaries (ended in 1997)
	Lions Clubs of Indiana and Lions Clubs International Foundation US Agency for International Development	Eye Bank Construction and Equipment Second Building Construction (2009); Solar Panels	

Tilganga is well known in the global field of international development, and staff have received humanitarian awards. For example, at Tilganga Institute of Ophthalmology, the director, Dr. Sanduk Ruit, and medical coordinator, Nabin K. Rai, are heavily involved with developing policy and national goals for both Nepal's Vision 2020 program. For his work in Asia, Dr. Sanduk Ruit has received the "Prince Mahidol Award of Thailand and the 2006 Ramon Magsaysay Award for Peace and International Understanding, known as Asia's Nobel Prize" (Ocular Surgery News Asia Pacific Edition 2010). The Tilganga Institute of Ophthalmology was a co-recipient (along with Lumbini Eye Institute and Nepal Netra Jyoti Sangh) of the 2013 Vision Award, a prize worth $1.3 million US Dollars, from the Antonio Champalimaud Foundation. Having worked throughout Nepal's long civil war to provide eye health care to Nepalese men and women, Dr. Ruit and his colleagues at Tilganga were experienced and well-networked to provide targeted relief efforts to the villagers most impacted by the 2015 earthquakes and landslides in the mountains (Healio 2015). Dr. Ruit received the Padma Shri award from the government of India for inventing small incision cataract surgical technique in 2018 (*Times of India* 2018).

Ophthalmologists from Tilganga frequently publish in prestigious Western ophthalmology journals; this also embeds them in the clinical ophthalmology network globally. Tilganga is eclipsed in terms of patient volume by the Lumbini Eye Institute of Nepal. The Lumbini Eye Institute was assisted through SEVA foundation to more directly adopt Aravind's "Robin Hood" model and is the highest volume cataract surgical unit in the country of Nepal. It is located in the plains region (the Terai) along the Nepal–India border and also serves many Indian patients who cross the border for eye health care.

Tilganga's work outside of Nepal (in Asia and Africa) is one example of how it is embedded in the subordinate network of community ophthalmology professionals within the global field of ophthalmology (see Chapter 7).

Tilganga uses cost recovery to provide 33% of its patients with free or subsidized care. Tilganga serves approximately 500 patients per day (Ruit 2003). It is a tertiary eye hospital and thus offers many ophthalmic specialties including: cornea, retina, oculoplasty, glaucoma, uvea, low vision, and pediatric. It also operates several community vision centers outside of Kathmandu in more rural areas of Nepal. Tilganga's The Fred Hollows Intraocular Lens Laboratory was the first ISO certified manufacturing facility in the country of Nepal. Tilganga sells its lenses to NGOs in Europe and Australia in addition to NGOs in other less economically developed countries. It is also distinct from these other community ophthalmology NGOs because of its highly regimented and standardized procedures for safe and efficacious cataract surgeries, "in the bush"; it conducts 10–20 outreach microsurgical eye camps in the Himalayan Mountains of Nepal yearly. Because of the poor technological infrastructure in Nepal, and the extreme conditions of the Himalayans, these outreach microsurgical eye camps are very expensive and are funded entirely through donations (primarily from foreign NGOs).

Please see Chapters 5 and 6, to learn more about the innovations that Tilganga incubated in their appropriate technology niche. Each appropriate technology niche shares an emergent radical rule set, but creates slightly different innovations. Tilganga goes farther than Aravind to empower patients. The original idea of cost recovery "of course" came from Aravind; they generate profits from patient fees. However, Tilganga's cost recovery method is distinct in that they have not sacrificed patient empowerment for Taylorist scientific management, Fordist "assembly line" principles or economies of scale. Patients at Tilganga choose their own surgeons regardless of caste (Mahadevan 2007). For example, before the end of the monarchy, a Beggar and the Queen unknowingly made use of the same operating table. In contrast, the separate hospital facilities (with and without beds, with and without private rooms, with and without air conditioning) structurally embed class and caste difference across the many Aravind Eye Care System campuses in southern India.

As shown above, Tilganga implements their cost recovery model differently than Aravind. However, the administrators at Tilganga, like those at Aravind, believe that the Robin Hood model allows them to serve more patients than they could through donations alone. This ability to serve more patients also made the Robin Hood model attractive to the nonprofit eye hospital in Kenya and the for-profit eye clinic in Mexico. The Nepal Ministry of Industry announced in 2017 that it would support the expansion of intraocular lens production by Tilganga The Fred Hollows Intraocular Lens Laboratory, with a subsidy of Rs 100 million ($990,000 US dollars; *The Himalayan Times* 2017).

11.2 Lions SightFirst Eye Hospital—Loresho (Nairobi, Kenya)

Like Tilganga, Lions SightFirst Eye Hospital, Loresho, started out as self-ruled but not self-sufficient, relying upon donations from one prominent global partner to pay operating expenses. Over time, it has experimented in its own appropriate technology niche and as a result has become completely self-sufficient.

Dr. Fayez Khan (an Asian Kenyan) and Dr. Omwakawe (an African Kenyan) started Loresho in 1997. Initially, Loresho relied upon financial assistance from the international charitable foundation Lions Clubs International Foundation (through their SightFirst Program) which, for a number of years, paid staff salaries and patient remittances. The hospital was built on a marsh that was a one-time donation (through a transfer of title) from the Kenyan government. The Lions Clubs International Foundation also supplied $1 million US dollars to build the hospital. Various NGOs also donated other equipment and instruments (see Table 11.2 and Fig. 11.2).

Loresho offers eye healthcare services through outpatient clinics and outreach eye screening camps. Potential patients are collected from the outreach camps in rural locations and brought to Nairobi for cataract surgery. Loresho has conducted 20,000 surgeries (approximately 6000 surgeries per year) from its opening in 1997 through October 2011.

Dr. Khan has been the chief executive officer for a long time. The hospital board chairman and the hospital manager have shifted over time from Lion Samson Ndegwa (African Kenyan) and Lion Mr. Shamsherali Datoo (Asian Kenyan) in 2011 to Lion Dr. Manilal Dodhia (Asian Kenyan) and Mrs. Rizwana (Asian Kenyan) in 2018 (Lions SightFirst Eye Hospital—Loresho 2011, 2018).

Table 11.2 Diverse revenue sources pay for expenses at the Lions SightFirst Eye Hospital, Loresho (Kenya)

Revenues from sales (+)	Revenues from donations (+)	Fixed expenses (−)	Recurring expenses (−)
"Executive Hospital Tier" Patient Fees	LCIF Subsidies (funding ended in 2011); Remittances from the Government's National Health Insurance (started 2018)	Building Construction (3 building Hospital Campus); Hospital Equipment	Hospital Consumables; "Camp Hospital Tier" No Cost Surgeries; "Walk-In Tier" Deeply Subsidized Surgeries; "Executive Hospital Tier" Surgeries
General Medical Clinic Patient Fees	INGOs (e.g., LCIF, SEVA, HCP, etc.)	Hospital Vehicles	Hospital Staff Training
Dental Clinic Patient Fees	Local: businessmen, community leaders, religious organizations, etc.		Staff Salaries
	Local Lions Club	Building Construction (Eye Bank and its Equipment)	Outreach Eye Camp
	Government of Kenya	Land Acquisition	

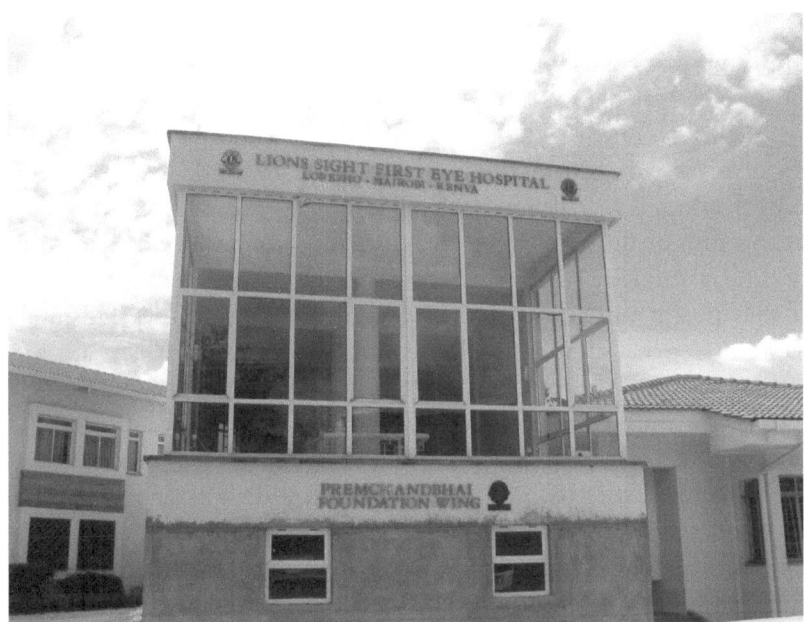

Fig. 11.2 Bright windows shine light onto the patient walking ramp between ground floor and first floor in the Lions SightFirst Eye Hospital, Loresho, Premchandbhai foundation wing (Photo by Logan D. A. Williams)

Loresho uses cost recovery to provide 75% of its patients with free or subsidized eye health care (see Chapter 3 for an explanation of cost recovery). Loresho offers eye healthcare services through eye screenings at outreach camps, where potential patients are collected from rural locations and brought to Nairobi for cataract surgery. It aims to eventually provide tertiary eye hospital services, but while (in 2011) it has the physical infrastructure, it has not yet developed specialties aside from cornea. With only three ophthalmologists and one ophthalmic clinical officer, Loresho must build human infrastructure in order to offer further specialties (e.g., retina, uvea, and pediatric). Thus, at the present time, it focuses on the very necessary eye-care service of providing cataract surgery to address the large backlog of people with cataracts in Kenya. The hospital administrators estimate that Loresho staff conducts 30–40% of the total cataract surgeries in the country. Additionally, Loresho's beautiful campus includes the first eye bank in East and Central Africa. The cornea preservative used in the eye bank comes from India.

Loresho is one of the three Kenyan institutions that might be described as part of the autonomous global network to eradicate and control blindness. It claims to be the best eye hospital in Kenya with the eye unit at the Presbyterian Kikuyu Hospital as its closest competitor. The eye unit at Kikuyu also performs high-volume cataract surgery, though not at the same quantity as Loresho. Sabatia Eye Hospital in Western Kenya also attracted Lions funding, although it is not a Lions hospital.

In East Africa, Loresho is well known in the global field of development because it is the site of the regional Lions services center covering several Lions districts across 7 countries. The doctors at Loresho present regularly at local and regional ophthalmology meetings, however Loresho does not publish enough (nor does it have enough specialties) to be considered part of the clinical ophthalmology network in the global field of ophthalmology. It was recently recognized by First Lady Margaret Kenyatta as a model of eye health care for the country, and for Eastern Africa (Official Website of the President 2018).

Now that Loresho is relying solely on patient user fees, it finds that its earlier deviation from a mission solely focused on blindness is helping to bring in surplus income. The additional dental clinic and general medical clinic create income necessary for Loresho to pay for free cataract surgeries for eye camp patients brought in from the smaller towns surrounding the Nairobi. Likewise, the Kenyan government's approval of cataract surgeries for the National Health Insurance Fund has incentivized patients to seek eye healthcare services (Official Website of the President 2018).

Next, I will discuss the for-profit organization Sala Uno. Juxtaposing Sala Uno's success, with the success of the three nonprofit eye hospitals described earlier, demonstrates that both a for-profit organization and a nonprofit organization can employ the principles of social entrepreneurship and share cognitive and normative rules, especially if these organizations share the same mission.

11.3 Sala Uno (Mexico City, Mexico)

Sala Uno started out as both self-ruled and self-sufficient. Over time, Sala Uno, like Aravind, has incorporated more diverse revenue streams from donations and investors, etc.

Sala Uno was started in 2011 by two engineers, Javier Okhuysen and Carlos Orellana. Javier and Carlos met when they both worked as investment bankers in Madrid, Spain, and London, UK (Hamermesh et al. 2014). Later, Carlos became a public health professional graduating from the University of California Berkeley's Masters in Public Health program. After touring a variety of social enterprise organizations around the world, they settled on the Aravind model as one which seemed feasible to reproduce (Mehta and Shenoy 2011).

They started Sala Uno with personal funds and the mentorship of faculty from the Lions Aravind Institute of Community Ophthalmology in India. The two friends put their savings together, approximately one million US dollars, for the initial investment into Sala Uno for the first year.

Sala Uno has a social mission similar to the nonprofit NGOs described in this book. Javier Okhuysen (unpublished interview, 2012) says,

> There are very few companies, especially in healthcare, that attend the 'bottom of the pyramid' in large masses in Mexico. And that do it very professionally. We believe that we can attend the 'bottom of the pyramid' with the best service, best quality. We want to provide an experience that is different than what might be expected for the money paid.

When he references "bottom of the pyramid," he is alluding to a popular concept that comes from a book by business scholars C. K. Prahalad's and Stuart L. Hart's frequently cited concept about multinational company driven innovation that decreases inequality by creating products for poor consumers (Prahalad 2005; Prahalad and Hart 2002).

Sala Uno partners with Fundación Cinépolis (Cinepolis Foundation) and also was certified in the Mexican government's health insurance scheme for informal laborers, Seguro Popular. Both Fundación Cinépolis and Seguro Popular provide a flat rate per patient in order to provide deeply subsidized care for low-income patients (see Table 11.3).

Sala Uno is becoming well known in the global field of ophthalmology. Just before I visited in 2012, CNN-Expansión gave them the Entrepreneurs of the Year award. Likewise, in 2012, the Latin America region of the Vision 2020 program was looking closely at how Sala Uno adapts the Aravind model for Latin America. In 2015, the World Economic Forum awarded them Entrepreneurs of the Year for Latin America.

Sala Uno has set up the first training program in Mexico for ophthalmology nurses. Their program is certified through Instituto Politécnico Nacional (National Polytechnic Institute). The chief medical officer of Sala Uno has also trained the other ophthalmologists in the small incision cataract surgery that he learned at Aravind.

The three most well-known eye hospitals in Mexico City that have been around between 30 and 40 years are: Nuestra Señora de la Luz; Hospital de la Ceguera; and Instituto De Oftalmología Conde de Valenciana. However excellent their clinical services and research may be, they do not approach the scale of Sala Uno's cataract surgical volume.

Sala Uno's small eye clinic entered a market already saturated with government hospitals and private eye clinics, but distinguishes itself because of its low cost for high-volume, high-quality cataract surgery. Sala Uno's emphasis on high volume makes it unique as one of few community ophthalmology organizations in Mexico. Sala Uno administers eye screening camps in rural areas, and an urban eye clinic with operating theaters. In the first 14 months of being open for business, Sala Uno screened 7000 patients in community outreach camps, 500 of whom then were scheduled for cataract surgery.

At Sala Uno, they have deliberately modeled themselves after Aravind; with cost recovery, 84% of patients receive free or subsidized eye healthcare services in 2012 (Freyria 2012). "In its first four years of

Table 11.3 Diverse revenue sources pay for expenses at Sala Uno (Mexico)

Revenues from sales (+)	Revenues from donations (+)	Fixed expenses (−)	Recurring expenses (−)
Wealthy Patients Fees; Deeply Subsidized Low-income Patient Fees	Remittances from the Mexican Federal Government's Seguro Popular (Popular Insurance) Domestic NGOs (i.e., Cineapolis Foundation)		Low-income patients Deeply Subsidized Surgery
			Low-income patients No Cost Surgery
			Wealthy Patients Surgery; Staff Salaries; Surgeon Bonuses
LabUno's sales of Aurolab Ophthalmic Consumables	INGOs (e.g.. LCIF, SEVA, HCP, etc.) Local: busiressmen, community leaders, religious organizat ons, etc. Personal Savings of Clinic Founders	Building Rental and Building Renovation; Hospital Equipment	Hospital Consumables
			Hospital Staff Training
			Outreach Eye Camp

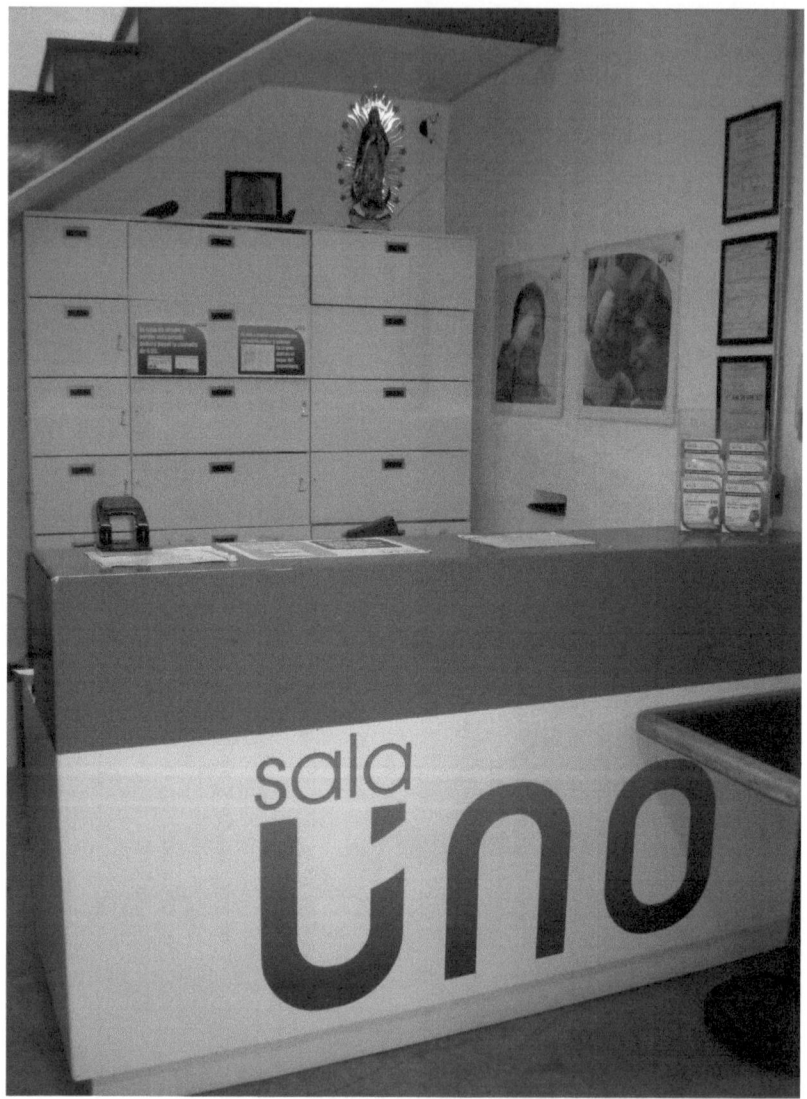

Fig. 11.3 Reception desk at Sala Uno (Photo by Logan D. A. Williams)

operation, Sala Uno has served over 100,000 outpatients and performed more than 12,000 surgeries," says Carlos Orellana in a personal communication in 2015 (Fig. 11.3).

Such a high cataract surgical total volume demonstrates both the commitment and the diligence of the Sala Uno staff. The co-founders credit their previous experience in the finance industry as essential to their new success with Sala Uno. The for-profit clinic now operates at the level of many millions of US dollars (Hamermesh et al. 2014).

Unsurprisingly, Alcon dominates the market for ophthalmic consumables in Mexico. Typically, the cost for an intraocular lens alone is $2600–$6500 pesos ($201.70–$504.25 US dollars). At Sala Uno, a patient typically pays $800 pesos ($62.06 US dollars) for a subsidized cataract surgery (to include intraocular lenses, laboratory fees, and transportation fees); this is compared to $17,600 pesos ($1365.36 US dollars) as the lowest market price for patients using health insurance at a government hospital. Sala Uno has come far since its start in 2011.

In addition to continuing their relationship with Fundación Cinépolis to provide free eye health care for the poorest Mexicans, Sala Uno has also attracted new partners such as Walmart, the BEST Foundation (Fundación BEST), and National Mount Piety (Nacional Monte de Piedad, a private nonprofit financial institution). These partners help direct patient referrals for eye healthcare to Sala Uno. Furthermore, Sala Uno has secured investment from two shareholders: Adobe Capital and International Finance Corporation (a World Bank group). This investment was used to build digital diagnostic centers in 2015 and a teaching hospital with a much higher surgical capacity in 2017 (International Finance Corporation 2017; Sin Embargo 2017). The diagnostic centers were smaller than surgical centers, with no surgical capacity, but unlike vision centers, included ophthalmologists in addition to nurses and technicians on the staff.

Sala Uno is incubating two innovations in their appropriate technology niche: their own manufacturing laboratory and urban vision centers. In 2012, Sala Uno began partnering with the city government in Mexico City which owns the retail spaces in every subway station. Sala Uno applied for and was awarded access to many of these vacant spaces and developed urban vision centers for eye screening (Williams 2012, October 3). The pedestrian foot traffic through these subway stations meant these centers resulted in more patients becoming educated about eye disease and having cataract surgery through Sala Uno.

In 2014, they ended their relationship with Seguro Popular because the federal government insurance scheme was being re-worked by policy-makers and was too costly in terms of smaller remittances and more time processing paperwork (Hamermesh et al. 2014). Also, they had not been paid for three months (Hamermesh et al. 2014). A large percentage of their poor patients were heavily subsidized by Seguro Popular. Therefore, ending their relationship with Seguro Popular meant a significant decrease in patient volume. The implications for their cost recovery model, and thus their operations, were stark: Having just finished optimizing patient referral from their twelve vision centers to their surgical center in 2012, they had to close them all and lay off many staff in 2013 (International Finance Corporation 2017). They re-instated Seguro Popular in 2015 (International Finance Corporation 2017).

The manufacturing unit, Lab Uno, is not yet up and running; instead, its manager focuses on sourcing low-cost high-quality intraocular lenses from Aurolab and other medical consumables from India, Mexico, and the USA. Lab Uno is the sole supplier of Aurolab products in Mexico (International Finance Corporation 2017).

The next organization I will discuss is an incorporated nonprofit in the USA whose mission focuses on global health education for North American college students and eye health services in the global south.

11.4 Unite for Sight, Inc. (New Haven, Connecticut, USA)

Unite for Sight's initial level of autonomy and financial independence is unknown. By 2015, Unite for Sight was both self-reliant and self-sufficient.

A US citizen, Jennifer Staple-Clark, started Unite for Sight in 2000 when she was a sophomore at Yale University. Unite for Sight, Inc. is registered as a 501(c)(3) nonprofit, non-governmental corporation in the USA. The corporation's office space in New Haven, Connecticut, was donated (Unite for Sight 2015). Otherwise, it is not commonly known how the corporation was originally financed.

Unite for Sight partners with eye clinics from less economically developed countries and volunteers from North America to provide free eye screenings and surgeries for low-income people. The North American volunteers are typically college students (but can also be professionals) and are called Global Impact Fellows. Unite for Sight's eye health service work is facilitated by the Global Impact Fellows collecting donations of money and eyeglasses to take on their volunteer internships at Unite for Sight partner clinics in the global south. Global Impact Fellows may choose to help with eye health education, work as ophthalmic assistants, or even conduct small research projects for a minimum of 7 days up to 10 weeks or more. The only scientific research studies that Unite for Sight produces are the small projects performed by the Global Impact Fellows, and the infrequent peer-reviewed publications published by founder Jennifer Staple-Clark.

In addition to two Ghanaian ophthalmologists, the remainder of Unite for Sight's nine-member medical advisory board is comprised of ophthalmologists from prestigious US medical institutions. One of the two co-founders of the US NGO Himalayan Cataract Project, Dr. Geoffrey Tabin, is on the medical advisory board. Jeffrey Sachs (PhD) is a premier international economist and the director of the Earth Institute at Columbia University; Sachs was a keynote speaker at the Unite for Sight Global Health & Innovation Conference in 2010 and 2011. Sachs oversees the United Nations Millennium Villages project where Tilganga does temporary eye camps in Africa. Both Tabin and Sachs connect Tilganga to Unite for Sight.

Unite for Sight is best known for its Global Health & Innovation Conference. This conference self-advertises on the Unite for Sight (2015) Web site as a "must-attend, thought-leading conference [that] convenes leaders, changemakers, and participants from all sectors of global health, international development, and social entrepreneurship." However, a review of previous programs indicates that a large percentage of the presentations are related to the problem of avoidable blindness.

Unite for Sight, Inc. is not an eye hospital, and it does not train domestic community ophthalmology professionals. However, the Global Health & Innovation Conference, the Social Entrepreneurship Institute, the Unite for Sight Global Impact Fellowship program, and the Global

Health University might be considered a source of training for community ophthalmology professionals: They primarily train US undergraduate college and medical students interested in issues of global health.

Unite for Sight has a unique model that engages North American volunteers to work with eye healthcare providers in the global south by emphasizing education, entrepreneurship, volunteerism, and fund-raising. The nonprofit corporation's model is similar to that of organizations such as Engineers Without Borders or Engineering World Health. However, it is more interdisciplinary.

Unite for Sight is more embedded in the global field of international development than the global field of ophthalmology. It partners with domestic eye clinics in India, Honduras, and Ghana. From 2005 until March 2013, it claims responsibility for facilitating 63,000 sight-restoring surgeries in India, Ghana, and Honduras. Unite for Sight (2015) charges $75–$350 or more for social entrepreneurship consulting. In the Unite for Sight Global Health University, an online certificate course costs $100 each, in topics as diverse as: social entrepreneurship, maternal and child health, community eye health, and cultural competency. It is likely from these, and other sources, that Unite for Sight pays the small core management team of five people. Meanwhile, all donations to Unite for Sight (2015) are used for eye health service provision for patients in India, Ghana, and Honduras. Corporate sponsorship and registration fees pay for the Global Health & Innovation Conference and the Social Entrepreneurship Institute. The nonprofit operates at the level of approximately two million US dollars (Unite for Sight 2015).

Unite for Sight incubates an anti-developmentalist approach to Western aid and Western intervention in global health. Approximately 25–33% of the Unite for Sight medical advisory board members and conference speakers are experts who are knowledgeable about global health because of their experience in providing global health care at their clinics and hospitals in the global south.

Unite for Sight is cognizant of the importance of building local capacity. In order to do this, it has broadened the problem statement of treating blindness due to cataract disease from a simple "lack" (of modern instruments or experts) to look at more of the complexities of care, in particular context-specific barriers. These barriers include: culturally expectations (e.g., if women need chaperones to travel, or if old people presume certain levels of respect from young medical care providers); opportunity costs (the family resources lost when an able-bodied family member misses work to take a blind family member to the hospital); travel costs, etc. (Williams 2008). In describing the activities of Unite for Sight, the ophthalmologists and organizers involved emphasize that each outreach eye camp starts with eye health education.

Instead of flying in Western experts to temporarily provide eye healthcare services, Unite for Sight creates long-term partnerships with private (for-profit and nonprofit) local clinics in order to build local capacity by providing them with a steady stream of patients. Unite for Sight is primarily focused on educating and treating patients (instead of infrastructure creation); therefore, it provides limited support for training local personnel in LEDCs.

References

Freyria, Sofia Garrido. 2012. Personal Communication, December 11.

Hamermesh, Richard G., Regina Garcia Cuellar, and Valeria Moy. 2014. "Sala Uno: Eliminating Needless Blindness in Mexico." 9-814-041. Harvard Business School.

Healio. 2015. "Ophthalmologists Spearhead Earthquake Relief Efforts in Nepal." *Ocular Surgery News U.S. Edition*, May 27, sec. Breaking News. http://www.healio.com/ophthalmology/ophthalmic-business/news/online/%7B9e2a50ac-6d75-4822-a879-2f52976c134a%7D/ophthalmologists-spearhead-earthquake-relief-efforts-in-nepal.

The Himalayan Times. 2017. "Nepal Eye Programme Gets Rs 100m Government Support." *The Himalayan Times*, June 2, sec. Business. https://thehimalayantimes.com/business/nepal-eye-programme-gets-rs-100m-government-support/.

International Finance Corporation. 2017. "Creating an Inclusive Market for Eye Care: Sala Uno: Committed to Eliminating Needless Blindness in Mexico." Case Study. International Finance Corporation, World Bank Group, Washington, DC.

Lions SightFirst Eye Hospital—Loresho. 2011. "Lions SightFirst Eye Hospital—Loresho About Us." Retrieved October 1. http://www.lionsloresho.org/index.php?page=aboutus.

Lions SightFirst Eye Hospital—Loresho. 2018. "Lions SightFirst Eye Hospital—Loresho—Board of Management." Retrieved May 22. https://www.lionsloresho.org/about-us/our-team.html.

Mahadevan, Ashok. 2007. "Miracles by the Thousands." *Reader's Digest*, January, 3–9.

Mehta, Pavithra K., and Suchitra Shenoy. 2011. *Infinite Vision: How Aravind Became the World's Greatest Business Case for Compassion*. San Francisco, CA: Berrett-Koehler.

Ocular Surgery News Asia Pacific Edition. 2010. "Surgeon Brings Innovative Techniques to Ophthalmologists Worldwide." *Ocular Surgery News Asia Pacific Edition*, June. Retrieved April 29, 2013. http://www.healio.com/ophthalmology/news/print/ocular-surgery-news-asia-pacific-edition/{8EC07D3B-A963-4A73-A770-0B06574FF9A0}/Surgeon-brings-innovative-techniques-to-ophthalmologists-worldwide.

Official Website of the President. 2018. "First Lady Applauds Lions Eye Hospital for Excellent Services—Presidency." Official Website of the President>Briefing Room>Latest News. February 26. http://www.president.go.ke/2018/02/26/first-lady-applauds-lions-eye-hospital-for-excellent-services/.

Prahalad, C. K. 2005. *The Fortune at the Bottom of the Pyramid: Eradicating Poverty Through Profits*. Upper Saddle River, NJ: Wharton School Pub.

Prahalad, C. K., and Stuart L. Hart. 2002. "The Fortune at the Bottom of the Pyramid." *Strategy+Business* First Quarter (26). http://www.strategy-business.com/article/11518?gko=9a4ba.

Ruit, Sanduk. 2003. "Dr Ruit: 'I Had a Puzzle to Solve' Interivew of Dr. Ruit by Puran P Bista." *The Kathmandu Post*, December 29, sec. Editorial. http://www.ekantipur.com/the-kathmandu-post/2010/02/16/Business/Tomatoes-at-Rs-1-per-kg/5230/.

Sin Embargo. 2017. "Sala Uno: Centros de salud visual para padecimientos en aumento." *SinEmbargo MX*, September 17. http://www.sinembargo.mx/17-09-2017/3299657.

Times of India. 2018. "Government Announces Recipients of 2018 Padma Awards." *Times of India*, January 26. https://timesofindia.indiatimes.com/india/government-announces-recipients-of-2018-padma-awards/articleshow_new/62653257.cms.

Unite for Sight. 2015. "Unite For Sight." https://www.uniteforsight.org/.

Williams, Logan D. A. 2008. "Medical Technology Transfer for Sustainable Development: A Case Study of Intraocular Lens Replacement to Correct Cataracts." *Technology in Society* 30 (2): 170–83.

———. 2012, October 3. Direct Observation Fieldnotes. Sala Uno Surgical Center, Mexico City, Mexico.

Organizational Charts for Four Community Ophthalmology Units

© The Editor(s) (if applicable) and The Author(s), under exclusive
licence to Springer Nature Singapore Pte Ltd. 2019
L. D. A. Williams, *Eradicating Blindness*,
https://doi.org/10.1007/978-981-13-1625-8

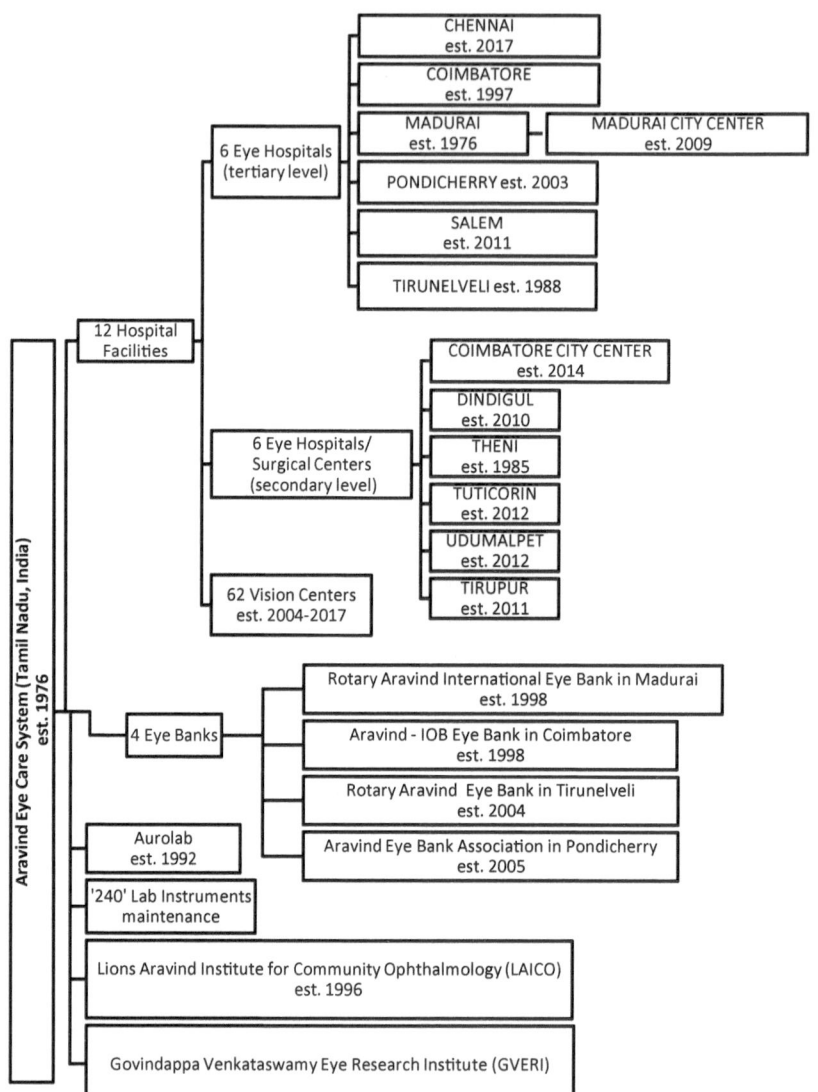

Aravind Eye Care System organizational chart

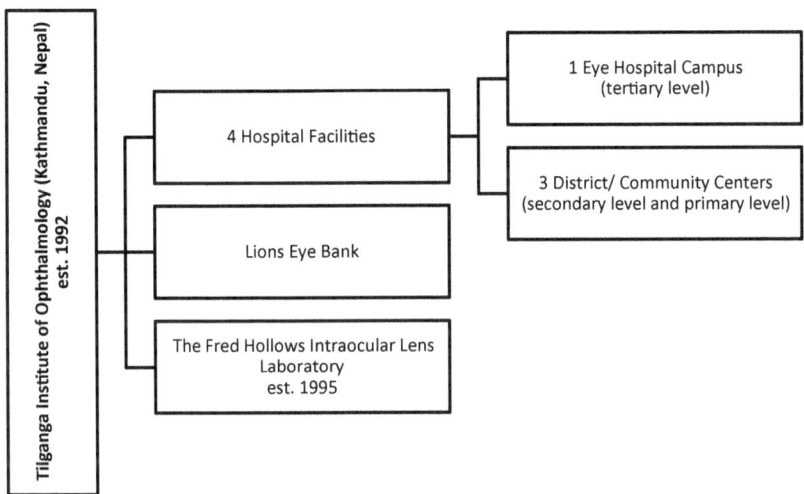

Tilganga Institute of Ophthalmology organizational chart

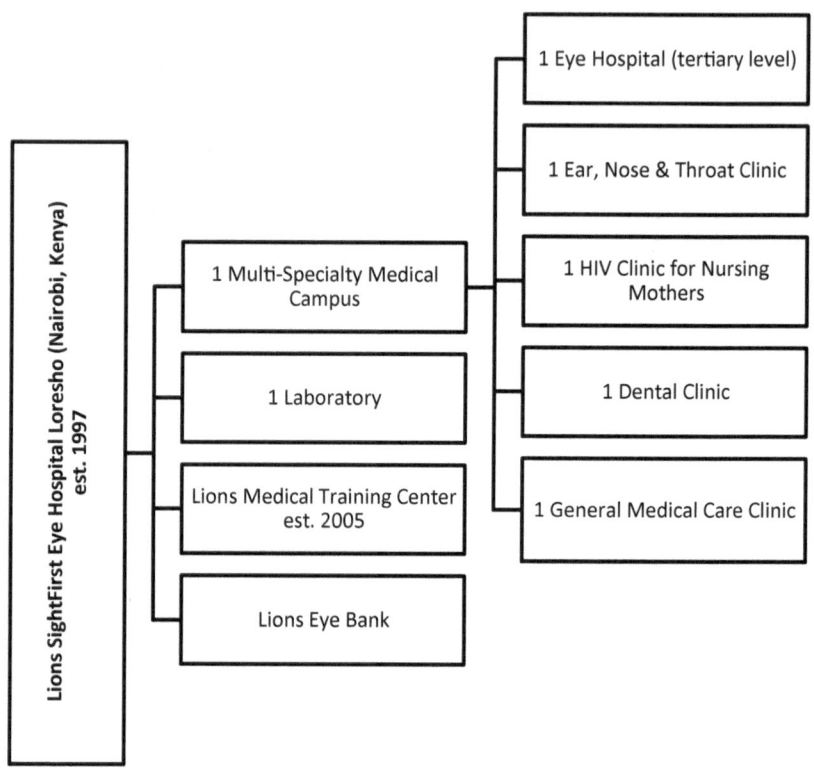

Lions SightFirst Eye Hospital-Loresho organizational chart

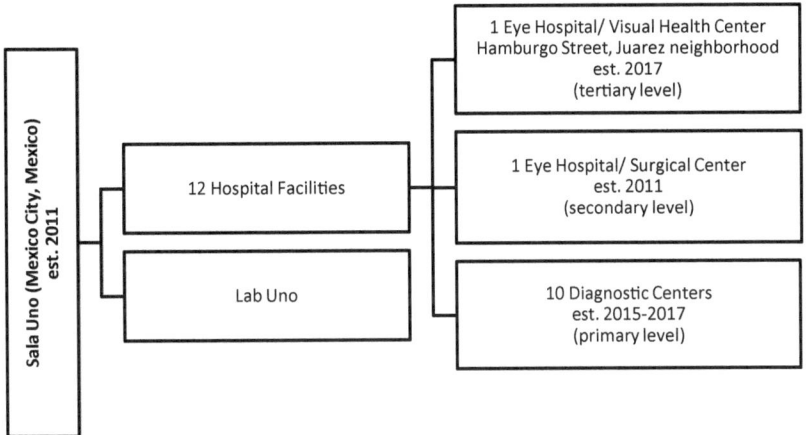

Sala Uno organizational chart

Glossary of Common Ophthalmology Surgical Terms

Quite a few terms that are commonly used by ophthalmologists are found in this book. The terminology that is most frequently repeated has been defined below.

Cataract A cataract occurs when the natural lens becomes opacified (i.e., cloudy). This cloudiness is visible to others looking into the eye and prevents the lens from focusing light properly into the back (posterior) of the eye organ.

Cornea The top layer of cells of the eye organ, like the natural lens of the eye, has an important role to play in focusing light properly into the posterior of the eye.

Couching This is an ancient surgical process by which a cataractous natural lens is displaced from its position, but remains inside of the eye organ. The patient then receives partial sight restoration (unless and until the dead natural lens tissue causes infection and loss of the entire eye). However, according to Western medicine, it has not been a reputable method of cataract surgery since the early 1900s.

Extracapsular cataract extraction (ECCE) A French ophthalmologist, Jacques Daviel, first published this novel method of extracapsular cataract surgery in 1748 (Rucker 1965). It is a manual form of cataract surgery where the natural lens is separated from the natural lens capsule (a thin translucent membrane or sac that is also called the capsular bag) and then the natural lens is drawn out of the eye. Extracapsular cataract extraction

L. D. A. Williams, *Eradicating Blindness*, https://doi.org/10.1007/978-981-13-1625-8

leaves the natural lens capsule predominantly intact and the intraocular lens is placed inside.

Intraocular Lens (IOL) Invented by Dr. Harold Ridley in Britain during the 1940s, this ophthalmic consumable mimics the shape and size of the natural lens used to focus light onto the retina located in the back (or posterior) of the eye (Apple and Sims 1996, Apple 2006). The natural lens is necessary for each eye so that a person's brain can produce images. However, this ophthalmic consumable is typically made out of stiff plastic called Perspex™ or acrylic (with the chemical name of poly-methyl-methacrylate). After surgery is performed to remove the natural lens, the ophthalmologist carefully places this plastic lens inside of the eye.

Intracapsular Cataract Extraction (ICCE) A British surgeon born in Jamaica, Samuel Sharp, first published this novel method of intracapsular cataract surgery in 1753 (Hubbell 1904). It was popularized in the 1920s by a British civil servant, the Irish ophthalmologist Col. Smith, who was working in the western part of British India (Knapp 1908; Smith 1910). Intracapsular Cataract Extraction (ICCE) is a manual form of cataract surgery where the eye organ is cut into, the entire natural lens capsule and natural lens is separated from the inside of the eye, and, then removed from the eye. Typically, patients are given aphakic cokebottle glasses to restore their sight after this procedure.

Laser-phacoemulsification (Laser-Phaco) Invented in 1986 by an African-American surgeon, Dr. Patricia Bath, this microsurgical technique uses a nanosecond laser probe to precisely disintegrate the natural lens in a process of emulsification (Croes 1987; Davidson 2005). Then, the lens pieces are removed from the natural lens capsule in a process of irrigation and aspiration. Typically, an intraocular lens is placed into the natural lens capsule after this procedure to restore vision. Laser-Phaco is not to be confused with LASIK.

Laser-Assisted in Situ Keratomileusis (LASIK) This is a surgical procedure that uses lasers to change the shape of the cornea to improve sight in a manner analogous to but more permanent than eyeglasses or contact lenses. It is mentioned here only to distinguish it from the cataract surgery procedures discussed in this book. LASIK, while commonly performed in high-income populations around the world to improve visual acuity, is not sight restoring (like cataract surgery).

Mini-nuc Mini-nuc was invented by Israeli ophthalmologist, Dr. Michael Blumenthal, in the early 1990s and is also a reinvention of extracapsular cataract extraction. In Blumenthal's (2002) technique, the natural lens is separated from the natural lens capsule and then removed from the eye through a small, self-sealing, sclera-corneal, tunnel incision.

Phacoemulsification (Phaco) Invented in 1967 by a Caucasian-American surgeon from New York State, Dr. Charles Kelman, this non-manual microsurgical technique uses an ultrasound probe to vibrate, break apart, and dissolve the natural lens in a process of emulsification (Hillman 2017). Then, the lens pieces are removed from the natural lens capsule in a process of irrigation and aspiration. Patients sometimes call it "the laser surgery," even though it does not use lasers. Typically, an intraocular lens is placed into the eye after this procedure.

Small incision cataract surgery (SICS) or Manual-SICS (M-SICS) Nepalese ophthalmologist, Dr. Sanduk Ruit of Tilganga Institute of Ophthalmology, first published this novel, manual microsurgical technique in 2000 (Ruit et al. 2000). It uses water pressure to break the natural lens into pieces in a process of hydrodissection. Then, the lens pieces are removed from the natural lens capsule in a process of irrigation and aspiration. Typically, an intraocular lens is placed into the eye after this procedure. SICS is a reinvention of mini-nuc.

Suture An ophthalmic consumable often made from very thin silk; this thread is used by ophthalmologists to sew surgical cuts closed.

Viscoelastic An ophthalmic consumable made from tinted soft plastic of similar mass and viscosity to the aqueous humour. Aqueous humour is a gelatinous substance inside the anterior chamber of the eye (the area in the front of the eye between the cornea and the natural lens). This soft plastic is often used during eye surgeries to maintain the correct intraocular pressure and the positions of various tissues within the anterior chamber of the eye.

References

Apple, David J. 2006. *Sir Harold Ridley and His Fight for Sight: He Changed the World So That We May Better See It*. 1st ed. Thorofare, NJ: Slack Incorporated.

Apple, David J., and John Sims. 1996. "Harold Ridley and the Invention of the Intraocular Lens." *Survey of Ophthalmology* 40 (4): 279–292.

Blumenthal, Michael. 2002. "Cataract Surgery." *Community Eye Health* 15 (42): 26–27.

Croes, Keith J. 1987. "Excimer Laser Probe "Phacoablates" Human Lens Through 1-Mm Incision." Ocular Surgery News, June 1 Retrieved November 20, 2010. http://laserphaco.net/content/osn87/osn87_1.html.

Davidson, Martha. 2005. "The Right to Sight: Patricia Bath." Lemelson Center Invention Features: Patricia Bath. Retrieved November 20, 2010. http://invention.smithsonian.org/centerpieces/ilives/bath/bath.html.

Hillman, Liz. 2017. "Phaco Turns 50." *Eyeworld*, April. https://www.eyeworld.org/phaco-turns-50.

Hubbell, Alvin A. 1904. "Samuel Sharp, the First Surgeon to Make the Corneal Incision in Cataract Extraction with a Single Knife." *Medical Library and Historical Journal* 2 (4): 242.1–268.

Knapp, Alfred. 1908. "On Extraction of Cataract in the Capsule: Report of a Visit to Major Henry Smith in Jullunder, India." *Arch Ophthalmol* 190 (37): 13–15. San Francisco, CA: The Foundation of the American Academy of Ophthalmology Museum of Vision & Ophthalmic Heritage.

Rucker, C. Wilbur. 1965. "Cataract: A Historical Perspective." *Investigative Ophthalmology & Visual Science* 4 (4): 377–83.

Ruit, Sanduk, G. Paudyal, Reeta Gurung, Geoffrey Tabin, D. Moran, and G. Brian. 2000. "An Innovation in Developing World Cataract Surgery: Sutureless Extracapsular Cataract Extraction with Intraocular Lens Implantation." *Clinical and Experimental Ophthalmology* 28 (4): 274–79.

Smith, Henry. 1910. *The Treatment of Cataract*. Calcutta, India: Thacker, Spink & Co. The Foundation of the American Academy of Ophthalmology Museum of Vision & Ophthalmic Heritage, San Francisco, CA.

Index

A

Actors
  dominant 2, 221, 257. *See also*
    Incumbent actors
  intermediate space 39. *See also*
    Challenger
  subordinate 2. *See also* Challenger
Pollock, Anne 3, 15, 16
Appropriate technology 3, 4, 6,
    17, 24, 26–28, 80–86,
    88, 98, 101–103, 113,
    114, 137, 139, 148, 152,
    156, 162, 174, 184, 206,
    208–210, 223, 256, 264,
    280, 290–292, 294, 296,
    298, 302, 305, 339. *See also*
    Intermediate technology;
    Kaplinsky, Raphael; Sussex
    Manifesto; Schumacher,
    Ernst F.; Willoughby, Kelvin
Arnold, David 14, 44, 86

B

Basalla, George 15, 219, 318
Bath, Patricia E. 9, 37, 54, 56, 203,
    326. *See also* Community
    ophthalmology, definition
    of; Laser phaco
Benjamin, Ruha 175, 306
Bourgeoisie 83, 114, 229, 259,
    261
Brilliant, Larry 44, 54, 55, 58, 59,
    117, 159
Buddhist economics 17. *See also*
    Limited growth economics;
    Middle path

C

Chakrabarty, Dipesh 14
Challenger 2, 14, 20, 22–25, 40,
    81–83, 114, 147, 148,
    184, 206, 222, 224, 255,

257–259, 281, 294, 297,
300, 302, 303, 306, 310

Circulation
bidirectional 184, 220, 276, 294
unidirectional 16, 102, 103, 125,
185, 233, 257

Clarke, Adele 196, 315

Clarke, James A. 117, 199, 234, 235

Collins, Harry 181, 205

Colonial exploitation 16

Community ophthalmology, definition of 9

Crystal Eye Clinic 117, 199, 235

D

Decolonialism 260, 261

Dependency 15, 16, 294, 302

Developmentalism 15, 146, 162,
168, 169, 261, 264, 280,
295, 317. *See also* Basalla,
George

Disinterested 115, 116, 123, 139,
261

Dotson, Kristie 275

E

Economies of scale 12, 98, 338

Economies of scope 12, 222, 305

Elite 16, 17, 39, 84, 85, 87, 102,
115, 233, 259, 260,
292, 303, 307. *See also*
Bourgeoisie; High status

Endogenous Development 3, 6, 86,
87, 104, 114, 139, 294, 295,
307

innovations from below 281

Enoughness 81–84, 293, 295, 308

Escobar, Arturo 7, 15, 16

Eye Hospital
Aravind Eye Care System 2, 6, 64,
77, 78, 80, 88–94, 96, 97,
99, 100, 103, 111–113, 116,
117, 119–121, 124, 126,
127, 129, 135, 151, 152,
162, 173, 194, 206, 207,
217, 218, 231, 237, 241,
242, 254, 270, 277, 290,
319, 323–326, 333, 338,
354

Crystal Eye Clinic 117, 199, 234,
235

Lions SightFirst Eye Hospital–
Loresho 5, 79, 97, 100, 231,
236, 245, 319, 324, 325,
339–341, 356

L.V. Prasad Eye Institute 64, 96,
136, 272

Madras Eye Infirmary 42

Nepal Eye Hospital 57–59, 150,
156, 164, 165, 172

Pacific Vision Foundation The Eye
Institute 309, 310

Sala Uno 5, 6, 79, 80, 88, 95, 97,
100, 122, 200, 201, 209,
228, 238, 239, 253, 254,
278, 281, 299, 300, 309,
319, 320, 324, 328, 329,
342–344, 346, 347, 357

Tilganga Institute of
Ophthalmology 1, 5, 6, 62,
64, 77, 79, 97, 113, 116,
124, 129, 130, 152, 181,
192, 202, 235, 245, 253,
262, 270, 274, 290, 318,
319, 324, 333, 334, 337,
355

F

Fanon, Frantz 16, 85, 260, 261
Feminist Science and Technology
    Studies 4, 14, 113, 116, 146,
    183, 218, 233, 256, 315,
    318, 319. *See also* Casper,
    Monica J.; Clarke, Adele;
    Dotson, Kristie; Harding,
    Sandra G.; Lorde, Audre;
    Pollock, Anne
Fred Hollows Foundation 99, 147,
    163, 164, 166, 170, 207. *See
    also* Hollows, Fred
Fujimura, Joan H. 219, 220, 247
Furlong, Kathryn 19, 20, 296

G

Gandhi, Mohandas Karamchand
    (Mahatma Gandhi) 79,
    84, 86, 210, 226. *See also*
    Inclusive
    sarvodaya 78–80, 88, 90, 92, 94,
        97, 98, 102, 210, 240, 246,
        293, 295
    swadeshi 79, 86–88, 94, 102, 333
    swaraj 79, 86, 88, 89, 94, 102,
        333
Geels, Frank 3, 4, 12, 13, 19–22,
    38, 81, 82, 102, 114, 148,
    207–210, 219, 222, 223,
    247, 257, 293, 297–304
Gilbert, Suzanne 45, 59, 150, 217, 225
Grasset, Nicole 44, 54, 55, 58–60

H

Harding, Sandra G. 3, 7, 16, 115,
    219, 220, 260, 261

Harris, Joseph 39, 65
Henke, Christopher 19
Hess, David J. 3, 18, 24, 39, 82, 83,
    134, 219, 256–258, 295,
    315
High status 83, 114, 229, 257, 259
Himalayan Cataract Project 99, 166,
    195, 236, 335, 349. *See also*
    Tabin, Geoffrey
Hollows, Fred 99, 124, 145–147,
    150, 151, 155–157, 163–
    167, 170, 175, 207, 263,
    324, 334–336, 338, 339
Humanitarian interest 115–117, 124,
    133, 138, 139

I

IAPB. *See* International Agency for
    the Prevention of Blindness
    (IAPB)
Inclusive 305
Incumbent actors 2, 11, 14, 20,
    22–25, 38, 40, 41, 81–83,
    103, 113, 146, 148, 174,
    184, 206, 208, 210, 222–
    224, 255, 257–259, 262,
    281, 290, 295, 297, 300,
    302, 303, 310
Innovation
    finance 3, 6, 23, 26, 27, 81, 289
    management 3, 6, 19, 27, 192,
        210, 218, 246, 289, 293
    science 3–9, 20, 21, 23, 27, 81, 82
    technology 3–9, 20, 21, 23, 26, 27
Intermediate technology 151, 174,
    291
International Agency for the
    Prevention of Blindness

(IAPB) 10, 37, 38, 45, 48,
51–58, 64, 65, 99, 122, 123,
153–156, 227, 298, 326
Interstitial 38, 52, 276, 281,
301–304
Interstitial space 52. *See also* Multi-
regime Interactions
Intraocular Lens Laboratory
Alcon 13, 14, 151, 172
Aurolab 147, 154, 157, 159–162,
168, 169, 173, 175
Tilganga FHIOL 167, 170–172

J

Jobs, Steve 59

K

Kaplinsky, Raphael 17, 18, 80, 83,
85, 97, 98, 100, 101
Kaplinsky's Dilemma 80, 83–85, 97,
98, 102, 104, 174, 291, 292.
See also Mass-participation;
Mass-production; Policy
dilemma
Kelman, Charles 11, 13, 183, 188,
189, 192, 193
Kleinman, Daniel L. 101, 134, 221

L

Large scale 17, 292
Laser phaco 189, 203
Less modest witness 113, 116, 117,
123, 137
Limited economic growth 82, 302
Limited growth 84, 148, 292. *See also*
Low profit margin

Limited growth economics 148
Lions Clubs International Foundation
10, 95, 96, 99, 124, 225,
227, 323, 339
Lorde, Audre 205
Low profit margin 292
Low status 83

M

Marginalized 7, 8, 88, 115, 116, 163,
182, 196, 259–261, 290,
292, 293, 296, 303, 305,
307, 310. *See also* Low status; Underserved; Unreached
Mass-participation 84, 86, 292
Mass-production 84, 86, 292
Microsurgical Technique
phacoemulsification 11–13, 26,
182, 183, 185, 188, 189,
191, 192, 194–199, 201–
205, 232, 247, 262, 269,
276, 277, 289, 294, 298
Small Incision Cataract Surgery
(SICS) 11, 175, 183–185,
190, 191, 193–195,
198–206, 208, 209, 231,
234–236, 247, 254, 263,
269, 273, 275–278, 290,
294, 299, 305, 308
Casper, Monica J. 196
Moore, Kelly 39, 275
Motivated truth 116, 124, 129, 138, 139
Multilevel Perspective
circular causality
appropriation 183–185, 205,
206, 294, 296
contestation 255–258, 262,
279–281, 294, 296

diffusion 18, 175, 294, 296
    Marianne DeLaet 256
    translation 218–224, 228–234,
        245–247, 294, 296
landscape
    landscape differentiation 298,
        299, 301
    stability 22
niche
    appropriate technology niche
        80–83, 101–103, 113, 114,
        137, 139, 147, 148, 174,
        184, 206, 208–210, 223,
        290, 291, 294, 298, 302,
        305, 338, 339, 347
    interlocking innovations 210,
        218, 219
    market niche 81, 83
    niche accumulation 218, 219,
        221–224, 245, 303
    technology niche 81–83,
        101–103, 113, 137, 139,
        147, 148, 174, 184, 206,
        208–210, 223, 289–291,
        294, 298, 302, 305, 339,
        347
regime
    dimensions 22, 293
    dual regime thesis 2, 4, 14, 20,
        21, 23–25, 28, 281, 290,
        291, 296, 298, 301, 302,
        305, 306
rules
    cognitive 38, 39, 64, 65, 78,
        80, 92, 114, 174, 209, 210,
        222, 295, 302, 303, 308
    formal 114, 137, 139, 209, 295
    guiding principles 222
    ideology 83, 210, 280

normative 38, 80, 222, 295,
    300, 310, 342
norms 38, 280
standards 38
transition pathways
    coexistence 299
    dealignment and realignment
        297, 300
    reconfiguration 22, 25
    technological substitution 22,
        299
    transformation 21, 22
Multi-regime Interactions
    competition 301
    interstitial birth 301–304
    symbiosis 301

N

Nepal Netra Jyoti Sangh 59–61, 65,
    164, 165, 170, 172, 337
Neutral 116, 117, 124, 139, 261

O

Objectivity
    strong 114, 115, 124, 139, 260.
        See also Humanitarian inter-
        est; Less modest witness;
        Motivated truth; Redfield,
        Peter; Harding, Sandra G.
    weak 115, 261. *See also*
        Disinterested; Neutral
Ophthalmic Societies
    American Academy of
        Ophthalmology 51, 195,
        234, 245, 274, 326
    American Society for Cataract and
        Refractive Surgery 197, 198

Asia Pacific Academy of
    Ophthalmology 2
European Society for Cataract and
    Refractive Surgery 270
International Council of
    Ophthalmology 51, 55, 186,
    274
the love and the hate 253
World Ophthalmology Congress 2

P
Padma Shri Govindappa
    Venkataswamy 45–49, 53,
    56, 59, 77–79, 89, 90, 92,
    94, 95, 116, 126, 150, 152,
    155, 157–159, 161, 169,
    222, 223, 225, 231, 242,
    247, 259, 260, 326
Padma Shri Sanduk Ruit 59, 62,
    116, 130, 136, 149–152,
    154–157, 163–167, 170,
    181–183, 185–187, 191–
    195, 199, 200, 202, 204,
    205, 235, 262, 263, 300,
    303, 334, 335, 337
Parthasarathy, Shobita 17, 148, 162
Phaco 11, 12, 183, 188, 198–204,
    206, 208, 308, 310
Pluralism, Epistemological 274
Policy dilemma 83, 291
Postcolonial perspective 15. *See also*
    Arnold, David; Benjamin,
    Ruha; Chakrabarty,
    Dipesh; Colonial exploita-
    tion; Decolonialism;
    Dependency; Fanon,
    Frantz; Furlong, Kathryn;

Wallerstein, Immanuel;
    Underdevelopment
Power
    asymmetric 79, 220
    bilateral 279, 294
    uneven 221
    unilateral 219, 221, 294
Prasad, Amit 162

Q
Quark, Amy A. 275

R
Redfield, Peter 116, 117, 123, 125,
    139
Ridley, Sir Harold 44, 149, 188
Royal Commonwealth Society for
    the Blind 37, 45, 47, 49, 64,
    153, 187

S
Scale-up 22, 210, 305. *See also*
    Economies of scale;
    Economies of scope; Large
    scale
Schot, Johan 12, 13, 19, 21, 22, 38,
    81, 207, 208, 222, 298, 300,
    304, 305
Schumacher, Ernst F. 17, 79, 82, 84,
    174, 264, 265, 292
Seely, Bruce 15, 17, 147
SEVA Foundation 55, 58. *See also*
    Brilliant, Larry; Gilbert,
    Suzanne; Grasset, Nicole;
    Jobs, Steve

Shrum, Wesley 94, 100, 233
Sightsavers International 37, 95, 99,
    153, 160, 187. *See also* Royal
    Commonwealth Society for
    the Blind
Smith, Adrian 3, 4, 18, 81–83
Socio-technical System. *See* Multilevel
    Perspective, Regime
Sovereignty
    epistemic 183, 205, 275, 276
    scientific 28, 175, 307
    technical 27, 147, 173, 175
Spivey, Bruce 186, 274, 279
Sussex Manifesto 17
Systemic technology choice 3, 21,
    255, 279–281, 290, 291,
    295, 305

T

Tabin, Geoffrey 78, 193, 195, 236,
    335, 349
Technological momentum 222, 247,
    303. *See also* Technological
    trajectory
Technological trajectory 13, 25, 81,
    82, 295, 303
Technology policy 87
Technology-practice 11, 114, 134,
    137, 150, 153, 154, 164,
    190, 218, 219, 246, 269,
    277, 280, 300
Thulasiraj Ravilla 241
Translation 3, 22, 25, 27, 218–224,
    228–234, 245–247, 280,
    281, 293, 294, 306

U

Underdevelopment 15
Underserved 51, 57, 62, 96
Unite for Sight 1, 117, 118, 199,
    234, 235, 240, 277, 319,
    324, 348–350. *See also*
    Clarke, James A.; Crystal
    Eye Clinic
Unreached 27, 56, 115–117, 125,
    130, 138, 161, 169, 308

W

Wallerstein, Immanuel 7, 15, 229,
    275
WHO. *See* World Health
    Organization (WHO)
Willoughby, Kelvin W. 17, 82, 84,
    174
Wilson, Sir John 10, 37, 45–49,
    52–54, 57, 121, 126, 134,
    187
World Health Organization (WHO)
    5, 9, 10, 16, 37–39, 42,
    45–61, 64, 100, 122, 145,
    147, 150, 153, 154, 158,
    172, 183, 192, 218, 229–
    231, 240, 245, 246, 295,
    298, 326. *See also* WHO